Executive Function Skills in the Classroom

The Guilford Practical Intervention in the Schools Series

Kenneth W. Merrell, Founding Editor
Sandra M. Chafouleas, Series Editor

www.guilford.com/practical

This series presents the most reader-friendly resources available in key areas of evidence-based practice in school settings. Practitioners will find trustworthy guides on effective behavioral, mental health, and academic interventions, and assessment and measurement approaches. Covering all aspects of planning, implementing, and evaluating high-quality services for students, books in the series are carefully crafted for everyday utility. Features include ready-to-use reproducibles, appealing visual elements, and an oversized format. Recent titles have Web pages where purchasers can download and print the reproducible materials.

Recent Volumes

Executive Function Skills in the Classroom

Overcoming Barriers, Building Strategies

LAURIE FAITH
CAROL-ANNE BUSH
PEG DAWSON

Foreword by Adele Diamond

THE GUILFORD PRESS
New York   London

Copyright © 2022 The Guilford Press
A Division of Guilford Publications, Inc.
370 Seventh Avenue, Suite 1200, New York, NY 10001
www.guilford.com

Printed in the United States of America

This book is printed on acid-free paper.

Last digit is print number: 9   8   7   6   5   4   3   2   1

The authors have checked with sources believed to be reliable in their efforts to provide information that is complete and generally in accord with the standards of practice that are accepted at the time of publication. However, in view of the possibility of human error or changes in behavioral, mental health, or medical sciences, neither the authors, nor the editor and publisher, nor any other party who has been involved in the preparation or publication of this work warrants that the information contained herein is in every respect accurate or complete, and they are not responsible for any errors or omissions or the results obtained from the use of such information. Readers are encouraged to confirm the information contained in this book with other sources.

Library of Congress Cataloging-in-Publication Data

Names: Faith, Laurie, author. | Bush, Carol-Anne, author. | Dawson, Peg, author. | Diamond, Adele, writer of foreword.
Title: Executive function skills in the classroom : overcoming barriers, building strategies / Laurie Faith, Carol-Anne Bush, Peg Dawson ; foreword by Adele Diamond.
Description: New York : The Guilford Press, [2022] | Series: The Guilford Practical Intervention in the Schools Series | Includes bibliographical references and index.
Identifiers: LCCN 2021047840 | ISBN 9781462548927 (Paperback : acid-free paper) | ISBN 9781462548934 (Hardcover : acid-free paper)
Subjects: LCSH: Educational psychology—Research. | Executive functions (Neuropsychology) | Teachers—In-service training. | BISAC: PSYCHOLOGY / Psychotherapy / Child & Adolescent | MEDICAL / Psychiatry / Child & Adolescent
Classification: LCC LB1051 .F23 2022 | DDC 370.15—dc23/eng/20211103
LC record available at *https://lccn.loc.gov/2021047840*

Illustrations by Trisha Highton (*thetinyscribbler.co.uk*).

About the Authors

Laurie Faith, PhD, works at the Ontario Institute for Studies in Education at the University of Toronto, Canada, where she teaches courses in special education and executive functions and coordinates a research center. Dr. Faith is the creator of Activated Learning, a self-regulated learning intervention that she continues to refine alongside a growing community of researchers, trainers, and teachers. She provides professional learning and training for individual teachers and school boards across Ontario, the United States, and the United Kingdom. Dr. Faith taught in special and general education classrooms for 17 years. Her website is *activatedlearning.org*.

Carol-Anne Bush, MA, is an executive function coach in the San Francisco Bay area. Ms. Bush's experience in K–12 education spans three continents and over three decades. After a long teaching career in the United States, the United Kingdom, and South Africa, she served in various leadership roles, including multiple assistant headships. Ms. Bush's expertise includes student, teacher, and parent mentorship; stakeholder communication; curriculum design; and whole-school strategy and steering. She is a certified Level III trainer in the Activated Learning approach, and is an ADHD-Certified Educator through the Professional Education Systems Institute. Her website is *www.mulberrycoaching.com*.

Peg Dawson, EdD, is a psychologist on the staff of the Center for Learning and Attention Disorders at Seacoast Mental Health Center in Portsmouth, New Hampshire. She also does professional development training on executive skills for schools and organizations nationally and internationally. Dr. Dawson is a past president of the National Association of School Psychologists (NASP) and the International School Psychology Association, and is a recipient of NASP's Lifetime Achievement Award. She is coauthor of bestselling books for general readers, including *Smart but Scattered, Smart but Scattered Teens, Smart but Scattered—and Stalled* (with a focus on emerging adults), and *The Smart but Scattered Guide to Success* (with a focus on adults). Dr. Dawson is also coauthor of *The Work-Smart Academic Planner, Revised Edition*, and books for professionals including *Executive Skills in Children and Adolescents, Third Edition*.

Foreword

In this book, Laurie Faith, Carol-Anne Bush, and Peg Dawson present an approach to teaching in which understanding executive functions (EFs) is central. The book is written by educators for educators from PreK through high school. There is much wisdom here. Several aspects of the approach stand out.

Students with weak EFs are often subject to harsh misattributions by peers, teachers, and themselves because their failures to follow instructions or the rules can easily be mistaken as being intentional and indicative of poor character. The approach described in this book provides a perspective and vocabulary for seeing learning and behavioral challenges in a whole new light, one that tries to identify the problem that is causing the learning or behavioral challenges and what the child can do to overcome that problem. For example, a student's paper might still be blank long after the class was given a writing assignment. Does the student not know the material, or could it be a problem with task initiation, organization, or with feeling what he or she writes must be perfect? Building basic EF literacy among children allows them to finally speak clearly about their experiences, challenges, and learning. Once the problem is identified, the whole class can brainstorm about what might be done about that. Usually other students have had problems with that too and can share what has worked for them. During whole-class discussions, the silence is broken and students see that their friends and even their teacher also experience difficulties. Not only do students learn they are not alone, but also as research shows, children and teens learn better from other young people than from adults. Often the challenges and strategies shared by peers seem more interesting, relevant, and useful than what adults offer.

The approach described in this book recognizes how much work teachers are expected to get through every day and that there is little time in the school day for adding anything else. Instead of proposing a new EF module, this approach incorporates EF training seamlessly into whatever the class is doing, whether that is math or recess. Not only do teachers not have time for freestanding lessons on EFs, but research shows that freestanding lessons are not best for improving EFs. Gains from such lessons too rarely generalize to life outside those lessons or to academic subjects.

Instead, Faith, Bush, and Dawson have students apply EF concepts during academic and social learning experiences. Research shows it is by using concepts that we truly learn them; otherwise we understand them only at an abstract, intellectual level.

This book is neither formulaic nor scripted. The authors recognize that one size never fits everyone. Each teacher, each student, and each class is different. Various strategies and a plethora of examples are provided to help teachers see how they can use this EF supportive approach in a way that feels thoroughly comfortable. Scripted lessons are easier, but research shows they are less effective—too easy for some, too difficult for others, too boring, and too out of touch with the reality in particular classrooms—and teachers are too bright and capable to be treated like robots who are to do exactly as they are told.

This book conveys a deep respect for both teachers and students, an acknowledgment that people get more benefit from any activity and enjoy it more if they have some say in how the activity is implemented, and the recognition that none of us is as smart as all of us collectively. Students and teachers discuss EF obstacles they face and co-create strategies. Central to this approach is the "Barriers and Strategies Protocol," which provides ways to strategize *with* students instead of *for* students, allowing them to be actively involved in the process of identifying problems and in developing suitable responses.

Because of this shared problem solving and brainstorming, no teacher needs to be an EF or strategy expert. Solutions arise through the communal discussion. Feeling they have to be the expert can be anxiety provoking or overwhelming for some teachers. There's no need to feel that way here; the authors provide many examples of possible solutions that educators can adopt or modify as they wish.

As I read, I kept writing in the margin, "I love it." This book contains so much wisdom and is written in a clear, engaging manner without any sense that the authors are watering things down too much. Real-life examples from the classroom greatly help to illustrate and elaborate points. I would recommend this book to all educators.

ADELE DIAMOND, PhD, FRSC
Canada Research Chair Tier I Professor
    of Developmental Cognitive Neuroscience
University of British Columbia, Canada

Preface

WHY WE WROTE THIS BOOK

We have given hundreds of workshops and talks. After each one, a school psychologist or educator will approach us to say, "This is what I have been waiting for! This is what my school (or district) needs! How can I take this back to everyone?" They tell us that the idea of teachers and students talking explicitly about executive functions (EFs) during instruction, feedback, and assessment feels like a missing link. We agree. In fact, while writing this book we often paused to wonder how we ever got along without these ideas. We remember how mysterious student behavior often seemed, and how ill equipped we felt to support their independence. We wish we could go back in time and give this book to our younger selves.

So, we offer this resource to school psychologists, principals, special educators, and mainstream teachers. We have filled it with a wide range of grounded, specific examples, tools, and approaches, and layered on just enough plain language research to support our advice. Our hope is that you will be able to use this book chapter by chapter with your colleagues to incorporate more EF support in mainstream education.

HOW WE WROTE THIS BOOK

We wrote this book with humor and insight about what really happens in schools and classrooms. Among us, we have spent almost 100 years in education—we've seen our share of baloney sandwiches, gummed-up scissors, and tearful parents. From this realistic and balanced perspective, we have compiled and edited a wide variety of approaches that were created and tested by practitioners for supporting the development of EFs at school. Nothing about this book is theoretical, or "best-case scenario," or something a researcher has conducted only under controlled conditions. Nor does it represent practices that only work for a certain kind of teacher or a specific type of student. The book offers guidance through stories from real classrooms. While many of the practical examples in the book are drawn from a community of early adopters in Ontario, Canada, the approach was created in collaboration with school board leaders, psychologists, principals, teachers, and students from all over Canada, the United States, and the United Kingdom. As you join our growing international movement, we hope you'll consider sharing your innovative ideas, adaptations, and improvements with our online community at *http://activatedlearning.org*.

HOW TO USE THIS BOOK

Don't just *read* about the approaches—roll up your sleeves and *do* the approaches. You can use the examples we provide like a springboard. Even better, gather your colleagues, a school staff, a bunch of special education consultants, or a crew of resource teachers and team up. Over the course of a school year, you can explore this book by working through it one chapter per month:

- Imagine launching your professional learning journey or book club by reading Chapter 1. The first chapter provides a vivid and grounded explanation of what EFs are and the role they play in day-to-day life and performance. Everyone should read this to get up to speed on the basics and to make personal connections to the impact of EFs on life. After taking a couple of weeks to read, if you're working with a colleague or small group, your team should come together to discuss what resonated with them. In our experience, this stage of the learning journey leaves educators rather shocked to discover that an issue they have been dealing with every day of their career has a name and an entire research literature to describe it. "I have learned that EFs *are a thing*," they tell us.

- Chapter 2 explains exactly how to teach children from grades K to 8 about EFs. It provides detailed examples across five different teaching contexts, including those in which the teacher is (1) in the early days with a class, (2) very time strapped, (3) seeking high structure, (4) hoping for a more free-flowing approach, or (5) managing a stressed group (see below). This means that the reading can be "jigsawed" among a team, with different people set off to read a different section of the chapter. For example, perhaps the grade 2 teachers will read about and apply *highly structured* methods for teaching children about EFs; the grades 1 and 4 teachers will read about and apply material related to a more *free-flowing* style of teaching children about EFs; the K, 5, and 8 teachers will apply methods for teaching EFs in the *early days* with a group of students; and the grades 3 and 7 teachers focus on how to teach EFs among *highly stressed* students. There are five different teaching contexts presented, so there will be plenty of options for everyone to choose from. When you come back together to discuss, your team will have a wide range of experiences and approaches to talk about. Perhaps you'll ask each team to briefly present what they have been applying in the classroom. What worked for the grades 1 and 4 teachers? What didn't work for the K, 5, and 8 team? How did the grades 3 and 7 students respond? How did the grade 2 teachers adapt and improve the approaches from the book? What are everyone's next steps? By the end of this month, your professional book club will have a lot of learning under its belt about how to build EF literacy. At this point, many educators reflect that they wish they had known about EFs sooner in their own education. "I wish I could turn back time and be a student in my own class," they tell us.

- In Chapter 3, you will learn a protocol for actually *using* the whole-class EF literacy that you have developed. There is nothing too technically fancy here—you'll learn to lead students in 5- to 10-minute problem-solving conversations about EF barriers and strategies. What you'll gain is an up close and personal sense for how, when, and why these conversations can be transformational. If you're working in a team, each member should read the introduction to the chapter, and then, once again, you can divide up the rest of the reading, perhaps each choosing a different context than the one you followed in Chapter 2. Mix it up! If the grades 3 and 7 teachers explored the "Highly Stressed" context in Chapter 2, they might like to split up and focus on something different for Chapter 3. At the end of the month, your whole team will have used the Barriers and Strategies Protocol to manage problem solving in a variety of different ways, and you should have a lot to reflect on and teach one another. Even with students as young as kindergarten, teachers tell us that creating space for barriers and strategies conversations is like opening the floodgates: "My students have so much to *say* about their learning!"

- By Chapter 4, you will have accumulated some expertise and confidence. You should be starting to notice a change in how you see and relate to your students. This is a perfect time to zoom in on the way EF literacy can improve the depth and quality of teachers' classroom observations. This chapter will explore a wide range of specific approaches for slowing down and tuning in to students' EF challenges and compensatory strategies. We stretch this guidance across the same five teaching contexts that we used in Chapters 2 and 3. By now, if you're working in a team, you will be in a rhythm and each member may know exactly which of the teaching contexts they want to read up on. Or, more likely, people will be way too curious to read only one. At this point, teachers comment on the increasing self- and other awareness growing among their students. "One of my kinders congratulated me for taking a deep breath to calm down when my coffee spilled. It was really rather lovely."

- Chapter 5 digs deeply into one of the most powerful teaching practices there is: feedback. We'll explore the issue of *drive* and explain how clear and precise feedback regarding the use of EF strategy is so intrinsically motivating. Money saved on stars, stickers, and other extrinsic incentives should be put toward the coffee fund because there will be a lot to learn, apply, and discuss! After reviewing motivation and some other key research, we'll dig into (once again) five different grounded examples for focusing both spoken and written classroom feedback on the use of EF strategy. In Chapter 4, you learned how to engage students in a process of problem solving and strategy use; they may now know when and how to be independent. In Chapter 5, we provide the extra motivational oomph needed to translate this knowledge into action. Teachers tell us that something kind of magical happens when they comment on EF strategy use. "It is like a trail of breadcrumbs that even my most disengaged students will follow."

- Chapter 6 focuses on everyone's favorite topic: formative assessment and report cards. This chapter explains how a day-to-day focus on students' process and EF strategy use can be balanced with high-stakes assessment, grades, and parents' expectations; we argue that both have an important place in education. Once again, we provide examples of practice across five different contexts, explaining how teachers gather summative data and then share that learning with administrators, parents, and students themselves. This chapter will be an asset to educators struggling to comment on students' learning skills or strategies. Discovering how to gather data relating to EF strategy use has left many of the educators we know feeling as if their reports "write themselves."

• Chapter 7 forms the first part of the conclusion of this book. We take a step back to consider how an EF-oriented classroom can support other educational priorities, such as closing the achievement gap, managing 21st-century learning, ensuring equity in multicultural classrooms, balancing individualized education programs (IEPs), using universal design, and mitigating teacher burnout. We present an overview of each of these challenges, a breakdown of the types of interventions and remedies typically recommended, and an analysis of how our approach may help. We included it because of the number of times we sat at a psychology or education conference on the edge of our seat thinking, "Oh! Our approach can help that problem." Essentially, we think many of these challenges emerge from the same deficiency in the way classroom teaching works: a lack of connection, understanding, relationship, and teamwork. We hope this will encourage you or your team to persevere with a whole-class, whole-child, EF-oriented approach, knowing the many other aspects of classroom life it affects.

• Finally, in Chapter 8 we sum up the learning we have done as partners, designers, and trainers. We include this because we've been asked many times how our EF-oriented teaching movement was conceived, took root, and grew. This section sums up the issues we faced (and continue to face), and we think it will help psychologists, administrators, and educators as they chart their own paths toward leadership in this field. It includes many practical tips that will likely be useful to those leading the charge.

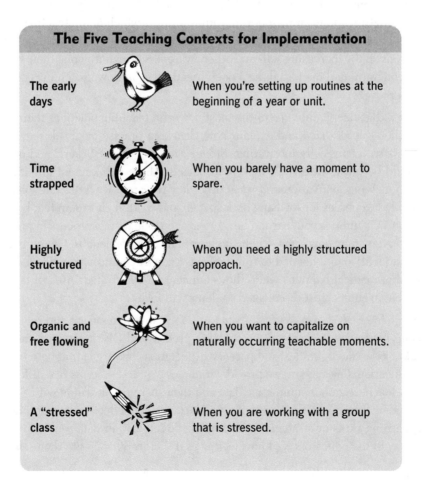

The Five Teaching Contexts for Implementation

The early days — When you're setting up routines at the beginning of a year or unit.

Time strapped — When you barely have a moment to spare.

Highly structured — When you need a highly structured approach.

Organic and free flowing — When you want to capitalize on naturally occurring teachable moments.

A "stressed" class — When you are working with a group that is stressed.

WHY THIS BOOK (AND YOUR WORK) IS SO NECESSARY

As far as EFs go, there are certain things that experts agree on and certain things that haven't yet been decided. Most psychologists agree that a typical day, in school or life, is loaded with EF challenge. In the morning, we all need to get up, eat a healthy breakfast, and arrive at our destination on time. Then, all day long, we need to interact with our peers, attend to expectations, and figure out how to respond to problems. Thanks to decades of painstaking research, we know that these essential skills don't develop fully without direct teaching and regular practice and that students who leave school with underdeveloped EFs will have poorer life outcomes. Considering all of this, it has become obvious that public education needs to support EF development. More recently, however, researchers have recognized just how challenging it is for teachers to do this complex work; because they are overburdened, overstretched, stressed out, managing extraordinary diversity, and struggling with EF challenges of their own, teachers need a heck of a lot more than encouragement and a basic knowledge of EFs to succeed. What experts don't agree on is what to do next. What can be done, knowing all that we know, to ensure that every child receives appropriate EF support and development?

On one hand, because the need for EF development is so acute, it is tempting to divert all resources toward targeted extracurricular programs, special counselors, private tutors, and small-group interventions. These programs are often well planned and executed, and they allow us to deliver the urgently required support to the most needy students. If classroom teachers simply cannot and will not ever be able to fully support EF development, then perhaps the infrequent, out-of-context support offered to a subset of students by an extracurricular program will have to do. On the other hand, do we really have to accept this? Across the course of a school year, we estimate that teachers have about a million highly meaningful opportunities to influence EF development in the children they teach. The good, old-fashioned classroom is a daily, intensive, personally meaningful, applied, and social pathway for delivering EF support—the exact type of pathway known to be the most effective. This is why we're so intent on driving a slow and steady, embedded, all-aboard, heart and soul transformation of education toward EF-oriented classrooms. Even though it seems hard, delivering EF support and development in the context of a mainstream classroom is not only the most equitable and efficient but also the very most effective way to do it. What's more, a student coming from an EF-supportive mainstream classroom stands to gain a lot more from any specialized (Tier 2 or 3) program to which they have access.

So, please read and *do* our book. It is a comprehensive playbook for embedding EF support into the daily operation of a mainstream classroom. It is built upon decades of insight from Dawson and Guare's books, including *Smart but Scattered Teens* and *Executive Skills in Children and Adolescents* (now in its third edition). It is an approach advocated by Adele Diamond, one of the world's leading neuroscientists and EF experts, and it is an approach that makes our teacher friends "love teaching again." Could *you* build whole-class EF literacy and use it to enrich your instruction, observation, feedback, and assessment? We truly believe you can. This book will provide the vivid examples, useful tools, and most relevant research you need to succeed.

Acknowledgments

We wish to acknowledge the inspired teachers, principals, and students from around the world who always had time, despite busy schedules, to talk to us about their practices and perspectives. Many of them come from the Trillium Lakelands District School Board in Ontario, which is bursting at the seams with innovation, community spirit, and love for children. We also owe so much of the joy and privilege of writing this book to the support and encouragement of our families. Thank you, Andy, Adam, Eli, Michael, and Steven.

Contents

> Purchasers of this book can download and print the reproducible figures
> and an appendix page at *www.guilford.com/faith-forms* for personal use
> or use with students (see copyright page for details).

CHAPTER 1

Executive Function and Learning

WHAT ARE EXECUTIVE FUNCTIONS?

Before we delve into a formal definition of EFs, we would like to place you firmly in your classroom. Think about your students. Recall the creative ones, the funny ones, the talented ones, and the ones who surprise you. They all, from time to time, have trouble setting and meeting goals. It may be Theo who struggles to *shift* from one activity to another or Juan who cannot help but *blurt* out while others are speaking. Consider Joanie who constantly *underestimates* how long a task is going to take or Samia who *forgets* there was even a plan to follow in the first place. These are just some of the many students we want you to hold in mind as you read this chapter. Every student you have worked with probably taught you something different about the way EFs affect performance. As an experienced teacher, you are the real expert on EFs in the classroom.

EFs are cognitive processes that work alongside our intellect and creativity to allow us to respond to challenges. They develop naturally throughout childhood and adolescence, maturing in our mid-20s. These skills are controlled by the prefrontal cortex in our brains and are the very reason we are able to remain focused, organize our time *and* follow through with a plan, meet challenges with flexibility and persistence, hold and quickly access information stored in memory, and retain self-control when the going gets tough.

If you look up "executive functioning" on the Internet, you will find a range of differing opinions. Experts hotly debate fundamental matters such as how many EFs there are, how to refer to them individually, and how to properly group them. Dr. Adele Diamond believes there are three core EFs (2013), George McCloskey's developmental model mentions 32 different capacities that support self-regulation (2013), while Dawson and Guare (2018) speak of 11. In 2012, Dr. Russell Barkley threw up his hands and pointed out that this lack of a common model among researchers had delayed a generally accepted definition of EF. Consensus continues to elude the top experts.

This focus on the details is important. Researchers are trying to understand how closely aligned EF weakness is with attention deficit disorder, for example, and how individual EFs, such as working memory, can be fostered in infancy. They wonder if certain EFs are disproportionately impaired by learning disabilities or if early intervention to support others could circumvent reading problems. They wonder if there are subsets of EFs that function differently from the others.

Despite the confusion among researchers, experts focused on mobilizing EF knowledge for classroom use have pushed forward with general definitions. If nothing else is perfectly clear, we can agree that EF is a good "umbrella term" to describe the processes involved in "purposeful, goal-directed, and flexible behavior" (Meltzer, Dunstan-Brewer, & Krishnan, 2018, p. 111). We take our lead from the list of 11 proposed by Dawson and Guare (2018), found in Table 1.1. After many consultations with teachers, we believe this is the most useful set of concepts for students to learn if they are to discuss their learning fluently.

TABLE 1.1. 11 Key Executive Functions

Response inhibition

The capacity to think before you act. The ability to resist the urge to say or do something allows us the time to evaluate the situation and how our behavior might affect it.

Working memory

The ability to hold information in mind and work with it when performing complex tasks. It incorporates the ability to draw on past learning or experience to apply to the situation at hand or to project into the future.

Emotional control

The ability to manage emotions in order to achieve goals, complete tasks, or control and direct behavior.

Cognitive flexibility

The ability to revise plans in the face of obstacles, setbacks, new information and possibilities, or mistakes. It involves adaptability to changing conditions.

Sustained attention

The capacity to attend to a situation or task in spite of distractions, fatigue, or boredom.

Task initiation

The ability to begin a task without undue procrastination, in a timely fashion.

Planning and prioritizing

The ability to create a roadmap to reach a goal or to compete a task. It also involves being able to make decisions about what's important to focus on and what's less important.

Organization

The ability to design and maintain systems for keeping track of information or materials.

Time management

The capacity to estimate how much time one has, how to allocate it, and how to stay within time limits and deadlines. It also involves a sense that time is important.

Goal-directed persistence

The capacity to follow through to the completion of a goal, even when it seems to take a long time, without being deterred by setbacks, mistakes, frustration, boredom, other demands, or competing interests.

Metacognition

The ability to stand back, take a bird's-eye view of oneself in a situation, or observe one's own problem solving. It also includes self-monitoring and self-evaluative skills.

Note. Adapted from *Executive Skills in Children and Adolescents, Third Edition,* by Peg Dawson and Richard Guare. Copyright © 2018 The Guilford Press. Reprinted with permission.

WHAT IS YOUR EF PROFILE?

We all have a variety of strength and weakness in our EFs; even the most capable students, and most adults, have one or two weak EFs that will impair performance to some extent. For example, think about the teachers at your school. We're pretty certain you have a great organizer, a task initiator who gets everyone started on new projects, or a super flexible teacher who always goes with the flow. You might also know someone who occasionally interrupts faculty meetings, or who, once a plan is made, needs plenty of reminders to refer to it again. You can bet that these individuals are, perhaps unknowingly, using strategies to manage the more critical impacts of these tendencies in their lives. Through experience, and some cringe-worthy mistakes, we smooth the roughest edges of our EF challenges so they don't wreak havoc in our lives. Our students are several years of maturity and many life experiences away from this adult level of self-management.

The children in our classrooms have much weaker EFs than we do for many reasons. We can easily understand that they are less cognitively mature, but there are other less obvious factors that put their EFs on unstable ground. Figure 1.1 shows the way modern life, a variety of different learning disabilities, and adverse childhood experiences can stack up to weaken EFs. Can you recall teaching a student who may have been affected by several or even all of these compounding factors?

We don't want to paint a picture of unrelenting doom and gloom. It is critical, however, for educators to understand the reason behind the variation in school behavior and performance. It is important to remember that, for some children, it is more mentally challenging to resist temptation, hold multiple ideas in mind, control emotions, or stay focused. While they may be able to demonstrate all of these skills for a few moments, or throughout first period, or when they are especially interested in something, managing them over the course of a long, demanding school day is a different matter entirely.

HOW DO EFs AFFECT LEARNING AT SCHOOL?

We all have a unique spectrum of EF strength and weakness, and we all have good days and bad days. Experts estimate that the individual differences in EFs explain over half of all the variation in school performance (Visu-Petra, Cheie, Benga, & Miclea, 2011). Take a moment to consider how EFs might affect a typical day in a teacher's life.

Bad EF Day

Imagine that you are at an interactive workshop on a topic you know little to nothing about. There are all sorts of interesting people attending. You should be excited, but you had a terrible night's sleep; you were up all night with a sick child whom you had to leave at home with a babysitter. This caused you to run late. Then, you missed the train, which meant you missed the breakfast, coffee, and chatter before the conference began. You look around and feel embarrassed. Everyone else seems to be happy, enjoying themselves, and on track. You start to think about the coffee and breakfast that you missed, and then the urge to check in on your son springs to mind. You look at the clock and realize the session is almost over. How will you report back to the staff at your school?

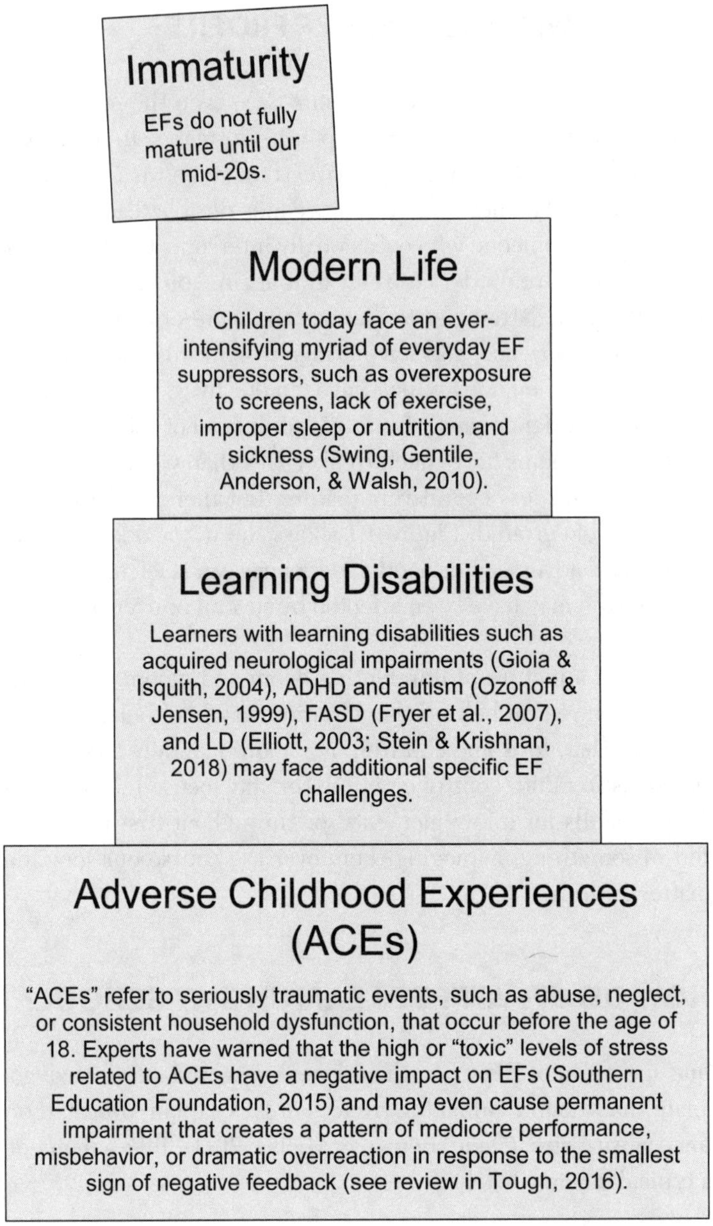

Immaturity

EFs do not fully mature until our mid-20s.

Modern Life

Children today face an ever-intensifying myriad of everyday EF suppressors, such as overexposure to screens, lack of exercise, improper sleep or nutrition, and sickness (Swing, Gentile, Anderson, & Walsh, 2010).

Learning Disabilities

Learners with learning disabilities such as acquired neurological impairments (Gioia & Isquith, 2004), ADHD and autism (Ozonoff & Jensen, 1999), FASD (Fryer et al., 2007), and LD (Elliott, 2003; Stein & Krishnan, 2018) may face additional specific EF challenges.

Adverse Childhood Experiences (ACEs)

"ACEs" refer to seriously traumatic events, such as abuse, neglect, or consistent household dysfunction, that occur before the age of 18. Experts have warned that the high or "toxic" levels of stress related to ACEs have a negative impact on EFs (Southern Education Foundation, 2015) and may even cause permanent impairment that creates a pattern of mediocre performance, misbehavior, or dramatic overreaction in response to the smallest sign of negative feedback (see review in Tough, 2016).

FIGURE 1.1. Additional challenges to EF.

Good EF Day

Attending a workshop in a neighboring city, you have a late dinner with a colleague and discover at midnight that your accommodations have no shampoo. You grudgingly set an alarm and plan to run to the store in the morning. When the alarm goes off you throw on sneakers and head to the store. Finding it closed, you end up jogging four blocks to the next one. The sun is rising, it's a lovely morning, and you take the long way home, jogging all the way. You get back, quickly shower, and feel surprisingly great, despite your poor sleep. Arriving at the conference, you're a bit late, but you feel energized, social, and optimistic. You feel deeply focused, and your mind quickly assimilates and extends the information you hear. You connect with another participant from your city. Though his school is slightly different than yours, you continue chatting during the coffee break about ways to start a project together.

Consider the impact of these good and bad EF days on the overall learning and performance of each teacher. The teacher having a bad EF day will not be able to give a good report to her colleagues. Organization, time management, attention, and emotional control impaired her ability to be successful. This failure may have a negative impact on her career, because she may not be chosen to attend the next conference. The teacher having a good EF day, however, through her emotional control, flexibility, attention, working memory, and goal-directed persistence, has shown leadership and will return to school with impressive news. Do you suspect that the teacher having a good EF day might just be more naturally curious, innovative, and generally successful? In fact, both of these stories are based on Laurie's (author) personal diary. They represent one and the same person. Can you appreciate how much our EFs, despite our intellect and creativity, can affect our learning and performance?

Students experiencing a "bad EF day" often do it in a very public forum, with no way to retreat or regroup, in front of peers and teachers who have become exasperated by them. If these bad days cause them to feel frustrated, depressed, and embarrassed, the situation becomes even worse. Stress is a disastrous condition for EFs. It floods our prefrontal cortex with cortisol and scrambles our ability to remember things, exercise discipline, and reason our way through problems. The feeling might be similar to experiencing stage fright, or being the new guy at a challenging job, or being lost in a big city during rush hour.

EF weakness has a greater impact on academic success than language or intellectual ability (Blair & Razza, 2007; Duckworth & Seligman, 2005; Espy et al., 2004). Forgive the harsh language, but EF challenges can make children look *and feel* lazy, naughty, or as if they simply aren't very smart. Below, we will characterize each of these types. At the end of Chapter 3 we provide even more detailed information about the impact of EFs on performance.

Students who drift off task, stall, or become disorganized are the ones who may appear "lazy." These are students with challenges in attention, task initiation, goal-directed persistence, and time management. Often these students have big ideas but are just so utterly overwhelmed by details that they don't know how or where to start. They might even be your gifted students but will often end a classroom period with nothing accomplished. Think of them as your "consultants"—you may notice them dropping in on other students' conversations with amazing ideas, enjoying a chance to do some thinking without having to manage any of the EF challenges. We wonder, why doesn't this student just start his own assignment if he has so much to say? In time, these students may become passive, discouraged, or even angry. Without an understanding of EFs and support to be strategic, they internalize the criticism that they are terribly wasting their potential or they decide they are destined to fail.

The "naughty" students are the hardest to ignore. These are the ones whose interruptions, rule breaking, stubbornness, and short fuse most likely caused you to buy this book in the first place. They can be very disruptive to other students and to your ability to conduct your teaching, and as a result may suffer the most severe consequences. For example, we know a student who spent March, April, May, and June working in a solitary wooden study carrel in the hallway of his school. Trust that we see this situation with compassion—no teacher begins their career hoping to exclude students, just as no student begins school hoping to become the enemy of his whole class. This unfortunate and unacceptable situation, instead, is a sure sign that a teacher and student are undersupported, out of ideas, and burnt out. These "naughty" students might like to know that, actually, they struggle a little more than usual with response inhibition, flexibility, and metacognition. Furthermore, they might like to know that emotional triggers are unusually powerful for them and cause all of their other EFs to fall apart. Research tells us that students with weak EFs are *often* subject to harsh misattribution from peers, teachers, and themselves because their challenges are mistaken for symptoms of poor character (Gaier, 2015) that seem intentional (Elik, Wiener, & Corkum, 2010). Unfortunately, because childhood includes plenty of intentional mischief and boundary testing, only the most well informed and sensitized can discriminate an EF weakness from layers of other typical behaviors.

Many other students struggle with EF challenges that directly affect deep thinking and reasoning skills. These are the ones who may look and feel as if they simply aren't very smart. Working memory and response inhibition, in particular, have tremendous impacts on math and reading ability (see review in Diamond, 2014). A weak working memory makes it difficult to hold the main idea of a story in mind while decoding difficult words. You've undoubtedly worked with students who have struggled like this; they get to the end of a paragraph and have no idea what they've read. Weak response inhibition, on the other hand, makes it very challenging to select only relevant information when making meaning in text. These are students who, when asked to summarize a chapter from their novel, will tell you every single detail from the first paragraph. Or this phenomenon may be due to weak metacognition, whereby these students have trouble connecting the dots and noticing the overall patterns and meaning in the material they read. Sometimes this "simply not very smart" type will have a cluster of strong EFs, so even though they seem organized, attentive, and disciplined, they just can't manage to nail their academic work. Though the EF challenges for these students are deep in their thought process, the situation is far from hopeless. We know many students who, through EF literacy and a strategic approach, have learned to manage working memory and response inhibition challenges.

How many "bad EF days" are taking place in your classroom? How will you know if the unexpected performance you're seeing really *is* due to EF challenges? It is easy to suspect that poor performance is intentional. For example, what if your class struggles to complete your mapping activity and then heads outside to recess and works away happily for 30 minutes, drawing elaborate maps all over the playground? Or can't understand a scientific concept but has no problem mastering the latest video game? It is important to remember that individual capacity for EF is heavily influenced by familiarity, experience, interest, comfort, and mood, not to mention sleep, nutrition, and illness. This is why the art teacher and the math teacher often have vastly different impressions of a specific student's abilities. American psychologist Ross Greene (2008) reminds us *kids do well if they can,* and he's right: When our students' EFs are working well, they tend to use them. Sometimes, however, EFs are mysterious, unpredictable, and conspicuously absent.

As you read and think more about EFs, you will find your senses become keener to their clues and you will learn to spot them. We sometimes refer to this as developing an "EF lens." It's like wearing a pair of glasses that gives you a different perspective on your learners. With this lens in place you may feel more compassion and understanding toward your students, and you might find your teaching muscles flexing as they haven't flexed in a long time. Finally, *seeing* the EFs in your classroom presents an exciting new range of responses, supports, and teaching opportunities.

HOW TEACHERS ALREADY SUPPORT EFs

Can you remember when the term "executive function" first hit your radar? Teachers are often exposed to this regrettably scientific-sounding label for the first time on the pages of a psychoeducational report. Given a few examples, however, they realize that EFs are very simple. By "EF" we mean, well, almost everything you notice about your *students' performance.* When we refer to "EF-supportive teaching," we are essentially talking about *everything a teacher says and does all day long.* Consider how your work with students is already so oriented toward EF support: We provide charts, planning webs, and tables to help students with organization. We give 10-, 5-, and 2-minute warnings to support time management. We create calming spaces to support emotional regulation. If you took a moment to jot down the 10 routine teaching moves that take the most time in your day, odds are you could connect each one to a lagging EF in your students.

For this reason, it often feels ridiculous to lecture classroom teachers on EFs. Much of what experts know in a theoretical, categorical, or statistical way is understood in a deep, practical, and dynamic way in the field. This contrast in approach makes teachers and researchers excellent partners. Working together, we can use the scientific names of different EFs to sort the behaviors we see and the approaches we use. Sorted into EF categories, both our students' performance and our teaching responses become easier to understand, compare, anticipate, and control. As with any messy, complex situation, a little bit of order goes a long way.

There are a wide range of styles of classroom teaching, but the most effective for building EFs strike a sensitive balance between support and demands. Experts agree that incremental, rigorous challenge in a calm, structured, stimulating, social, and joyful environment will best support EF development (Diamond & Ling, 2020). It's a bit like Goldilocks and her porridge, so let's explore the different flavors, textures, and presentations that make up a "just right" recipe.

First, let's discuss the rough quantities of support in classroom teaching. On one hand, we shouldn't aim to scaffold and support our learners every step of the way. Imagine second-grade students who have had the same "jobs" for 6 months, who require classical music playing softly in the background and an adult "hush" in the air all day, and who barely interact with one another because they are so comfortable in their routines. While this feels relaxing, and you may want to incorporate short periods of respite during your teaching day, a classroom that is comfortable all day is too mushy and bland. It will not be stimulating and challenging enough to promote the normal, healthy growth of EFs in your classroom. On the other hand, neither is it advisable to create an EF war zone by removing all structure, rules, predictability, and order. This is too extreme, and just isn't conducive to learning.

Japanese classrooms might provide an example of a good balance. In studies comparing Japanese teaching to that in the United States and Germany, Stigler and Hiebert (1999) noticed a big difference. In Japan, teachers delivered a new mathematical concept and wrote a problem on the board. No other instructions were given; the students struggled, strained, and stressed as they attempted to figure it out. After a generous period of time, students were gathered up for a supportive discussion about their process, ideas, and strategies. In the United States, a very different situation was observed. The teachers went over a few problems on the overhead, made sure everyone understood the new concept, and gave the students a number of similar problems to solve. They provided guidance all the way, ensuring little to no confusion or frustration. While there is a time and place for structured, fail-proof teaching, it should not be the only approach happening in your classroom.

Apart from core instruction, teachers do many other things at school that either build EFs directly or provide the type of context in which children are most receptive to the direct builders. All of the little extras we do at school are important. As it turns out, our commitment and generosity are not for entertainment, or babysitting, and nor are they cute examples of the eccentricity of experienced teachers—they are powerful factors in the support and development of EF. Consider the research-based direct and indirect builders of EF presented in the left column of Table 1.2. When we ask teachers how they already tap into these builders in their classrooms and schools, they respond heartily. The right column lists just a few of their examples.

There is one additional important factor in the support and development of EFs in your students: you. Remember how EFs are optimized with good sleep, nutrition, health, and regular exercise? This is true for teachers too. The end of Chapter 3 describes how EFs can affect your work, but seriously, have you ever attempted a day of teaching on 2 hours of sleep, or without eating all day, or with a migraine? We don't recommend it, but it's a great way to understand what an EF blackout feels like. You may be short tempered, disorganized, constantly missing the point, firing off ill-advised emails, or terribly inflexible with your class. You can do a lot of damage to your relationships, self-esteem, and reputation on days like these, so if you find yourself in this position, it's best to lay low. Trust us, we've been there. Over the long term, exhausted teachers can experience *burnout cascades* whereby student behavior problems lead to teacher stress, which leads to suboptimal teaching, which leads to further student behavior problems, and on it goes (Maslach & Jackson, 1981). Research suggests, however, that teachers with better EFs experience less stress, tending to report feeling less irritated by children and more in control (Friedman-Krauss, Raver, Neuspiel, & Kinsel, 2014). Optimizing your EFs may protect you from a downward spiral at work.

Conversely, you might remember days when you've managed really well. Perhaps you put your phone away at 9:00 P.M. and got a brilliant night's sleep, or you managed to make breakfast and pack a good lunch. Sometimes it's the simplest things, such as having walked part of the way to school, or having stumbled into a funny conversation with a student that lifted your mood. On days like these you might feel a little magical. You might feel highly attentive, emotionally tuned in, able to handle multiple demands, and capable of exercising good judgment. You might project calm and happiness. For your students, this professionalism and maturity will be an inspiring, and, for some, life-changing source of security. Students who go home to a chaotic environment will benefit especially from the stability and nurturing you provide. Think of yourself as the fifth wall of your classroom. Your health and happiness are so important to your own EF. Don't forget to make time to nourish your own body, mind, and soul.

Teachers, through their support of EF development, play a crucial role in the success of their students. On a day-to-day basis we set a tone of good self-control; perceive many different intellectual, emotional, and social needs; and respond with a "just right" balance of challenge and support. This is heavy-duty work, and why teachers are often exhausted at 3:30. Have you ever had the frustrating experience of having a non-teaching partner or friend explain to you all the ways you should make your work easier? "You're so tired because you do all that extra stuff! Stop taking on so much. Keep it simple. Just get your work done and get out of there." The next time this happens, maybe you'll feel a deeper sense of satisfaction knowing that the extra effort you put in really makes a difference.

TABLE 1.2. EF Builders and How Teachers and Schools Already Use Them

Ways to build EF according to research	Examples of things teachers regularly do
	Direct builders
Evolving structures and rules in the classroom	• Provide a classroom jobs board that changes weekly. • Teach a science unit that requires students to partner up. • Organize new table groups every month. • Have special expectations and rules for a field trip.
Organized, social activities with rules	• Coach basketball or house league dodgeball. • Teach games in gym class, and then encourage students to play them on the playground. • Lead martial arts club and dance club.
Frequent/varied practice using EF for tasks	• Help students organize their essays and math problems. • Help students calm down and resolve disagreements. • Teach students to pay attention to schedules and clocks. • Emphasize steps to use in problem solving.
	Indirect builders
Happiness, familiarity, comfort	• Greet students enthusiastically at the classroom door. • Decorate the classroom so it feels warm and inclusive. • Maintain friendly contact with last year's students. • Participate in schoolwide spirit activities.
Experience, interest, connection	• Include students' interests in learning. • Assess prior knowledge before starting to teach. • Provide examples students can relate to.
Appropriate level of academic challenge	• Conduct preassessments to determine proper level of challenge. • Check in regularly with formative assessment. • Change assignments slightly in response to student success.
Sleep, nutrition, exercise	• Keep homework light and meaningful. • Run active clubs and teams at the school. • Thank parents for balanced lunches and early bedtimes.
Self-confidence	• Make easy opportunities for success and belonging, such as jobs or helpers, or highlighting special accomplishments. • Make sure there are achievable goals for all students.

Note. Based on research by Diamond and Ling (2020) and Bethell, Newacheck, Hawes, and Halfon (2014). Teacher examples generalized based on teacher responses during EF training workshops.

CHAPTER 2

Laying the Foundation
Building Whole-Class EF Literacy

BUILDING EF LITERACY FOR FREE

Traditionally, "literacy" is defined as the ability to decode, understand, interpret, create, and communicate; it takes place across a continuum of growth. This definition often refers to the complex skills required to read and write, but EF literacy can be thought of in much the same way. It involves vocabulary ("goal-directed persistence") and rules (EFs don't mature until our mid-20s). We use it to decipher, demystify, and relate to the people around us and, with practice, we become more fluent and adept. We will talk a lot about EF literacy in this book: the way it can influence relationships and self-understanding, as well as the way it can change instruction, feedback, and assessment. We will use the term to describe teachers, students, principals, and whole school communities who see and respond to one another through an EF lens.

We prioritize building EF literacy in children for several reasons. Most important, we do it because it helps them keep challenges in perspective. *Self-complexity theory* suggests that students with a complex and multifaceted understanding of themselves are more emotionally safe. When they make a mistake, their hard feelings about those negative events don't "spill over" and encompass their entire self. Rather, using knowledge of the many EFs that they have and use, they can attribute the challenge to only one or two specific facets of a big, broad identity (Linville, 1985). It is a little like having a diverse financial portfolio: If one stock tanks, you don't go broke. Thus, boosting self-complexity by teaching students about their EFs allows a student handing in a late report to think, "I didn't plan my time properly" or "I struggle with attention and missed the deadline information" rather than "I'm a total loser and will never succeed at report writing." This makes a big difference.

Teachers often assume that the best path to EF literacy is a formal, whole-class, spiral-bound or computerized program. Many of these types of programs exist for teaching EF strategy (see

Appendix A), but do they get used? Look behind your teaching desk. Amid the binders and books, overstuffed file folders, and piles of last years' assessments, can you find at least one great program that you simply didn't have time to apply? Can you find five? Bet you can. If you search the Internet or ask a colleague, you will find many formal programs that touch upon student self-awareness or EF. These can be very powerful, but they are often time-consuming and restrictive. Meanwhile, research tells us that teachers try new things most enthusiastically when they feel a sense of control (Le Fevre, 2014) and when the "new things" don't feel too intrusive (Kazdin, 1980; Reimers, Wacker, & Koeppl, 1987). Sound familiar? As frontline users, teachers know an awful lot about the context and timing factors that will determine the success of what they are attempting. So, before you rush off to buy a formal program, you might like to consider taking a do-it-yourself approach. It might work just as well, if not better!

Most great classrooms are a balance between curricula that the school purchases and supplemental materials that teachers add in. On any given day we may use something as structured as a scripted remedial reading program and as open-ended as an inquiry-based social studies program. In our experience, teaching students about EFs is straightforward enough to be done simply, creatively, and for free. Don't get us wrong—heavily researched curricula have their place—but we've seen hundreds of teachers build whole-class EF literacy, and not one of them used a commercial program. Let's talk about why this makes sense.

First, while it is interesting and satisfying for children to learn new EF knowledge and vocabulary, we believe the best learning happens during the authentic and meaningful learning situations that you can't find in a formal program. For this reason, we believe teachers should introduce basic EF knowledge and concepts as quickly as possible and then dive right in to actually speak the language of EFs. With only a basic introduction to EFs, your students can begin to engage in classroom discussions about the EFs in everyday work. We often describe the initial, brief, direct teaching of EFs like the setting up of conceptual "buckets" in children's minds. We then plunge our students into real-life EF experience, so these buckets can be filled in a meaningful way. Their applied conversations about EFs will provide rich context and meaning, and their understanding will blossom naturally. This process of becoming EF literate is like mastering any language: You practice just enough to get by, and then immerse yourself in the culture of the language so the real learning can happen.

Also, teaching children about EFs is just too delightfully fun to leave your creativity and autonomy at the door. If done with compassion and understanding, building EF literacy is a special opportunity for teacher and students to learn about each other, connect deeply, and share a laugh or two. You'll want to be fully engaged, inquiring, curious, and active in this learning right along with your students. Trust us, this is not too complex to undertake on your own.

Enough preamble—let's get down to specifics. If you want to teach your whole class to be functionally EF literate, your learning objectives are a simple *knowledge* + *skill* + *concept* combination. Table 2.1 lists the key learning outcomes for our EF-literate students.

Almost every single teacher we have worked with starts by printing a set of posters to capture these key ideas in an anchor chart. Figure 2.1 shows a snapshot of some of the many teacher-created materials that you can access and print on our community website (*http://activatedlearning.org*), but there are many other kinds of EF posters available at little to no cost online. A general Google search will yield useful results, and Pinterest has many interesting options (*https://pinterest.com*). Also, websites such as Teachers Pay Teachers offer many different low-cost paid options (*https:// teacherspayteachers.com*).

TABLE 2.1. Key Learning Outcomes for Students Who Are Becoming EF Literate

Knowing . . .	EFs work alongside our intellect and creativity to help us respond effectively to challenges.
	Names and definitions of 11 EFs.
Being able to . . .	Notice and name the impact of specific EFs in everyday performance.
Understanding . . .	EFs are a natural, normal, growing, and controllable part of everyone's performance.
	Our EFs allow us to express our creativity and intellect.
	We all have a unique pattern of EF strength and challenge—even adults.
	We should feel proud of our own unique profile of strength and challenge.

With these basic materials printed and posted, the teaching of EFs can be done in a variety of different ways. How you choose to teach EFs will depend on your own personal style and preference, the time of year, the group of students you're working with, and how much time you have available. Throughout the remainder of this chapter, as well as in Chapters 3, 4, 5, and 6, we'll give specific information about how to implement what we're discussing in *five different contexts*. These contexts describe different dynamics you might experience with students, and you may find yourself in several of them throughout your teaching day. For example, you may feel time strapped when addressing your class on a field trip, huddled on a busy downtown street, but you may feel more structured when teaching those same students later in math class. Or you might be a single-subject teacher who instructs group after group of students who couldn't be more different. We hope that, across these contexts, you'll find something useful—an example to modify, an idea to explore, or an approach that you love enough to use "as is."

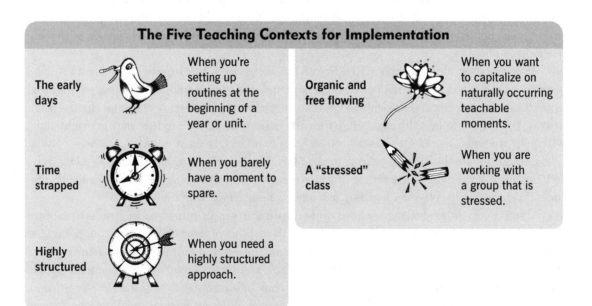

The Five Teaching Contexts for Implementation

The early days — When you're setting up routines at the beginning of a year or unit.

Time strapped — When you barely have a moment to spare.

Highly structured — When you need a highly structured approach.

Organic and free flowing — When you want to capitalize on naturally occurring teachable moments.

A "stressed" class — When you are working with a group that is stressed.

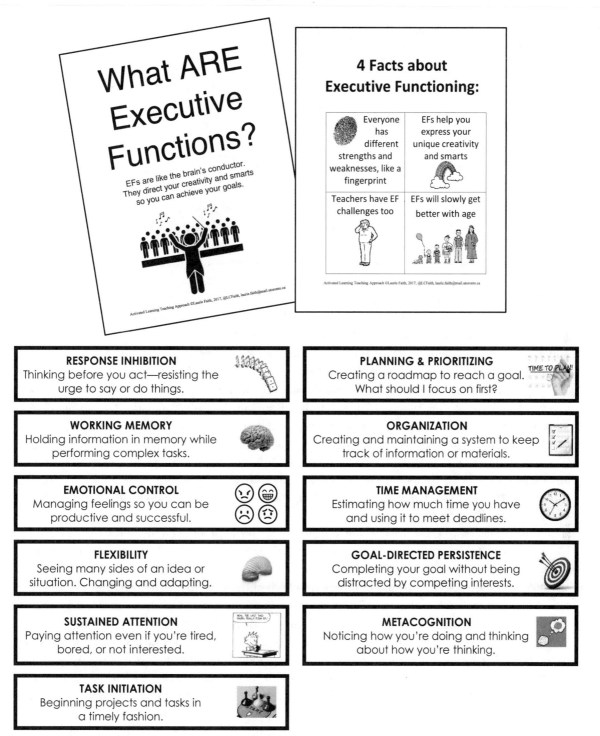

FIGURE 2.1. Classroom posters developed to display key knowledge and concepts about executive functioning. The posters "What Are Executive Functions?" and "4 Facts About Executive Functioning" were created by Laurie Faith in consultation with other teachers. The small EF posters were created by Stephanie Walker at Scott Young Public School in Lindsay, Ontario, Canada. All posters can be downloaded from *http://activatedlearning.org*.

How to Teach EFs: *Early Days*

The *big idea* here is that teaching students about EFs aligns nicely with the classic "early days" work of getting to know your class and setting a positive tone. In this section, you'll learn more about how to do the following:

- Create a simple EF bulletin board in your classroom.
- Do an informal EF survey right along with your class as a getting-to-know-you activity.
- Encourage students to keep their EF strengths in mind.

The early days of a school year have a special rhythm. Most teachers spend a week or so going over classroom expectations, reviewing routines, and conducting "getting to know you" activities. Even the most overprogrammed and highly structured classrooms do this, because in addition to being welcoming, setting the right tone, and teaching everyone how to use the restroom pass, it unearths crucial information about our students as learners.

We (the authors) remember this tradition well: Every one of *our* teachers quizzed us about our favorite colors and favorite foods in September. We tried the activity as adults and discovered that Laurie's favorite food is spaghetti, Carol's is a good curry, and Peg's is a lobster roll. We aren't sure, however, if knowing these preferences really brought us closer together, and we can't imagine how our teachers used this type of information to help us learn.

If you're planning to start teaching your students about EFs in September, you're in luck. You can comfortably cover the basics of EF before the academic year starts and also tick off many of your September goals: getting to know your students, allowing them to get to know you and each other, and setting a positive and inclusive tone. The self-discovery and discovery about others you facilitate will go way beyond favorite foods and colors. It will begin a compassionate relationship among your class that is based on a deep understanding that we are all unique and have different profiles of strength and challenge. And the information you discover as individuals and as a team will be useful all year long.

Many teachers we know use the simple materials we have gathered on the Activated Learning (AL) website (*http://activatedlearning.org*) to launch their September getting-to-know-you conversations. They start by posting a set of EF posters and administering an informal EF survey. To use the survey, children work through a two-page list of prompts, rating themselves on three indicators for each of 11 different EFs (Figure 2.2). For example, in the response inhibition section, they must decide if they always, often, sometimes, rarely, or never "rush into assignments before fully understanding instructions" or "blurt stuff out in class." This activity can help students build knowledge of the impact of EF on school performance, and they enjoy discussing their responses. We know teachers who introduce the activity by presenting their own results on the teacher questionnaire (available on *http://activatedlearning.org*). This is a great opportunity to model self-understanding, self-acceptance, and self-compassion. And you can help students feel connected to you right away with an honest comment like "You've only just met me, but you'll see that I have to work really hard to stay organized. Maybe you can give me ideas for keeping my desk tidy? The good news is that I'm really flexible, so I'll be excited to try your ideas!"

After spending about 30 minutes helping students understand and complete their own surveys, some teachers encourage their students to fill in a graph to visualize their profile of strengths and challenges. By creating a graph, students can quickly notice which of their EFs are the stron-

1 Always	2 Often	3 Sometimes	4 Rarely	5 Never

EF Checker for Kids

Item	RESPONSE INHIBITION	Score
1	Even if I'm full, I just can't stop eating and nibbling.	
2	I blurt stuff out in class: "I know!" or "Pick me!"	
3	I start work before I've heard all of the instructions. I just rush off.	
	Total Score for Response Inhibition	
	WORKING MEMORY	
4	I forget what I am saying halfway through.	
5	If I get too many instructions, I can't remember them all.	
6	It's hard to hold a few things in my head at once (like rules of a game).	
	Total Score for Working Memory	
	(Continues for 11 sections to represent 11 EFs.)	

FIGURE 2.2. A portion of the "EF Checker for Students of All Ages" available at *http://activatedlearning. org.*

gest, and in which areas they tend to struggle. It can also help them appreciate personal growth when completed in September and June. In Figure 2.3, you can see two different student graphs. Notice that Student 1 is a natural planner, while Student 2 discovered that planning and prioritizing was an area of weakness. Meanwhile, Student 1 struggles with response inhibition, while for Student 2 this EF is not as challenging. These students certainly have a lot to learn from each other, and they might be helpful partners!

We know a few teachers who display these graphs to stimulate conversations among students about EF diversity. "Wow!" a student commented, "This is cool to see. Each of us has strengths, and our needs are so different!" Imagine standing next to this student. What a lightbulb moment! Would you say, "Interesting, Kaylie . . . organization is a strong EF for you. Do you use it to help you with time management?" or "Look, you and Zev are both so flexible! Have you ever worked in a group with him?" or "Emotional regulation is tricky for me too, but I use my strong planning skills to help. Do you?" Looking at evidence like this helps students realize that, while they do have challenges, they also have a few powerful resources. We know classrooms in which the students were so proud to discover their EF skills they decided to create strength badges to stick onto their desks; a teacher, substitute teacher, or peer walking by would know right away that Zev was highly flexible and Kaylie was a super organizer. Completing an EF survey (and graphing the results) also helps students to appreciate the huge variety of strength and challenge among their classmates. They may discover a peer with a similar skill or one whose skills are complementary to their own. After the students have gone home, teachers confide that seeing a pile of 20–30 completely different looking graphs helps them understand their students, and really confirms the complexity of the work they do to support them.

Bar Graph of EF Strengths and Challenges: Student 1

	RI	WM	EC	CF	SA	TI	PP	O	TM	GDP	M
15											
14											
13							▓				
12							▓				
11							▓				
10			▓				▓			▓	
9		▓	▓	▓			▓		▓	▓	
8		▓	▓	▓	▓		▓		▓	▓	
7		▓	▓	▓	▓	▓	▓		▓	▓	
6		▓	▓	▓	▓	▓	▓		▓	▓	
5		▓	▓	▓	▓	▓	▓		▓	▓	
4		▓	▓	▓	▓	▓	▓		▓	▓	
3	▓	▓	▓	▓	▓	▓	▓	▓	▓	▓	▓

Bar Graph of EF Strengths and Challenges: Student 2

	RI	WM	EC	CF	SA	TI	PP	O	TM	GDP	M
15											
14											
13										▓	
12										▓	
11	▓				▓					▓	
10	▓		▓		▓	▓				▓	
9	▓	▓	▓		▓	▓			▓	▓	
8	▓	▓	▓	▓	▓	▓			▓	▓	▓
7	▓	▓	▓	▓	▓	▓		▓	▓	▓	▓
6	▓	▓	▓	▓	▓	▓		▓	▓	▓	▓
5	▓	▓	▓	▓	▓	▓		▓	▓	▓	▓
4	▓	▓	▓	▓	▓	▓		▓	▓	▓	▓
3	▓	▓	▓	▓	▓	▓	▓	▓	▓	▓	▓

FIGURE 2.3. Student graphs to show the relative EF strength and challenge discovered using the "EF Checker for Students of All Ages." These are similar to those created by Stephanie Walker's grade 4/5 learning strategies students at Scott Young Public School in Omemee, Ontario, Canada. Blank copies available at *http://activatedlearning.org*. Used with permission.

Homeroom teachers aren't the only ones who can launch the year with EF literacy. In Ontario, we know a group of music, drama, and visual arts teachers who are also focused on EFs.[1] In one of their music classrooms, for example, students began the year by exploring the impact of EFs on music making. Figure 2.4 lists many examples generated by a group of grade 8 band students. This activity occupied a whole period at the beginning of the year but was invaluable for understanding the many ways different students experience musical challenges. This teacher encouraged students

---

[1] This group's work can be found on Twitter at @ArtsActivated.

to celebrate their strengths as individuals and to offer "shout out" feedback about the strengths they saw in others.

Teachers who have time for a more extensive introduction to EFs can use our more in-depth materials. The "EF Basics" lesson series found in Appendix B provides teachers with 30–40 minutes per function of definition, discussion, and immersive EF experiences. The activities suggested use ordinary materials, such as playing cards, paper, markers, and clocks, or use resources readily available on the Internet. Many teachers choose to cover one function per day to kick off the school year. For example, your class can explore how goal-directed persistence feels by trying to build card houses for 10 minutes without giving up. Teachers tell us that this activity helps students

---

How Do EFs Impact Grade 8 Band Class?
(Student Ideas)

Response Inhibition	Don't start playing before being asked Hold rests for long enough
Working Memory	Remembering notes Watching conductor, instrument, and sheet music
Emotional Control	Staying calm when you mess up Not getting upset when you don't know how to play a song
Flexibility	Adjusting to change of instruments, songs, or groups Working well no matter who is in your group
Sustained Attention	Waiting to start playing Practice even when others are practicing their different parts
Task Initiation	Taking out your instrument at home to get going with practice Learning a new song when it feels overwhelming
Planning and Prioritizing	Meeting deadlines Writing down your next playing test
Organization	Keeping track of your sheet music Knowing how the sheet music works—which parts repeat
Time Management	Getting your instrument set up in time to play Scheduling enough practice time each week
Goal-Directed Persistence	Playing your instrument even if there are distractions Continuing to play even if you make a mistake
Metacognition	Noticing how you're playing Remembering which are the hard parts to focus on in practice

FIGURE 2.4. Created during a band lesson at Central Senior School in Lindsay, Ontario, Canada, by Holly Smith. Used with permission.

notice that some EFs work together because, for example, staying calm or focused or organizing the area in which they are building may help support their ability to persist.

If you're at a school that hosts a well-attended parents' night in September, consider sharing EF literacy with your greater community. Our friends, Ontario teachers Jer, Julie, and Sallie, hosted the families of their grades 7 and 8 students at a special "EF Bootcamp for Parents" event. During an action-packed 45-minute session, they provided everyone with a basic definition of EF, conducted a special "Parent Survey" (available at *http://activatedlearning.org*), and led the group in a discussion of the types of EFs that might affect their child's ability to keep a clean and tidy bedroom. They discovered that, after only a brief introduction, parents could be much more understanding and insightful about their children's performance. Among the group, parents came up with five EF challenges that might underlie their children's messy bedrooms. Not bad! The day after their parents' night, Jer, Julie, and Sallie repeated the discussion about EFs and clean bedrooms with their students, and they came up with a whopping 13 potential EF challenges. You can see both the parents' and the students' ideas in Figure 2.5. Building basic EF literacy among children and their parents allows them, finally, to speak clearly and learn from one another about the EF barriers they engage with every day.

How to Teach EFs:
Time Strapped

The *big idea* here is that teaching students about EFs needn't happen in dedicated, formal lessons. Rather, it can take place in the context of everyday "teachable moments." In this section, you'll learn more about how to do the following:

- Keep your eyes peeled for great teachable moments and indulge in a noticing and naming conversation with your students when they occur.
- Work an EF activity into things that are already happening, such as homework assignments, assemblies, or curriculum nights.

You have *literally no time* for anything extra. We get it—teachers have a million priorities. Even without dedicated lessons or activities; however, you can still make a huge difference in how your students understand their learning. This section will present a few options for time-neutral EF teaching in your classroom.

First of all, formal, dedicated lessons about EFs are not always necessary to develop EF knowledge in students. You can build EF literacy using a more casual approach. To do this, find an empty bulletin board, a door, or a chunk of wall and bang up some EF posters. We recommend hanging the "Basic EF" definitions and the "EF Ideas" posters that you can find on *http://activatedlearning.org*. This will cover the basic knowledge and concepts your students need to become educated and empowered. Then, let the words and ideas seep into your room as part of your everyday conversations about learning. You will quickly realize there are many natural opportunities to talk about EFs. Consider the commonsense approach shared by this experienced teacher:

"I'm confident in my EF teaching, but I don't use a lot of fancy laminated material or checklists. I believe a lot of EF information can be incorporated with little time and effort. This year, my monarch caterpillar chrysalis hatched on day one. Not the best situation, but I told the kids that we would let it go after the assembly. Our plan fell through, so we let it out at the end of the day. I pointed out flexibility and congratulated all of them. Each day thereafter I briefly connected an EF to a situation. Yesterday I had the students write a paragraph on the monarch life cycle. The topic sentence was on the board. I kept checking in with Megan who was not writing anything and was looking increasingly frustrated. In the end she finally did it. I told her, 'You're obviously a good writer, but it looks like you have a hard time getting started.' I pointed out task initiation, told her it's a problem for me too, and told her we'd find strategies

How Do EFs Impact Our Teenagers' Ability to Keep a Clean Bed Room (Parents' Notes)

Sustained Attention	Becoming distracted by their phones
Planning/ Prioritizing	Making room cleaning a priority over other activities
Task Initiation	Putting it off "until later"
Flexibility	Insisting they prefer it messy and that they are used to it
Emotional Control	Feeling overwhelmed by the mess

How Do EFs Impact Our Ability to Keep a Clean Bed Room (Teenagers' Notes)

Sustained Attention	Becoming distracted by our phones Feeling lazy or tired
Planning/ Prioritizing	Thinking we should do homework or have a snack first Wanting to spend time with friends
Task Initiation	Putting it off "until later"
Flexibility	Feeling that we prefer it messy and that we are used to it
Emotional Control	Feeling overwhelmed by the mess
Goal-Directed Persistence	Getting started but then becoming distracted Didn't really commit to cleaning the room in the first place, so easy to quit
Org	Not enough space/storage
Working Memory	Managing multiple directions Forgetting the last steps

FIGURE 2.5. Parents' versus their teens' ideas about EF demands in household work. These charts were created at a grade 7 and 8 parents' night activity facilitated by Jeremiah Beggs, Sallie Byer, and Julie Kuiken from Central Senior School in Lindsay, Ontario, Canada. Both parents and their children were asked to describe the way EFs might affect a teen's ability to keep a clean bedroom. Used with permission.

to help her. I swear I saw her body language show relief." (J. Rhude, personal communication, September 8, 2018)[2]

As teachers, our days are filled with opportunities such as these. EF challenges fill our classrooms and dominate our work with students. For example, we support students as they struggle to *start* on writing assignments, *organize* their ideas, or pay close enough *attention* to catch every error while editing. In social studies, we may find ourselves urging students to explore multiple theories or work with partners *flexibly*. Or, have you ever marked arithmetic with a student, noticed missing steps or dropped numbers, and suggested they write down every step clearly? The truth is, you are already talking about EFs all day long. With posters up, your conversation about writing down every step of a math problem can become one of many quick lessons about *working memory* and *organization*.

EFs are complex concepts. They change slightly in response to different challenges and may even look different from day to day based on sleep, nutrition, and mood. This is why it makes sense to build EF literacy in context. Would you try to teach a young child about the concept of a tree in a windowless room? If you're lucky, you can go outside and see a variety of different sizes and types, feel the texture of papery and rough bark, smell pine sap, and taste what happens when maple sap is boiled down into syrup. Building a concept slowly with practical examples from real life allows for a full, nuanced understanding and deep learning.

You may also consider putting some of your "transition time" to work. By printing an extra copy of the EF posters and simply cutting the title away from the definition, you can make a matching activity or memory game. Students can amuse themselves with this while the classroom administration is happening in the morning or between subjects. This seems very simple, but it will help your students build vocabulary, fluency, and familiarity with the concepts.

Another efficient option is to "flip" your teaching of EFs into a task that takes place either after school or during a special schoolwide event. To flip it into an at-home activity, send a student EF survey (available at *http://activatedlearning.org*) home for homework and have your class make a quick report on what they discovered the next day. Depending on your parent population, you may wish to send home the parent EF survey as well. Involving parents works best if your school administration is supportive of your classroom work on EFs. We have seen many easy in-class follow-ups to EF homework. After assigning the EF survey, one teacher we know asked her students to decorate classroom EF posters by placing two pink paper hearts on their strengths and two blue paper hearts on the EFs that were most challenging for them. An activity like this can add dimension and a bit of structure to your everyday efforts to notice and name.

Or, many schools organize special themed days on which normal classes are canceled and the whole population engages in special, spirit-building activities. This would be a great time to distribute the EF mini-lessons (Appendix B) among different stations and have students rotate through them during the day. Several schools we work with have made EF literacy a whole-community priority and have made great strides toward educating all teachers, students, and families with special events, newsletters, and curriculum-night workshops. Having a background in EFs will ensure that your community responds supportively when discussing strengths and challenges with their children.

---

[2]Janet Rhude teaches at Scott Young Public School in Lindsay, Ontario, Canada. Used with permission. Student name changed to protect privacy.

The saying goes that anything worth doing is worth doing well. Perhaps, though, anything *really* worth doing is worth doing in whatever way you can—no matter how limited your resources and how short the time. Exposing your students to even a few key concepts about EFs plants a seed and is so much better than nothing. So, have no fear. Feel no shame. We believe that a time-strapped education in EF literacy is a darn fine place to start.

How to Teach EFs:
Highly Structured

The *big idea* here is that teaching students about EFs can be done in a routine and structured way. In this section, you'll learn more about how to do the following:

- Teach each EF in a systematic way using the 11 lessons provided in Appendix B.
- Engage your students in a variety of projects related to EFs, including posters, pamphlets, storybooks, or magazines.
- Add an EF component to classroom routines you already have up and running.

Many teachers decide that EFs will be a major focus in their classroom and adopt a highly structured approach. By this method, EF literacy is built up slowly as EFs are introduced one by one throughout a portion of the school year. By this method, attention may be covered in the first 2 weeks, time management in the second, and so on. Or you may choose a weekly or monthly pace. While this doesn't front-load EF literacy quickly, it does allow students to fully explore each EF in a systematic way. It is important, however, that this learning is not relegated only to separate mini-lessons. You need to reinforce the ideas in casual discussions and encourage your students to make connections during meaningful academic and social learning experiences for this approach to be truly powerful.

Stephanie Walker's fifth-grade classroom is a good example of how this can work.[3] She introduces one EF per month, preparing a wide variety of different activities to deepen her students' understanding. Stephanie's lessons often begin with a four-square Frayer model (Figure 2.6). In the first square, she provides a clear definition for the EF they are focusing on. In squares 2 and 3, she encourages her students to come up with written and drawn examples of its impact on their performance. Finally, in the last square, students think of a strategy that helps them manage the EF being discussed. With this basic understanding established, she conducts other activities, including reflective bulletin boards created with the help of students, poster making, journaling, podcasts, songs, and daily bell work. For an additional mini-unit on working memory, her class created a variety of fun working memory games and hosted a fair for other students at the school. Students leave Stephanie's classroom with very well-established EF literacy.

To support Stephanie's work, we created a series of 11 mini-lessons, which are available in Appendix B. For each EF, you will find a blank Frayer model and a sample of how it may look when filled in. As well, we've described several quick, hands-on activities that will allow your students to play with the ideas and bring each EF to life. These lessons are designed to cover one EF per teaching period but could be extended across several lessons. Or if you don't have time or the need for all of them, you may find the material useful as a way to deepen understanding in one or two

---

[3] Stephanie teaches at Scott Young Public School in Omemee, Ontario, Canada. Used with permission.

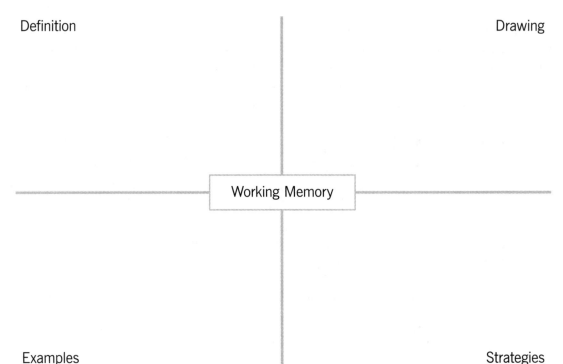

Definition   Drawing

Working Memory

Examples   Strategies

FIGURE 2.6. One of 11 Frayer models used by Stephanie Walker at Scott Young Public School in Omemee, Ontario, Canada, to discuss each executive function. Used with permission.

key areas. The activities are straightforward, suitable for any age, and highly adaptable. Teachers in one Ontario school have used the lessons for schoolwide EF teaching, agreeing that every classroom will designate one 45-minute teaching period per month to launch an EF. Then the "EF of the month" is discussed in school assemblies and in the school newsletter. The timing of highly structured teaching is predictable, so this approach is compatible with collaborative teaching, either between classrooms or among whole schools.

Several teachers we work with facilitate in-depth projects relating to EFs. Students in Julie Hough's grade 7/8 class worked in groups to create articles for a magazine on EFs for their parents.[4] Each student researched and wrote a short piece describing an EF and how strategies can be used to support it. This project did double duty—both supporting student learning and bringing parents up to speed! Some classes create "EF passports" or portfolios over the course of the year. Students created small booklets in which each EF is listed along with their personal strengths, challenges, and most effective strategies. When created inside a small 5 × 7 photo album, these booklets are heavy duty enough to travel with students from class to class, and they become an invaluable part of a students' transition plan when graduating to a new grade, school, or program, or even when a new teacher joins the faculty. These in-depth projects require planning and time but can be very rewarding.

Teachers already using social and emotional learning programs, such as Zones of Regulation, restorative practices, or community circles, may find that the teaching of EFs falls nicely into the

---

[4]Julie Hough teaches at Woodville Elementary School in Woodville, Ontario, Canada. Used with permission.

structures and routines they have already set up. You can add on to your Zones bulletin board, for example, because Zones tackles emotional regulation, and this is itself an executive function. If your class is already self-aware, self-compassionate, and strategic regarding their emotional regulation, building these attitudes and skills around other EFs will be second nature. Other teachers incorporate discussion prompts relating to EFs into their community circle conversations. Colleen Eagle's grade 7 class uses a ring of task cards that she purchased on Teachers Pay Teachers through a vendor called Pathway 2 Success.[5] The cards may ask, "You have a lot of homework, but you have practice at 6:00 P.M. What can you do?" or simply, "What does it mean to prioritize?" Students pick an EF to focus on, choose a question, and explore ideas together. This simple material encourages students to engage in reflective, authentic dialogue about the ways that EFs relate to their challenges in the classroom. EF teaching can be tacked on to structures you already have in place.

We know plenty of highly structured EF teachers that are particularly *data oriented.* Is this your style? If not, buckle up because things are about to get intense. There is a certain type, who after working through an EF survey (available at *http://activatedlearning.org*) with their students, simply can't resist entering that data into a spreadsheet. Once entered, this data becomes a delightful playground for making graphs and charts, aggregating groups of students according to areas of strength, and planning whole-class lessons based on common areas of challenge. Charlene Chapman's grade 4 class was organized into expert groups based on an Excel spreadsheet of EF survey data.[6] These groups then consulted with other students to better understand how strength and weakness in a particular EF might feel. On a day-to-day basis, data-hungry teachers can use widely available apps such as Plickers (*https://plickers.com*) to quickly snapshot, chart, and display data on EFs that students feel are most affecting their performance for specific tasks. Organizing your teaching around data is always a good idea, and it certainly fits a highly structured teaching approach.

Delivering highly structured EF lessons builds deep understanding, compassion, and perspective, especially if you can provide ongoing reinforcement in your classroom. Your students will become fluent in a language of learning that they can return to throughout their lives. So, even if you are the only person at your school who is interested in EFs, and suspect that your class will not have any further training with next year's teacher . . . persist! Your work will be an enduring gift.

How to Teach EFs:
Organic and Free Flowing

The *big idea* here is that the teaching of EFs can take place during everyday classroom challenges and experiences. In this section, you'll learn more about how to do the following:

- Capitalize on unexpected or unwanted behavior to make a connection to an EF.
- Share your thinking about your own EFs with students to help them learn.
- Look for EF challenges in the stories you read aloud using the mentor texts we list in Appendix C as a starting point.

---

[5] Colleen Eagle teaches at Scott Young Public School in Omemee, Ontario, Canada. Used with permission.

[6] Charlene Chapman teaches at Queen Victoria Public School in Lindsay, Ontario, Canada. Used with permission.

When you are in tune with your class, you can approach the teaching of EFs in a way that capitalizes on naturally occurring teachable moments. There are so many perfect opportunities. For example, imagine a fall day at around 10:30 in the morning. Your class is outside for recess, and you've managed to make a cup of tea. The bell rings, the heavy double doors at the end of the hall burst open, and you hear your class arguing as they hang up their coats. (They tried to invent a hide and seek game but couldn't agree on the rules.) You can respond in several ways. You can tell them to leave playground issues on the playground. You can suggest they all go outside and come back in again quietly. Maybe you'll sit them down and explain the proper rules for hide and seek. Or— aha!—perhaps this is the perfect time to call them to the carpet to introduce the idea of flexibility.

Let's think of an example a little closer to the classroom: Your students are lined up and heading to the gym. They are quiet and orderly, but as they go down the hall, they drag their little fingers along the walls, wiping away words written on whiteboards and ruffling art displays. You remind them that this is destructive and ask them to stop but turn around to find a few students still at it. Again, you have many possible responses. You can stop the group, stand quietly before them, and comment seriously, "I am so disappointed." You can loudly thank the students who have followed your instructions, or name the students who have not. But what if, in a flash of inspiration, you reflect on the science of EF and the fact that it is harder for some children to inhibit impulses? You may realize that this is the perfect opportunity to introduce the term "response inhibition," and to explain that we all have different strengths and challenges. "Response inhibition is hard for me too," you might say. "When I have an itchy mosquito bite, it is so hard to stop myself from scratching it!" From here, the conversation can flow more naturally into the different ways we sometimes feel tempted to do the wrong thing, and how we can work strategically to make sure we are in control of our impulses.

Let us provide a final example that is nestled right inside the four walls of your classroom. Imagine your class has been researching animal adaptations for 2 weeks. Each student has a file full of notes that will be useful for writing a short essay, and today is the day they are to begin. You've given a good lesson about sorting the research idea into structured paragraphs. Your students are excited about their research and ideas, but nothing is happening. Nobody writes very much. They chat with each other and doodle, and after 20 minutes some haven't managed a single word. You might feel disappointed and frustrated. Your responses could include an exasperated sigh, a calm warning that tomorrow everyone will be placed at separate tables away from friends, or a generous reiteration of the lesson. In response, your students might look hurt or angry, and someone might declare, "I hate writing!" In this way, even our most disciplined and effortful teaching responses may compound problems with students. Consider how a knowledge of EFs enables different approach. For example, you could say to your students, "I see everyone in the room struggling with this work, and I don't know why. Is this an organizational challenge? Or are you worried about making your writing perfect in the first draft—is it emotional regulation? Or are you just having trouble taking the first step to initiate the work?" In conversations like these, you will discover something new about your students' learning, and they will learn to apply their EF literacy to their everyday challenges. By capitalizing on naturally teachable moments, it is possible to structure your EF teaching around the shared experiences of the students in your class.

This organic approach to teaching EFs takes place naturally in a language arts classroom. In the upper grades, we have observed literature units focused on themes of "hero versus self" in which classes spend weeks searching for evidence of goal-directed persistence, emotional control, and flexibility. In the lower elementary years, we have observed classrooms filled with stories that either indirectly or directly focus on EFs. The "What Do You Do?" series by Kobi Yamada includes three books on the topic of choice, control, self-awareness, and goal-directed persistence. Julia Cook has several books that tackle specific EFs, and one of our favorite feel-good, you-can-do-it books is *Jabari Jumps* by Gaia Cornwall. You will find a complete list of great stories organized by grade level in Appendix C at the end of the book.

People often wonder how complex ideas like EFs can be a part of the daily chatter in a room of very young children. In fact, kindergarten is a perfect place to start. At this age, so many of the children's experiences are dictated by their emerging EFs, from limited flexibility to sometimes explosive emotional control and to completely unpredictable response inhibition. Paula Barrow capitalizes on daily teachable moments to introduce each EF in her primary classroom.[7] When an opportunity arises, such as a heated disagreement over whose turn it is to use a certain material, she stops her class to teach the students about which EF is being challenged. "You had a hard time controlling your emotions," she tells them. Then, referring to a display of EF posters, she says, "That is one of the executive functions. Emotional control is important because it helps us stay calm and work together." Finally, with the help of her students, Paula creates a poster to represent the idea of emotional control. Guided by her students, she searches for pictures online, scrolling through different options on the SMART board until the group agrees on just the right one. In the case of emotional control, her students decided that a picture of a brain holding hands with a heart made sense because it showed the way you can think about your feelings and choose how to express them. While not every classroom has access to a SMART board, we think this idea would work just as well using simpler materials to draw the representative images.

Teachers often worry that EF concepts will be too complex for their students to fully understand. On one hand, they are right. Even adults learning about EFs will notice that their comprehension deepens slowly over many years. We, as authors of this book, feel as though each student we meet teaches us something new. On the other hand, our experiences suggest that the acquisition of basic EF concepts may come *quite* naturally to children, even at a very young age. We suspect this is because their daily work at school is so novel, challenging, and heavily affected by the limitations of their emerging EFs. Kindergarten children being included in a discussion about "response inhibition," for example, often lean in intensely, become very animated, or look at us as if to say "Duh! What took you so long to talk to us about this? We struggle with this stuff all day long!" Conversations about EFs often feel personal to students, and make typical school tasks feel more interesting. Once you start teaching EFs organically throughout a school day, you'll wonder what in the world you were doing before, and you'll never look at your students in quite the same way again.

How to Teach EFs:
Working with a "Stressed" Class

The *big idea* here is that teaching students about EFs is a wonderful way to build trust, acceptance, and openness. In this section, you'll learn more about how to do the following:

- Show students that it is safe to be vulnerable and honest.
- Intentionally plan the EF challenges that will be involved in lessons and activities and discuss them with your students as they arise.

---

[7] Paula Barrow teaches at Fenelon Township Public School in Cameron, Ontario, Canada.

Our classrooms can be intense places, and many teachers worry that EFs will be too personal, too "touchy-feely," or too triggering to discuss with their students. You might, for example, teach children who always seem stressed—tightly coiled springs ready to explode at the smallest disappointment or perceived slight. Will they feel offended at the idea that their ability to pay attention, say, might be slightly less acute than that of a classmate? Or perhaps you have a class that is very distracted and impulsive and can only manage the basics. Can this group be trusted with the vulnerability of their classmates? Other teachers tell us that their ability to try new things is dictated by one or two volatile students. They feel bad for the rest of the class but generally avoid anything unusual or special because it might cause a meltdown. Many of the teachers we work with use the Zones of Regulation program and refer to these students as "red zone" students or "high fliers." If you find yourself in one of these situations and are concerned about delving into EFs because your students might feel threatened, overwhelmed, or angry, this section might be particularly useful.

How can we help students feel safe, relaxed, and engaged during conversations about EFs? We can start by being sensitive to their reality, both past and present. Remember that many of our students' past experiences of EF challenge will have been negative. A failure to plan, for example, may be associated with getting into trouble, failing to meet expectations, or feeling embarrassed in front of peers. Students with weaker attention may be used to the frustrated sighs of their classmates when they ask *another* question that has already been answered. Struggles with emotional regulation may be a reminder of tearful, traumatic moments and subsequent shaming responses from family, friends, and others. Almost everyone has difficulty managing one or two EFs. Can you think of what is most challenging for you? Can you remember a moment from your life at which this weakness made you feel embarrassed, not smart, or unkind? Our most stressed students are often those who have significant difficulty in several areas and have well-established habits of avoidance and helplessness. These students would rather go anywhere than into a conversation about behavior that might result in punishment or embarrassment.

Because of this rocky past with EFs, stressed students often perceive our EF teaching as a clear and present danger. Compared to others who are often willing to trust us and talk openly about EFs, our stressed students may seem stubborn, willfully self-destructive, and intentionally unsuccessful. Sound familiar? Unfortunately, our most needy students may not have room in their self-esteem budget to make risky and vulnerable moves at school. For example, let's say a student in your class doesn't start daily math assignments because her working memory is unreliable, and she can't always recall the instructions. If she admits this, will everyone roll their eyes? Will she be the only one to admit to a difficulty? Or will her teacher be mad at her for not asking about the instructions? Furthermore, will these reactions make her feel angry and sad and out of control? This student may have only one or two friends to socialize with during recess or break; will these precious friends turn away and find someone else to spend time with? For these reasons, a legitimate and adaptive response for this student may be to pretend she doesn't care about math or create a wide range of different distractions. By making such a choice, she can control the situation, appear strong in front of her peers, and experience a predictable outcome. School isn't easy for our most vulnerable learners. To deliver our EF teaching, we need to make it a safe and in-control option.

Once you are tuned in to the experience of your most vulnerable students, you can get active with an approach that will calm them down. Experienced teachers of EF tend to rely heavily on modeling self-understanding and self-acceptance. To do this, teachers need to understand their own EF spectrum and may find the teacher survey available at *http://activatedlearning.org* helpful. From there, teachers can reinforce the message that they themselves are capable and successful despite a few lagging EFs. We hear them say things like "Organization is not my strongest EF, so I have a red lanyard on my keys"; "You know me; I can't hold anything in my working memory in a noisy room. Can someone shut the door please?"; or, in a more serious mood, "I think we're all upset about what happened yesterday. I know I'm not feeling very calm or flexible. Maybe we can all try to be extra patient and considerate?" We can even have a laugh at the unique qualities that make us special. "I was working on my reports with Ms. Brown who also loses focus easily. We got ourselves in a terrible muddle until we agreed on a few strategies and set some goals." The message to students is that "It's okay if you're not perfect." In this context, we can accept and appreciate our differences, and believe that no matter the obstacle we face, we can be bright, creative, and powerful.

There are many playful ways to model positive feelings about EFs. Feast your eyes on Figure 2.7, in which two teachers asked their students to guess their identity based on EF behaviors. While students were initially worried about embarrassing Ms. Kuiken and Mrs. Tomlinson, they were quickly reassured that it is okay to have strengths and weaknesses. In this way, the teachers worked together to model humility, self-understanding, and self-acceptance for their students.

One of the most effective teachers of stressed students we have ever seen is Stephanie Walker.[8] When we met her, she had already been teaching her students about EFs for years, working with smaller classes in a strategy-focused environment. While she comes across as a strong and clear-thinking person, she frequently shares her own struggles, limitations, and life hacks with students. During one of her lessons, she presented her own EF profile of strengths and weaknesses and revealed that planning and prioritizing was a challenge for her. She then provided her students with copies of her daily to-do list and asked them to help her prioritize it. Her students were delighted with the trust she had placed in them, cut the list into strips to manipulate each task more easily, and engaged in animated conversation about what makes a task higher in priority.

Guess Who → Mrs. Tomlinson, Mrs. Kuiken, or BOTH?
• I keep detailed to-do lists for every aspect of my life.
• I don't like leaving jobs unfinished; sometimes I'll even forget to eat when I'm focused on finishing something.
• I have a filing cabinet where I keep manuals and important receipts.
• When I work out, I often forget the number of repetitions I have completed.
• If something didn't go well, I get upset with myself and have a hard time putting it behind me.
• I don't like when plans change at the last minute.
• People describe me as someone who "doesn't have a filter."

FIGURE 2.7. Classroom activity to reinforce self-understanding and self-acceptance. Sam Tomlinson and Julie Kuiken displayed this provocation for their grade 7/8 students. Used at Central Senior Public School in Lindsay, Ontario, Canada. Used with permission.

---

[8] Stephanie Walker teaches at Scott Young Public School in Omemee, Ontario, Canada. Used with permission.

John Bianco takes a calculated and deliberate approach to teaching EFs in his mixed grades 6–8 classroom.[9] Part of the planning he does each day is to loosely estimate the amount and type of EF challenge his assignments will place on students. For example, familiar tasks will be straightforward, but group work will demand organization, flexibility, and emotional control. Because many of his students follow a modified curriculum that is tailored to their developmental level, he sometimes throws them a curveball to ensure they will experience a specific EF challenge and a slightly higher stress level. For example, he might omit a useful piece of information in a math problem to create an opportunity for his students to persist without it. Or he might ask them to organize their own groups. Once, he tightened a deadline to challenge his students' time management. These challenges are sometimes intentionally fabricated, but he often just forecasts the type of EF demands that will already exist in his planned activities and assignments. Could you do this? What if you added the prompt "Predicted EF Challenge" to the top of your written plans and tried to fill it in for each lesson or activity? Or what if you wrote your predicted EF challenge on the board and then covered it with a paper called "EF Mystery"? Your students might enjoy guessing which EF you were trying to challenge as their daily learning unfolded.

Fabricating EF challenges? This may sound a bit extreme, but we like it for several reasons. First, John's class knows he is trying to develop their awareness of EFs. He has warned them there might be special challenges in their work and that he's excited to discuss them as they arise. Using this approach, he has meaningful conversations with his students about EFs every single day. Finally, because his students know the challenges were premeditated, both John and his students feel a greater sense of security. "This was planned," they many think. "We are in control, and we are learning something important." For a volatile class, this calculated challenge is like a controlled burn to prevent a forest fire, or a driving teacher asking a nervous student to steer onto a gravel shoulder to see how it feels. This approach takes finesse and trust, but we like the way it deliberately targets EFs and encourages students to be conscious of their responses.

Teaching stressed students is double the work—twice as much planning, twice as much patience, twice as much adaptability, and yet twice as much risk that everything will go sideways. We persist because our stressed students are already so compromised; we don't want them to get behind academically, or suffer socially, so we work overtime, day after day, to scaffold and ease our core academic program. We propose that the delivery of information about EFs may provide a more permanent scaffold. Teachers who model self-understanding and self-acceptance create a safer environment for risk taking. In this climate, a confused student may feel okay asking for clarification, a traumatized student may feel comfortable opening up, and a disorganized student may take the opportunity to work with others to get back on track. Breaking through to your trickiest students with an education in EFs might be the most productive thing you do all year.

---

[9] John Bianco teaches in an alternative program in Kawartha Lakes Ontario, Canada. Used with permission.

CHAPTER 3

How EF Literacy Can Improve Instruction
A Simple and Versatile Approach

MOVING SUPPORT INTO THE MAINSTREAM

As you become more informed about the impact of EFs on performance, your approach with students will undoubtedly change. You may see your students with fresh eyes, feel more empathy, and change the way you provide support. And while you will continue to collaborate with a broad range of colleagues that you respect and admire in many different ways, your deeper understanding of EFs may not be shared by very many of them. Students rarely encounter EF-literate teachers, and when they do it is usually after they have been streamed into a smaller-group context to receive special education. Studies conducted in the United Kingdom and North America show that most qualified teachers have not been prepared to fully understand and address the needs of students with poor attention, inhibition, organization, or emotional regulation (Bekle, 2004; Bussing, Gary, Leon, Garvan, & Reid, 2002; Jones & Chronis-Tuscano, 2008; Martinussen, Tannock, & Chaban, 2011; Gilmore & Cragg, 2014). For example, when asked what was important to mathematics learning, only the most experienced teachers named factors such as the ability to store and manipulate information in one's head, focus on relevant information, and avoid distractions. And as of 2014, fewer than 20% of all U.K. teachers had heard the term "executive function." Knowing this, you might wonder if EF-literate educators belong only in intensified, remedial contexts. Don't give up just yet! Let's talk about why EF support belongs in the mainstream.

First, EF challenges are a huge problem in the mainstream. Even teachers with no training in EFs will tell you that *something* more than a lack of intelligence is bogging down almost every one of their students. We limp home after long days of playing an EF version of "whack-a-mole." A typical day might look something like this: First, we're bent over a group of disagreeing students in the hallway (emotional control); then it's back into the classroom to help another group get organized (organization); after that, we're over to the group by the window where a certain student has forgotten the timeline (time management); next, off to the corner group who hasn't started at all (task initiation); and finally, back to the hallway where the principal has swooped in to help. Only 15 minutes has gone by. As soon as we resolve one problem, another one pops up.

With 25–35 unique students to support per lesson, we are literally wearing out the soles of our shoes just to accomplish the basics. We, authors of this book, chuckle at the memory of bewildered spouses, children, and friends asking how our work in schools could possibly be so exhausting. "Just do independent reading!" they'd suggest. "Just tell them to write in a journal!" Or in kindergarten, "Don't they just *play* all day?" Research tells us that EFs cause widespread impact on academic success (Visu-Petra et al., 2011) and it's not wrong. We move from child to child all day, providing external support for their EF weaknesses. We can't move every student into a special education program. EF challenges are in the mainstream to stay.

The second reason EF support belongs in the mainstream is that it is actually, according to research, best delivered there. Forgive us if you already know this, but there are "tiers" of intervention. Generally, Tier 1 represents student support taking place in a mainstream, whole-class context; Tier 2 represents a small-group context; and Tier 3 represents a one-on-one context. This system is often illustrated by a triangle, as in Figure 3.1, to represent the ideal number of cases at each level and the relative intensity of intervention. As we respond to student need, we are meant to use resources from the bottom up, only escalating when our attempts prove unsuccessful. So, a

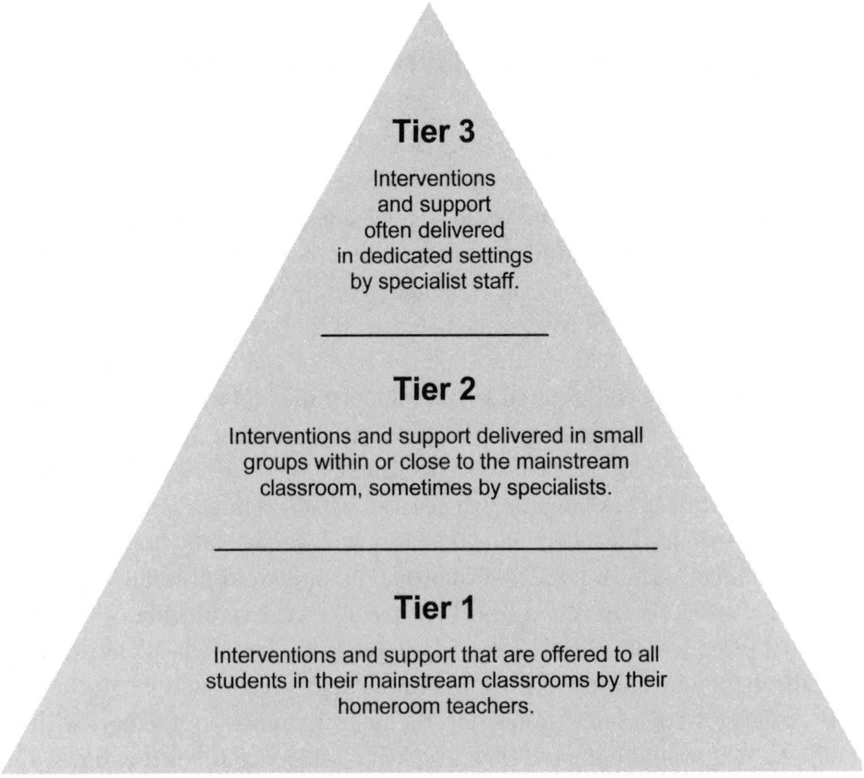

Tier 3

Interventions
and support
often delivered
in dedicated settings
by specialist staff.

Tier 2

Interventions and support delivered in small
groups within or close to the mainstream
classroom, sometimes by specialists.

Tier 1

Interventions and support that are offered to all
students in their mainstream classrooms by their
homeroom teachers.

FIGURE 3.1. Tiers of support provided to students at school.

child who simply cannot learn to manage emotions in a Tier 1 context may be offered small-group Tier 2 support for 20 minutes, four times per week. If this doesn't work, ideally, that student would progress to one-on-one support, but this may only be available in mini-lessons twice per week. We know, however, that the best way to teach EF skills is not in isolated mini-lessons but as integrated into meaningful and authentic tasks throughout a mainstream day (Diamond & Ling, 2020; Far-rington et al., 2012). Isn't EF intervention important enough for all teachers to learn about and try to tackle as part of their core program? Longitudinal studies of EF weakness conclude that interventions yielding even small improvements to individual capacity for EFs could dramatically improve society (Moffitt et al., 2011, p. 2694). Given the amount of time children spend at school, surely the everyday work of teachers—a sizable corps of public service employees—should con-tribute to that improvement.

Third, boosting EF support in the mainstream would ease the burden on Tier 2 and 3 resources. Think about your school's special education program; while some of you may reflect upon a system that is providing targeted and effective support to students with specific challenges, some of you tell us your special education department has become a bit of a muddled dumping ground for students with behavioral problems. Often, these programs are clogged with extremely discouraged students who have been unsuccessful and seem "impossible to teach" in the main-stream. Indeed, students with EF challenges may be highly sensitive, overreactive, disorganized, and inflexible. They can be overwhelming for classroom teachers, difficult to work with, and hard to relate to. Furthermore, their maladaptive behaviors are often mistaken for symptoms of poor character (Gaier, 2015), and they are frequently regarded as intentional (Elik et al., 2010). For this reason, many students with EF challenges find themselves at odds with their classroom teachers and streamed to Tier 2 or 3 contexts. If we could more effectively understand and support EFs in the mainstream, from the very first day of school, we might free up some time and space in our precious special education programs.

Also, an EF-supportive mainstream is more equitable and fair for all learners. Because we know that EF challenges are often intensified in children from traumatic and low socioeconomic backgrounds, we can be clear eyed about what is happening when this group of children keep winding up in our "alternate" programs. Getting our mainstream classrooms properly set up to serve this prevalent group must be a top priority because, while being removed from the main-stream can be very beneficial, it often invokes troubling side effects for students. Children in alternate programs often feel stigmatized, disconnected, and embarrassed, and they lose access to the influence of a wider peer group. In the case of intensive and effective reading remediation, for example, these side effects are often worth it. But if the alternate or Tier 2 option is so oversub-scribed and poorly resourced that it has, in fact, become a muddled dumping ground, the situation is quite concerning. In many ways, we have a moral imperative to make our mainstream programs as EF supportive as possible. While we may not be able to serve every student at Tier 1, we can probably serve more.

A NEAT TRICK: DISCUSSING BARRIERS AND STRATEGIES

Teaching is a very busy job. Managing the many competing demands and priorities of a classroom is like juggling with a large number of different sized balls . . . if the number of balls kept changing and they sometimes needed to be chased down the hall. It is not surprising that even the best "jugglers" among us often drop a few balls to the floor. On challenging days, the sheer volume of unaddressed problems can make your classroom feel like an IKEA-style ball pit. You wade, hip deep, through below-grade readers, forgotten math homework, and dissatisfied parents. On better days, we efficiently *rotate* the dropped balls, spreading our attention as evenly as possible among the many diverse students we serve. Knowing we won't be able to meet every student need can be stressful. It is no surprise that as we gain experience in the classroom we develop tricks, habits, and routine responses that make us more efficient.

Some of our routines and tricks serve us well. Classroom management systems, such as organized libraries, well-established cues, and shared responsibilities, make us more efficient in the best possible way. Some of our habits, however, may have unintended results. Experts tell us that all humans, even the very smartest ones, use certain mental shortcuts to think and work more efficiently. In the classroom, these shortcuts speed us up, but they can also cause us to miss important information, jump to conclusions, and sometimes take unhelpful action. Table 3.1 characterizes the kinds of thinking errors teachers may be making. Each one leads to a *teaching error* that we'd like to address.

Can you simply stop committing these thinking errors and thus avoid the teaching errors we describe? Maybe, but it will be an uphill battle. After years of unrelenting stress in the classroom, you have probably developed a lightning-quick draw and an itchy trigger finger with these efficiencies. They will be very hard to notice, let alone change. Instead, we recommend you try to momentarily interrupt your habits with a *semi-structured teaching protocol*. Table 3.2 presents the **Barriers and Strategies Protocol (BSP)**, which is probably the biggest and most important idea in this book and will be referred to continuously throughout the upcoming chapters. It essentially asks teachers to gather students to discuss, first, "What are your/our barriers to this work" and then "What strategies can we use to be more successful?" It will give you a rare opportunity to function outside of your habits.

Let's get technical for just a moment. Under the "hood" of the BSP is a powerful metacognitive process called "mental contrasting with implementation intentions" (Oettingen & Gollwitzer, 2010). Mental contrasting refers to the process of contrasting one's goal with its specific obstacles. When accompanied by the formation of an "*if* this happens, *then* I will do that" plan, this contrast has been shown to boost success in goal achievement by helping individuals to act more quickly (Gollwitzer & Brandstatter, 1997), deal more effectively with cognitive demands, and execute planned strategies with less effort (Brandstatter, Lengfelder, & Gollwitzer, 2001). These if–then conversations stimulate metacognitive monitoring and metacognitive control, the fundamental processes at the root of self-regulated learning (Corno, 1993; Winne, 1995, 1996, 1997). Sound cool? It is. The researchers responsible for it have created an app called "WOOP" (by Gabrielle Oettingen) that allows individuals to use the process for personal goals.

The BSP will force you out of your routine long enough to slow down, do things you usually wouldn't, see things that you might otherwise miss, and understand your students more fully. It is effortful and structured, but let us compare it to being locked in a room with a window that is a little too high. If you want to catch a glimpse of what is typically hidden from you, you will have to expend some extra energy, jump up and catch the sill, and struggle to hang on for a moment or two. Though you can't hang there all day, the insight you gain from even a quick peek through this ordinarily inaccessible window may change the way you see and support your students. Like many protocols, this one is worth the effort.

TABLE 3.1. Unconscious Thinking Errors That Often Lead to Teaching Errors

Thinking error	Definition	Example from the classroom	What we might be missing	Teaching error
Race to action	Jumping to action before considering all possibilities and fully understanding problems.	A student hasn't finished her writing assignment in the allotted time and is off track. We assume she needs more ideas, ask her to summarize her story orally, and then compose and scribe the first few sentences.	This student has a lot of ideas she is passionate about and is excited to share. Her actual problem is the *organization* and sequencing of these ideas. Our scribing support is discouraging for her because we don't quite capture what she means.	Taking over students' creative control and thinking
Confirmation bias	Automatically paying more attention to information that confirms what you already think about something.	A student in math class is very rude when asked to contribute to the class discussion. We assume he needs discipline and ask him to leave.	Students who are rude *do* need boundaries and to be reminded of our high expectations. This student might *also* have reduced *working memory* or *attention* that impairs his ability to keep track of what is happening in class discussions and contribute without saying the wrong thing.	Missing the lagging skills that underlie poor performance
Vividness bias	When something is loud, intense, or salient, we see it as the norm, overemphasize its importance, and give it more attention.	Our students are passionate about the environment, so we assign a poster/essay in social studies. Several students are way behind on Day 1, and several are not managing to collaborate, so we cut the essay requirement.	The students' poor performance may be due to executive functioning challenges—*task initiation and emotional control.* While these challenges are often very loud and vivid, they don't have anything to do with essay writing skills. We may overreact and eliminate academic challenges that are appropriate and important for our students.	Reducing expectations unnecessarily
Illusory superiority	The belief that you hold a broader, more objective, and more accurate perspective than most people.	We know that biases and thinking errors exist but believe we are the exception and can accurately understand and appreciate the challenges experienced by our students.	We can never appreciate what is missing from our perspective. If we struggle with *goal-directed persistence* ourselves, we will probably assume our students struggle in the same way. We may spend a lot of time on interventions that are not the most efficient or effective for our students.	Wasted effort for both teacher and student

Note. The idea of intentionally interrupting biases in teaching is based on ideas from Katz and Dack's book *Intentional Interruption: Breaking Down Learning Barriers to Transform Professional Practise* (2013).

TABLE 3.2. Administering the BSP Before, During, or After Student Difficulty

Step in process	How it can sound	How it is documented
Clearly identifying academic goals (SMART goals)		
Duration: 1 min. Teacher identifies **S**pecific, **M**easurable, **A**chievable, **R**easonable, and **T**ime-specific learning goal before, during, or after student difficulty. This learning goal can be differentiated for students with accommodated or modified programs.	<u>If done before difficulty</u> TEACHER: We are going to do some math problems today. The expectation is that you will complete 12 of them (or modified number) accurately during this period. <u>If done during difficulty</u> TEACHER: You seem to be having difficulty with these math problems. Just a reminder that the expectation is for you to complete 12 of them accurately during this period. <u>If done after difficulty</u> TEACHER: You had some difficulty completing 12 math problems accurately during this period.	On a flip chart, whiteboard, or any other display, teacher writes the agreed-upon learning goal clearly.
Discussing barriers		
Duration: 4 min. Teacher asks students to describe their challenges and "barriers," helping students identify the EFs that may underlie each challenge. Teacher encourages a broad range of different possible underlying EFs.	TEACHER: What are our barriers to success? What will stop us from succeeding? STUDENTS: We're rushing and forgetting to do certain steps. TEACHER: That sounds like *inhibition.* Am I right? What else? STUDENTS: For me, it is hard because my numbers get all out of line. TEACHER: That sounds like **organization**. Am I right? *(Further discussion: Teacher elicits other obstacle ideas and encourages class to connect them to a broad range of EFs.)*	On the same flip chart, whiteboard, or other display, teacher creates a "T-chart" with two columns. The word "Barriers" is written above the first column, and student ideas are recorded in point form, along with the name of any EFs they are able to connect to their barriers.
Discussing strategies		
Duration: 3 min. Teacher asks students to think about good strategies to overcome these barriers. Teacher encourages a broad range of different strategy ideas for each problem. Teacher informs students that their use of strategy is important and will be assessed.	TEACHER: What strategies can we use to overcome these barriers? *(Discussion, during which teacher charts a variety of strategy ideas created by the student[s].)* TEACHER: You have suggested several strategies that might work. I will be watching to see which strategy you choose and use. I will be making notes about your choices.	On the same flip chart, whiteboard, or other display, teacher adds the label "Strategies" to the right-hand column of the T-chart. Student strategy ideas are recorded in point form.

The BSP uses a metacognitive conversation that helps students notice their challenges and respond strategically. When used in a classroom, it interrupts several teaching errors. Refer again to Table 3.1 and consider how a process like this might slow down our race to action. The protocol asks us to explore our challenges from all sides, soliciting many different opinions and perspectives about what might make them tricky. This *slower processing* of problems is, according to research, the hallmark of expert performers who seem to linger, poke around, and really get to know the problem before jumping to action (Dronek & Blessing, 2006).

The BSP asks us to share a thorough process of problem analysis *with students.* By doing this, we radically improve our chances of avoiding confirmation bias (attending to information that confirms preconceived ideas) and vividness bias (attending to information that is most salient or perceptible). Teachers using this protocol are often quite surprised by what they find out from students. For example, in math class you might have assumed your students were struggling because they didn't understand the math. By this assessment, you might have reduced your expectations and eliminated several of the more challenging questions. Using the protocol, however, you might discover that two students are in a fight, three are hungry because they didn't have breakfast, four are confused by the instructions, nine don't know where to find the materials, and the rest didn't pay attention to the lesson. You might be amazed at how diverse your students' problems are. Working together, you can plan several different strategies for students to use to tackle these different problems. Regularly checking your assumptions with a roomful of people, especially when they are your students, can add tremendous clarity to your understanding, assessment, and intervention.

After you apply this protocol a few times, you might feel a little wiser and more self-aware. That will be a clue that your illusory superiority, the sense that you alone possess the ability to see the world clearly and without bias, is starting to erode. Without being too dramatic, using a protocol like this might help you develop a greater sense of compassion and humanity. When you look at a roomful of people, you might be more likely to assume they hold different opinions, challenges, and perspectives from your own. And if the use of this protocol can be so powerful for you as an adult, imagine what could happen if we were trained to think this way from an early age.

A formulaic approach to teaching should be used judiciously. We think, however, that the BSP is a wonderfully efficient little tool for driving EF literacy beyond lip service and bulletin boards. It can help us replace empty cheerleading of the "You can do it if you keep trying!" variety with a deep understanding of the practical problems and challenges of learning at school. With your team of EF-literate students, you will have everything you need to analyze problems as experts and craft targeted, diverse solutions.

THE BARRIERS AND STRATEGIES PROTOCOL (BSP): STRATEGIZING *WITH* STUDENTS INSTEAD OF *FOR* STUDENTS

Most teachers believe it is important to develop independence and problem-solving skills in their students (Perry, Hutchinson, & Thauberger, 2008). We bet you do too. In the research world, this independence is referred to as "self-regulated learning" (SRL). It is thought to require motivation, metacognition, and cognitive skill, and to take place in a cycle of planning, monitoring, and reflecting (Zimmerman, 2002). While everyone—parents, teachers, and researchers—seems to intuitively know that the ability to self-regulate learning is essential, there is about a century of research confirming its association with academic success and better life outcomes (Winne, 2017).

It isn't easy to teach a large and diverse group of students to be motivated, metacognitive, and capable; each student has unique needs, and the process seems to require an endless array of different supports. Research tells us that, in general, teachers struggle to support SRL in real classrooms (Dignath-van Ewijk, Dickhäuser, & Büttner, 2013; Kistner et al., 2010; Spruce & Bol, 2015). Even the most well-trained teachers do not engage students in SRL as often as they say they'd like to (Spruce & Bol, 2015) because it just doesn't seem to work for them. Properly supporting students' SRL seems to require constant individual attention from teachers and seriously competes with other curricular demands (Winne, 2010).

So, how can one teacher help dozens of students find strategies to move forward when the going gets tough? Because it is so efficient, adaptable, and pocket sized, we believe the BSP may be the solution. Think about how you support your students. Depending on the grade you teach, you may move around your classroom, kneeling, bending over, pulling up a chair, or sometimes even kicking off your shoes and sitting with students on the floor. Or maybe you work through lineups of students from your desk. The point of these interactions is to determine, first, *How is this student struggling?* followed by *What does this student need in order to move forward?* and, later, *Did our plan work, or should we try something different?* In this way, with many different students all day, we move purposefully around the cycle of SRL presented in Figure 3.2. This is very important work because the development of SRL is so essential to success in school and in life.

There is a big difference, however, between teaching strategies and teaching SRL. To teach SRL, you have to involve students actively in the metacognitive part of the process, identifying problems and choosing and monitoring suitable responses. If you're like most teachers, you probably rally your students to be involved in these steps as much as humanly possible—when you have time. For example, during first period you might have time to settle in with a student who is having difficulty with math problem solving in an effort to inspire some thinking about exactly how he is struggling. "What's happening here? What is making this so tricky for you?" From there you can work with him to devise strategies that closely match the problems he is experiencing. By Period 4, however, you might be firing through a backlog of "stuck" students a mile a minute. "Make a list!

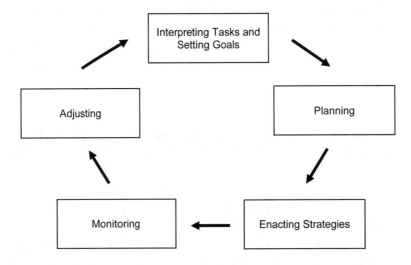

FIGURE 3.2. A cycle of self-regulated learning. This diagram is based on conceptualizations proposed by Winne and Perry (2010) and Butler, Schnellert, and Perry (2016).

Next! Read it to a partner! Next! I see six mistakes; go and fix them! Next! Take 10 deep breaths and put on headphones! Next!" As we quickly assess problems and churn out strategies, we dearly wish our students could be a little more independent.

The irony is that the less independent our students are and the more they need us, the faster we have to go while helping them and the less time we have to involve them in an informed process of SRL. This shifts the process toward *external* learning regulation and deprives students of important learning about why and when certain strategies should be used (Veenman, Van Hout-Wolters, & Afflerbach, 2006). Teachers describe the way their students sit waiting for help, hands up, sometimes seeming to grow frustrated at the delays to service. In fact, to a large extent, this is what we've trained them to expect at school. "Hello, 911? I'm trapped on a broken escalator." It's a bit like that.

This escalator rescue work takes a lot of patience, attention, care, and time. A classroom with 28 students may have 28 unique and perplexing problems to be quickly understood and solved at any given time on any given day. And the work you do with Sally on Day 1 might not even be useful on Day 2. We often describe the range of problems experienced by any one child as kaleidoscopic, because if you change the context or challenge even slightly, like turning the handle of the kaleidoscope, the issue transforms into something completely new. So despite the tremendous energy spent and the very best of intentions extended, this high volume of diverse and ever-changing student need means that when conducted one-on-one, a full, inclusive process of SRL may only reach a handful of students per day.

For this reason—because they are overwhelmed and looking for a way to be more efficient and effective—teachers often plan and deliver whole-class strategy lessons. Imagine a teacher—let's call him Mr. Jackson—who noticed that he spent a lot of time on Day 1 of an essay-writing project providing one-on-one organizational support. On Day 2, therefore, he may decide to begin class with a group lesson on how to use a planning template: "My friends, yesterday we seemed to have some difficulty with our essays. I thought about it long and hard, and realized that you are all having trouble with organization. I figured out a strategy to help with this—let me show you!" This whole-class strategy instruction will allow Mr. Jackson to support his entire class at one time and will teach his students how to use a certain planning template, but did you notice who is doing the metacognition? Mr. Jackson! This means that only *he* really noticed being stumped, only *he* wrestled with the problem of being stumped, and only *he* devised a strategic approach. While his students learned a useful cognitive strategy, they traded the metacognitive aspects of self-regulated learning for the relatively less creative work of strategy implementation.

Over the course of a year, in response to many different problems, imagine how Mr. Jackson will benefit from practicing this resilient, "dukes up" approach. Research tells us that as he devises strategic solutions to a wide variety of different real-life problems, his ability to be strategic will become more automatic. This is why, at holiday gatherings or family reunions, if something unexpected happens and you have an unusual problem to solve, you'd be well advised to call on the teachers in the family. They are guaranteed to be your strategic thinkers. Our goal, however, should be to move more of this well-practiced resourcefulness *toward our students.*

Could the use of the BSP solve these problems, or is this just more starry-eyed, out-of-left-field thinking learned from a teaching book? It's certainly ambitious; when compared to status quo SRL teaching, both whole group and one-on-one, it appears to be much more efficient, dynamic, and inclusive (Table 3.3). But is it just too unusual to become a regular part of what teachers do? On the contrary, the teachers we work with often point out that—well, thank you for the grand idea—but

TABLE 3.3. Classroom Options for Teaching Self-Regulated Learning

	One-on-one	Whole-class strategy lesson	BSP[a]
Number of students involved in each individual SRL interaction	1	Whole class	Whole class
Approximate number of students who may receive SRL support per day in one subject/class	4–6	Whole class	Whole class
Total teacher time required to provide daily SRL support in one subject/class	5 interactions × 5 min. each = 25 min.	1 interaction × 10 min. = 10 min.	1 interaction × 10 min. = 10 min.
Metacognitive monitoring of task is conducted by . . . ("What am I struggling with?") or ("What are they struggling with?")	Student	Teacher	Whole class as a team
Strategy created by . . . (person getting practice creating strategies)	Student	Teacher	Students (peers)
Strategy chosen for implementation by . . . (person getting practice choosing and using strategies when facing challenge)	Student	Teacher	Students
Chance that SRL support is sufficiently tailored to target problem actually experienced by students	High	Low	High
Chance that SRL support is offered in a timely way, right when students need it	High for some, low for most	Medium	Medium

Note. [a]BSP, Barriers and Strategies Protocol.

the components of it aren't actually all that new. "Why is this hard for you?" and "What strategy can we use to be successful?" are questions we have been asking for years, all day every day, in our one-on-one interactions with students. All the protocol does is transfer into *group* conversation an interaction that is already taking place. "It's the weirdest thing," they tell us. "I've never done it this way, but it is so powerful."

THE BARRIERS AND STRATEGIES PROTOCOL (BSP): A POWERFUL WAY TO CONNECT

Not too long ago, an Australian researcher named John Hattie conducted the largest ever meta-analysis of research on what affects learning in school. Many of the most powerful effects he found were related to metacognition, monitoring, and problem-solving, and, you guessed it, could be stimulated using the BSP. Of his 18 teaching or learning strategies with the potential to "considerably accelerate" student achievement, five of them are essential components of the BSP; you'll find these explained at the top of Table 3.4. It is worth noting that many of the other important factors

TABLE 3.4. The Barriers and Strategies Protocol (BSP) and Hattie's "Visible Learning"

Teaching factor	Effect size	How it relates to the BSP
Cognitive task analysis (CTA)	1.29	Research shows that helping a learner to analyze the cognitive skills, steps, and approaches required to accomplish a difficult thinking task helps them to succeed. Within the BSP, students work together to examine problems and generate lists of possible skills, steps, and approaches. The BSP is collaborative CTA.
Transfer strategies	0.86	The BSP incorporates problem monitoring at a high frequency, during regular whole-class conversations. This contributes to students' familiarity with different types of problems and the solutions they tend to prefer; it supports their ability to quickly devise appropriate strategies or transfer ones that were previously used.
Class discussion	0.82	Within the BSP, teachers regularly gather all students together to respond to two prompts: "What are our barriers to this task?" and "What strategies can we use to be successful?"
Planning and prediction/ self-judgment and reflection	0.75/0.75	The BSP asks students to predict barriers and plan strategies in a group setting on a regular basis. This allows individuals within the group to steadily notice and reflect upon what is unique about their own challenges and preferred strategies.
Focus on problem-solving/ metacognition	0.67/0.58	The BSP integrates metacognition into the fabric of everyday problem solving. Again and again, over many short BSP interactions, students are scaffolded into the habit of monitoring problems for barriers and experimenting with creative strategies.
Feedback	0.64	The BSP helps students identify important process steps (strategies) for any task. Teachers (and students themselves) may then easily recognize and provide formative feedback on these steps because they have been co-constructed and are very clear to both teacher and student.
Cooperative vs. individualistic learning	0.55	The BSP takes place during a group conversation in which students work together to actively consider and support other perspectives and ways of learning.
Teacher–student relationship	0.48	The BSP creates a regular opportunity for teachers to express interest in and make connections with students. During a BSP, teachers find out about students' experiences, thoughts, feelings, and good ideas, which builds a strong relationship.

Note. From *www.visiblelearningmetax.com* (2018). When reading effect size, remember that, generally, 0.5 is a medium effect and 0.8 is large.

that Hattie found are also supported by the use of the BSP, including feedback, cooperative learning, and good teacher–student relationships. Hattie's work is available online, and if you're curious, it's quite easy to access at *www.visiblelearningmetax.com*.

In addition to lining up well with the factors on Hattie's meta-analysis, the BSP makes a lot of sense for developing healthy learning mindsets. All students, and especially those with exceptionalities such as learning disabilities, sometimes struggle with negative emotions and a sense of powerlessness. Left to their own devices, many students tend to believe their failures and successes are caused by fixed factors that cannot be controlled. This is the "I'll never amount to anything; I'm just not smart" mindset. Not only does this feel terrible, but also it leads to maladaptive coping strategies (Elliott & Dweck, 1988) such as avoidance and distraction. Pausing your classroom for an open discussion about barriers to learning and strategies to be successful interrupts this pattern in two ways: It helps students to see that many of their challenges are natural, normal, and shared by their peers, and it trains them to look for and act upon sources of control. Let's discuss this in more detail.

Using the BSP within a socially shared process of learning regulation, learning challenges are normalized. When students work together to brainstorm the many different reasons a task may be difficult, they learn they are not alone. During these whole-class discussions, the silence is broken, and students can see that their friends and teachers also experience difficulty. Instead of a guilty secret that individual students experience alone, learning challenges become a source of camaraderie and connection. In fact, by placing opportunities to engage in self-regulated learning into the social context of whole-class conversations, the BSP stimulates "social contagion," which *boosts* strategy use (see review in Jones, Alexander, & Estell, 2010). This idea, that motivation for strategy use can be "caught" from peers like a virus, was mentioned by two grade 8 students from Central Senior School in Lindsay, Ontario, Canada. After engaging in communal problem solving using the BSP, Hunter Sidsworth commented on how reassured he felt to be cooperating with his peers:

> "Now that we all learn and we all help each other through this, I think everybody's on the same gears. We all work together to solve it. I think it's really important that teachers take this into consideration of students, because students who aren't doing as well can benefit from this."[1]

Kylie Archer-Alfred, meanwhile, provided an extraordinary comment about how energizing it can be to create strategies among peers:

> "It's hard for me to use strategies, but when I see that other people in my class—and it helps them—it gives me the motivation to use it too, and it helps. When you come up with strategies as a class, it's more useful to me. When it's just me and a teacher talking about it one-on-one? It's just . . . I think, yeah, yeah, I think that'll be really useful, but it just goes straight through and I just completely forget about it and don't apply it to anything."

This is not to say teachers don't have an important role to play in normalizing everyday difficulties. Time and again we see teachers setting a tone of self-understanding and acceptance. For example, when using the protocol to discuss math problem solving, a teacher might say, "I often make small mistakes too. For me, it's all about organization. I struggle to line up my numbers

---

[1] Quotes from Hunter Sidsworth and Kylie Archer-Alfred used with permission.

neatly. I know that for some people the problem is attention. They don't copy the numbers carefully enough. What is it for you?" Students working with a teacher like this will understand that a wide range of underlying causes will be acceptable, and that there is nothing to be ashamed of. The message is *We've all got something to work on and that's okay* and *We're all on each other's team*. This message comes across implicitly and often explicitly. As the trust builds, and more positive sharing occurs, a ripple effect takes place and the class become more cohesive and cooperative. In this increasingly supportive context, even your trickiest students may begin engage in the BSP.

As students become more motivated and strategic, teachers can step back from external learning regulation (and their "escalator rescue" work) and take a more attentive and facilitative role. Instead of being focused on doing, they can focus on encouraging and appreciating how their students *do*. Within this context, a huge diversity of student personality can be expressed, and the feeling of being known, valued, and included by peers can make its considerable impact on engagement and learning (Deci & Ryan, 2000). And as more students share, there is more chance others will find not only common ground but also a strategy that will work. Students discussing the obstacles to writing an essay, for example, may suggest several different possibilities. For one student, the problem is task initiation; for another, organization. Yet another student may struggle with perfectionism and conclude that the lagging EF is emotional control. Each of these obstacles may resonate with a handful of different students in the room when suggested, as will the compensatory strategies that the students discuss and list. Students often tell us that the challenges and strategies shared by peers seem so much more interesting, relevant, and useful than what is offered by adults.

The BSP lessens the experience of stigma and shame, but it also boosts students' feelings of control. When students practice breaking down problems and finding solutions, they get in the habit of responding to challenges as though nothing is impossible. Even something as stubborn as dyslexia, for example, can be supported using goal-directed persistence to self-advocate for access to technology, organization to keep personal copies of anchor charts and other visual supports, and emotional control to stay calm in the face of frustration. In this way, our students can learn to be adaptive, getting in the habit of moving obstacles from the "impossible" pile to the "I can handle this" pile. Scientifically speaking, teaching children to recognize and use sources of control is a powerful approach. When students are struggling, decades of research suggests we should de-emphasize innate, internal, and fixed factors such as character or intelligence. Rather, we should steer students to focus on external factors that can be controlled. This shift in focus has been shown to consistently boost performance (Andrews & Debus, 1978; Chapin & Dyck, 1976; Dweck, 1975), change students' expectation of success, reduce debilitating emotions such as shame and hopelessness, increase positive emotions such as hope and pride, and make the use of strategic approaches more likely (Hall et al., 2007; Haynes, Ruthig, Perry, Stupnisky, & Hall, 2006; Menec et al., 1994). These findings are most pronounced for students with performance worries (Van Overwalle & de Metsenaere, 1990; Wilson & Linville, 1985) and poor past performance (Menec et al., 1994; Perry, Stupnisky, Hall, Chipperfield, & Weiner, 2010).

At a time when everyone is so reliant on technology, the BSP is a refreshingly down-to-earth and old-school approach. Just as it moves students toward empowerment, it also helps them to understand themselves and each other. They realize, I can help you and you can help me. Making time to share reflections and insights on learning distracts students from their never-ending quest for an experts' opinion and right answers and nudges them back toward developing their own capacity for problem solving.

THE BARRIERS AND STRATEGIES PROTOCOL (BSP): PLANNING LESSONS THAT CHALLENGE EFs INSTEAD OF MAKING THINGS EASY AND COMFORTABLE

We have described the way the BSP injects a socially shared process of learning regulation into the school day. It can be an efficient, effective, collaborative, and unifying way for students to learn strategy and independence. We would like to touch on one more important benefit: the way the BSP helps us move children out of their EF comfort zones and how very gratifying and healthy this actually is.

First, let's characterize the "EF comfort zone" and how it might feel to be there. This is the zone where our EF abilities easily match or even exceed the demands being placed upon them. A great place to see children dip in and out of this zone is a family restaurant. Odds are, when you look around, over half of the children you see will be sitting perfectly still and will stay that way for as long as they are permitted: perfect angels. Others might be enjoying themselves and eating a meal with their family, but also doing some noisy or disruptive behaviors such as talking a little too loudly (inhibition), knocking over drinks (attention), or fighting with their siblings (emotional control). The difference? Mom or Dad took the iPad away. Most video games are set up to very quickly and generously reward a player's efforts, and thus nestle those players in a very comfy and cozy EF zone. We can all agree that children relieved of all EF struggle are a good deal easier to supervise and manage.

In classrooms, the EF comfort zone is sometimes created using an iPad, but not always. Teachers may create this zone by either steering away from EF challenges or quickly patching over them to get students closer to academic targets. Imagine a teacher assigning a set of math questions. How will she respond when students get a little noisy and distracted in their struggle with EF demands? Her students might stall, become distracted, miss details, present disorganized answers, or experience performance anxiety. Feeling pressure to move her students though this math unit, she might reduce her assignment to fewer questions, or provide students with additional examples and increasingly straightforward algorithms. Before long, students will be tucked back into their comfort zones, able to complete the assignment without applying any organization, attention, or emotional control to their performance. With this support, they will do their math quietly, calmly, and without disruption for as long as they are allowed. When the principal, a parent, or a colleague walks by, they may stop and smile and think, "What a great class."

Let's face it—students who are out of their EF comfort zone can be challenging to manage. They often become distressed because it seems as if something is going wrong. Meanwhile, everyone appreciates a teacher who is flexible, adaptable, and responsive, so it seems perfectly reasonable to announce, "Guys, most of you haven't finished the questions, so let's just do half of them, okay?" or to size up the situation and find ways to do students' EF work for them. Unfortunately, when we smooth over all EF challenges for our students, we may be eliminating the very thinking, problem solving, creativity, and autonomy that makes learning gratifying and supports motivation. By stripping away these challenges, even a complex math assignment can be made as straightforward and mindless as a video game.

If you recall, motivation is one of the big three components in SRL, alongside metacognition and cognitive strategy. For this reason, it is worth knowing a little bit about the theory of motivation, which has an awful lot to do with a sense of self-determination—the ability to control oneself and make one's own choices. When we exercise self-determination, we fulfill three basic human needs: (1) competence (the need to feel effective and masterful), (2) autonomy (the need to control our choices and behavior), and (3) relatedness (the need to feel present in relationships with others). When these needs are met, we experience intrinsic motivation, interest, enjoyment, and satisfaction. When these needs aren't met, we may feel unrelated to our work, experience a lack of control, feel incompetent, and require rewards and punishments to persevere (Deci & Ryan, 2000). We'll talk a lot about autonomy, competence, and relatedness as we progress through the book. For now, just hold in mind these foundations of motivation.

As EF-literate teachers we have special powers of perception: We can see and understand the lagging EF skills that underlie our students' performance. This power can be used in two ways. On one hand, we can use this ability to become even more efficient at patching up or steering away from EF challenges. Thus, we can become expert scaffolders, designing a whole system of organizers, planners, routines, and supports to move students safely through EF challenge. Teachers do this in a variety of subtle ways. For example, we might offer summaries of what we think a student is thinking so they can get started on a writing task. "How about writing this . . . ?" we prompt. Or "This is what you mean, right?" When supervising group work, we might circulate around the room, gradually nudging each group forward by offering our strategies and solutions to their problems. These approaches often yield bewildered looks from students and escalate the frustration for everyone. It is exhausting for a teacher to do seven projects at once, and, let's face it, it's pretty boring for students to be at school when a teacher is doing all of the creative thinking. Constantly patching EF challenges may ease the stress in our classrooms and keep everyone moving forward with academic content, but it will not develop independence or support a feeling of autonomy and competence.

On the other hand, we can use our EF literacy to consciously move out of the EF comfort zone into another zone just beyond it called the "zone of proximal development" (Vygotsky, 1978), where students will come into direct contact with EF challenges and *will* have to exercise their autonomy and competence. This zone is the optimal place for students to grow—it offers challenge that can be managed with just a little bit of guidance. As long as we're equipped with the BSP, taking 20–30 slightly distressed kids into this more challenging arena isn't actually all that crazy. As we usher them in, and the tensions starts to rise, we can say, "Hold on, don't panic. We're going to tackle this together. Now, let's figure out what is standing in our way . . ." In the zone of proximal development, the BSP provides a sensible process to help everyone manage.

Teaching students to be autonomous, independent, skilled, and strategic is important to their ability to meet the expectations of school and life, but it is also important for their mental health and happiness. As described above, self-determination just *feels good.* Consider the kindergartener who can put on and do up his own coat, or the third grader who at first struggles through a math problem and then becomes the classroom expert on it. As students get older, competence, autonomy, and independence become a lifeline. Consider the delight of an eighth grader who provides just the right kind of support to a classmate experiencing an embarrassing moment or knows exactly how to troubleshoot a new technology at school. People who know how to take the bull by the horns and solve their own problems feel powerful, motivated, and satisfied.

The idea of taking a whole class of students outside of their EF comfort zone, we admit, sounds a little scary. Suddenly, things aren't running quite as smoothly; students are a little agitated and stressed, and work isn't getting done as quickly. Whose idea was this, anyway? We propose that this discomfort is necessary for the growth of EFs and that by using the whole-class BSP you can not only handle it but also learn to love it. When we gather our students for regular whole-class troubleshooting, we work with them to learn how to navigate discomfort and ambiguity. We create an opportunity in which the skills necessary for academic success, independence, self-determination, confidence, and happiness can grow. Equipped with the BSP, we can embrace EF challenges not as unwanted side effects to be actively minimized and avoided but rather as great opportunities to learn. Einstein famously said, "The measure of intelligence is the ability to change." Indeed, the ability to adapt and cope may be the most portable and valuable skills we can impart at school.

How to Facilitate the Barriers and Strategies Protocol (BSP):
Early Days

The *big idea* here is that neither you nor your students need to be EF experts to start using the BSP. You can start right away! In this section, you'll learn more about how to do the following:

- Use barriers and strategies conversations to build whole-class expertise about EFs.
- Use the BSP to discover new things about your students, and to help them discover new things about you.

The BSP is a dandy tool for establishing routines and getting to know a new group of students. You can use it on Day 1 without doing anything to prepare and you will be richly rewarded with important information about how your students think and what they are feeling. Picture this: After everyone arrives, unpacks their materials, and exchanges a few nervous hellos, you gather the group together to ask, "What was tricky about getting yourself here today?" With this question, you have begun the first step of the BSP. You may choose to jot down their answers on a chart, or you may decide to simply enjoy the moment. Regardless, in the following conversation, students may reveal challenges about finding lost items, avoiding distractions, or managing their frustration with siblings. You might share similar experiences, telling your students about having to backtrack to pick up a forgotten item, or about how you almost fell out of bed when your alarm went off. Soon you will all know a lot more about each other, and your most nervous students will realize that mornings can be tricky for their friends too. By giving them a chance to voice their challenges right away, you will have cemented the first layer of your new relationship with common experience. We hope you will delight in each other and have a few laughs.

The next step in the BSP is to get students thinking about strategies for success. You might ask, "Who has a trick for managing? Who knows how to overcome these challenges? What strategies do you use?" Scanning from face to face, you might see a little smile, or a twitch of a hand, or a knowing look. If you wait, your gaze may fall on someone who is bursting to share an idea. Or you may be met with a quiet room—your students not quite feeling safe enough to take a risk yet. At this point, you might encourage them by clarifying how *good* it is to be strategic. You can support their confidence by saying, "Oh, last year everyone was nervous and then one person shared an idea and it was like the floodgates opened!" or "I was just talking to a few older students about what they do, and I wondered if any of you did the same thing," or "I just *bet* we have a 'morning person' in here. Who is going to be our morning expert? There's one in every crowd and we need your help." If there's a really popular older student or teacher at the school, you can mention something they do as an example. It's all part of the process of using social connections to normalize a strategic and self-aware stance. The message is this: There's nothing wrong with struggling, working hard, and being open about it.

In addition to bonding your students, easing first-day jitters, and making space for good humor, using the BSP on Day 1 could provide crucial diagnostic information. Through the BSP, your students can deliver important context for how they feel, how they will behave, and what they need from you. You'll know who is tired, hungry, sad, or frustrated. Or in this case, if you're asking about the challenges of getting to school, you might find out that a student missed breakfast that morning, found a dead mouse on the street outside of their house, or got elbowed in the nose 2 minutes before the bell rang. Whether you're discussing math, science, English, or a field trip, you'll hear a great deal about what your children are experiencing in those domains, some of which may even surprise you. Regardless, this knowledge and understanding is a gift. It will make your students' unplanned-for responses a little less of a shock, allowing you to respond in a more tailored and sensitive way.

And it works in reverse. Contributing to a BSP conversation with information about yourself will provide the raw materials your students need to behave in a sensitive and compassionate way toward you. When we asked teachers of the BSP about their relationship with students, we got responses so full of kindness and warmth they sounded more like stories from a family: students offering to read aloud the last chapter for a teacher they knew to be emotional, students providing a fidget toy for a teacher they knew to struggle to pay attention during staff meetings, or students taping little reminders around the classroom for a teacher who was open about working on her organizational skills. One teacher commented, "They know flawed is okay." We suspect that the truth is just one step further—that the little "flaws" a teacher reveals are the texture that allows students to get a grip and hang on to in a caring relationship. These close, positive dynamics are deeply satisfying and also a key ingredient for social development, engagement, and achievement (Rimm-Kaufman & Sandilos, 2015).

We hope you agree that this "early days" use of the BSP is too valuable to hold off on until your class is EF literate. Don't wait! While you may have big plans to teach your students about EF, not only can you start using the BSP before you mention anything about EFs, but also it can really help you get started. Figures 3.3–3.6 provide the notes gathered during four different BSPs in four different classrooms. Each one takes a different approach to the integration of EFs, showing how an understanding of EFs can emerge naturally alongside these Barriers and Strategies conversations. In Figure 3.3, the BSP was used in a primary classroom with no explicit mention of EFs at all. Rather, while discussing "Getting Dressed to Go Outside Quickly," Danielle and Nikki chose to boost students' confidence and sense of mattering by typing their ideas on the overhead with student initials next to each contribution. You will notice that the themes of emotional regulation and organization are present in several of their comments. As a result of this conversation, these teachers chose to pick up and directly teach the idea of organization.

The "Organization of Materials" BSP in Figure 3.4 integrated an EF as an overarching theme. This was an unplanned 5-minute booster that Julie used to quickly support her grade 6 students' management of the papers, equipment, books, and other materials in their shared spaces. She began by suggesting that the overall problem was organization and then recruited students to explore why disorganization had become such a problem. You might notice that time management is a factor in many of the barriers they mention, and also in the strategies they propose. This was a nice "aha" moment for students to discuss. They realized they could be more organized if

Getting Dressed to Go Outside Quickly	
Barriers	**Strategies**
Not enough room (AB)	Move to another space with more space (CJ)
Bumping into other people (HR)	Use your words if someone pushes you (AB)
	ork it out before getting a teacher (CS)
Talking (EN)	
It is too loud (IP)	Calming down or taking a few breaths before you go out there (LP)
	Ask people to be quiet (RW)
We are being too silly, getting distracted (AB)	
Getting distracted because friends are talking and making you stop doing your jobs (KS)	
Size of the person; can't move as fast (FB)	
Winter was hard because we had a lot of stuff to put on (FB)	Hanging up your stuff (MM)
We didn't know where our stuff was (EN)	Put hat and mittens in sleeve (CA)

FIGURE 3.3. BSP: "Getting Dressed to Go Outside Quickly." Created by Danielle DeRusha and Nikki Reese at King Albert Public School in Lindsay, Ontario, Canada. Used with permission.

the teacher provided a little more time—so she did! An approach like this performs double duty, as it engages students in some metacognition and self-regulated learning, and also helps them to explore the many facets of one single EF.

The "Focus: Finish Your Work on Time" BSP featured in Figure 3.5 also concentrated on one EF (time management). This chart was created by a teacher hoping to address what seemed like a dreamy, slowpoke kind of problem, but quickly realized the issue was much more related to student stress and emotional regulation. Through this conversation with her class, Paula was able to help them elaborate on calming strategies such as self-talk and self-advocacy. These strategies turned out to be useful for resolving disputes at the cubbies and on the playground, and so this teacher decided to explicitly teach the idea of emotional regulation. A casual conversation about barriers and strategies provided the perfect teachable moment.

Finally, the "Submitting Work on Time" BSP in Figure 3.6 was conducted by grade 7 students with a good basic understanding of EFs. As they described their challenges, Mrs. Pearson encouraged them to connect these challenges to EFs. As their conversation progressed, they began to notice that, for different students, the same issue was borne out of different EF obstacles. So, for example, forgetting work may be related to time management for a student who wakes up late and rushes though their packing, organization for a student with a messy desk who loses the homework in a pile, and planning for a student who leaves the work at a friend's house. Through this conversation, the students (and their teacher) learned how diverse they all were, and accordingly how diverse the strategies would need to be in order to meet their needs.

Barriers	Strategies
too many loose papers	- "loose paper folder"
I don't know where they go	- ask peer/teacher
ready to move on too fast	- sort before putting things away
rushing	- 5 min warning
not using duotangs properly	- give yourself a consequence
bringing too much	- bring what you need
bored	- gamify - music
forgetting	- piles for now and later
not asking	- post-its
	- ask for materials

FIGURE 3.4. BSP: "Organization of Materials." Created by Julie Hough at Central Senior School in Lindsay, Ontario, Canada. Used with permission.

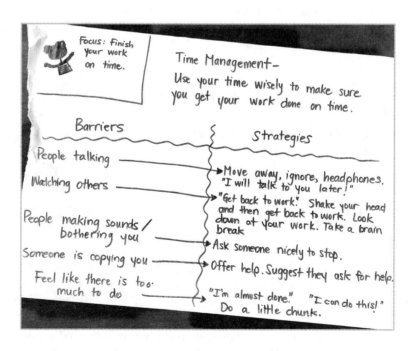

FIGURE 3.5. BSP: "Focus: Finish Your Work on Time." Created by Paula Barrow from Fenelon Township Public School in Cameron, Ontario, Canada. Used with permission.

Submitting Work on Time	
Barriers	**Strategies**
Not done (TI)	Make a schedule
Didn't start yet (TI)	Chunk the assignment into small parts
Started really late (TI)	Advocate for help
Too busy (PP)	Use class time
Didn't understand the task (RI/SA)	Use bus time or car rides
Distracted during work periods (SA)	Ask to stay in at recess
Don't have materials (SA/O)	Go to homework club
"What assignment?" (SA)	Ask for clarification
Tech difficulties	Ask for a repeat of the instructions
(F/GDP)	Find a quiet spot to work
Lost it (O)	Set a reminder or use the calendar
It's at home (O/P)	Create a special binder, folder, or list
Forgot (TM/O/P)	

FIGURE 3.6. BSP: "Submitting Work on Time." Created by Nicole Pearson at Ridgewood Public School in Coboconk, Ontario, Canada. Used with permission.

A short, simple BSP can be used to great effect at the very earliest stages of working with a group of students. In 5–10 minutes, it will allow you to inject self-regulated learning, metacognition, self-awareness, and strategic thinking into your teaching day. And contrary to what you might think, it is not easier to use in a small group, or with an EF-literate group, or with a group who already know each other. All you really need is the willingness to listen to your students. You can bet they will be curious about each other, and delighted by the knowledge that, in your classroom, their experiences, feelings, and ideas matter.

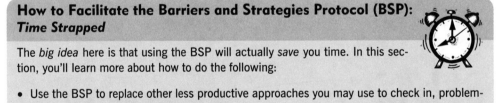

How to Facilitate the Barriers and Strategies Protocol (BSP): *Time Strapped*

The *big idea* here is that using the BSP will actually *save* you time. In this section, you'll learn more about how to do the following:

- Use the BSP to replace other less productive approaches you may use to check in, problem-solve, and get students started on work.
- Reuse your Barriers and Strategies charts by returning to them for reference, continuation, or adjustment.

While every teacher has moments of feeling "time strapped," some of us make a career out of it. Whether you rush from room to room to teach a language, receive different groups of students all day as a specialist, or work in a religious or cultural school and balance the basics plus extra lessons, we realize there will be readers of this book who feel they have exactly *no* extra time. It's no easier for teachers in typical settings. There are so many things that take a bite out of active learning time. Consider the way a 45-minute period might be used: Usually, we begin by putting out the behavioral fires; then we establish order, teach a small lesson, make sure students have understood the lesson, and finally give instructions for activities. This "fires-to-instructions" process might take 10 or 15 minutes, but what happens next? We're betting that, on many days, you spend the rest of the period repeating almost every one of the steps you've just finished. You may follow up with students who weren't paying attention, who had questions but didn't ask them, or for whom the expectations required a slight modification. While you're tied up recapping and troubleshooting with those individuals, or with small groups, you might otherwise be standing back to observe your students, providing feedback or making useful assessment notes. So, how can you avoid this duplication and make your precious teaching time more productive? You guessed it: A time-strapped context presents a great opportunity to use the BSP.

Even the busiest teachers probably already do something similar to a BSP. Let's say you're a Spanish teacher asking students to write a paragraph about a cultural celebration. After conducting your fires-to-instructions teaching, you might say, "Okay—we have about 20 minutes to work on this. Before we get started, do you have *any* questions?" Silence. You might then nudge your students further by asking, "Anything? Are you sure? You're completely ready? You've got your research? Everyone? So, when I pass out the materials, we're all set to go? José? You good? Sami? Yes? Ahmed? *Really?* Okaaay . . ." It is amazing how quickly things can fall apart right after a check-in like this. In fact, you may find that José missed half of the instructions, Sami is stumped by a spelling word, and Ahmed has no idea where to start.

A more productive line of questioning might have been "What will be tricky about this? What barriers could many of *us* come up against? How will *we* struggle?" Questions like these ease a student's sense of being *the only one who doesn't get it.* Instead, they allow the students to come together and answer as a team; they can reflect on personal experience, but they can also make a prediction or consider the experiences of their classmates. This is the first step of the BSP, and if you want to keep it really short, you can simply ask students for one or two barriers. In response, Sami might feel comfortable suggesting that a number of classmates tend to get stuck on the spelling of Spanish words.

Depending on how much your group knows about EFs, and how time strapped you really are, you can mention EFs by name or not. Either way, their impact will probably be evident. You might glance at an anchor chart posted in the room and ask, "Is it just hard to keep going?" (goal-directed persistence). Perhaps Sami will agree, or perhaps she'll say, "Not quite. I start to feel overwhelmed and worried when I don't get the spellings right" (emotional regulation). Or perhaps she'll tell you that when she can't spell the words perfectly, she doesn't even want to give them a go (flexibility). As you're chatting with your students about the assignment, EF connections will come up naturally.

Before you even ask for strategy ideas, José might point out that there are Spanish/English dictionaries on the shelf, Ahmed might mention that there is a word list in the front of the text, and another student might suggest that when she can't spell a word, she just tries her best, underlines it, and comes back to it later. Another student might suggest using self-talk to manage stress, and another might suggest working with a partner. Before you know it, you'll have a list of good suggestions for how to manage this particular problem, and the second part of your BSP (strategies) will be well on its way. At this point, you can circle back to ask about another barrier, but because the conversation has already been so rich, you could also just wrap it up by saying, "Great. So today I'll be watching to see how you use these strategies." If you've charted their ideas, you will have created a valuable resource that you can pull out or refer to any time you ask students to do a piece of writing.

In just a few minutes a day, you can work with students to tackle many different areas of performance. For example, after dealing with the spelling barrier, this Spanish teacher could tackle the challenge of students missing half of the instructions—why is that happening? Or perhaps she'll deal with the issue of students not knowing where to start. The BSP is a worthwhile process in even the most time-strapped classrooms. Day by day, common barriers will become better understood, strategy ideas will accumulate, and after the fires are out and the instructions are delivered, you might just notice that your students are getting things done.

How to Facilitate the Barriers and Strategies Protocol (BSP): *Highly Structured*

The *big idea* here is that a BSP can be used to create structure and discipline in daily work, small assignments, or big projects. In this section, you'll learn more about how to do the following:

- Use a more involved BSP for a larger project.
- Help your students pursue high standards by using the BSP to tackle the barriers that are holding them back.

In this section, we will present a highly structured application of the BSP for a rather unstructured "21st-century" task. You will see how even a teacher taking his or her first steps into student-centred, inquiry, or design-based learning can bring order and specificity to the development of problem-solving skills. We share this type of example because we know many teachers are struggling to meet the demands for a 21st-century education with a student body that is largely devoid of 21st-century skills. How can we set complex problems, release control, and let students practice adaptive skills before they actually *have any?* It is very much like the chicken and egg quandary, or the paradox of "I can't get a *job* because they want me to have *experience.*" In our case, we often feel our students can't do complex work because they don't have the ability, but they can't develop the ability without being immersed in complex work. The BSP offers the missing link between our ambitious projects and the tools students need to complete them.

These ambitious projects typically take place over a few weeks, offering us a chance to focus on thematic topics and dig deeply into the potential of our students. In kindergarten this can look like a weeklong project in which everybody brings in cereal cartons, kitchen towel tubes, and tissue boxes, and figures out how to stick them together to create a robot. In grade 4, it may be a monthlong project working in teams to design a disaster-proof house. In grade 8, it might be an eight-page careers project and class presentation. No matter how many days you've dedicated to these projects, we'd like you to imagine allocating a considerable chunk of time to creating, and then continually adding to, a BSP. We suggest dedicating a full period at the outset and then revisiting it daily as the project evolves. We have seen that this is time well spent, a stitch that definitely "in time saves nine."

Our friends' experience with a "makerspace" provides a good example. In case you're not familiar, in a makerspace, students can use all sorts of different tools and materials to construct objects they themselves design. Dawn, Steph, and Roger, a team of grade 3, 6, and 8 teachers who opened a space like this in their school, used an EF-based approach and the BSP to help it run more smoothly.[2] They told us about their ambitious beginnings: planning exciting challenges for their students, gathering all the necessary materials, freeing up a generous amount of time, and securing the support of their administration. They noticed, however, that even though they had planned "design" activities that should have been very creative and engaging—brainstorming, developing ideas, planning, and prototyping—students often weren't as productive as they had hoped. Rather, the children often seemed overwhelmed and frustrated. What to do? Should they reduce their expectations? Remove components from the project? Step in and do parts of the work *with* students? They wondered how to help without taking over the very creativity and independence that the makerspace was designed to support. They were fine tolerating a little chaos, but they felt their problem went beyond noise and disorder. Their students seemed to be lacking the essential skills that they needed.

These teachers wanted to support their students' ability to plan, organize, manage time, stay calm, and pay attention to details, so they initiated a BSP. After clearing a space amid the sawdust, tools, and drawings, they spent a good 25 minutes reflecting with the students. "What is happening?" they asked. "What is stopping your progress?" Their first conversation, captured in Figure 3.7, included the kinds of challenges one might face on a real construction site: how to manage the use of valuable tools when they are in demand by different teams, how to ensure each builder's time is used optimally, and of course, how to minimize the natural distractions arising from task avoidance and fatigue. During that short conversation, the students created systems they would continue to refine and improve upon throughout the course of the project. Roger, Dawn, and Stephanie made time for short follow-up conversations on a daily basis to allow students to update the list of good strategies or add more dimension to the types of barriers they faced. This list became the backbone of the project.

After construction wrapped up, the teachers shared several observations. First, many of the students who had previously been reluctant to speak up in front of classmates were the ones to step up with the most strategy ideas. We have heard this before. Research tells us that students with a wide variety of learning difficulties often struggle to respond strategically to challenging tasks

Our biggest barriers for completing our house have been . . .	Executive function	Our strategies to overcome these barriers
Waiting for tools	Flexibility, planning, time management	We can each have the tool for 20 minutes and then switch, work with something else, or see if the same tool is somewhere else.
Taking too long on one task	Planning, task initiation, time management	Two of us can work on one thing, and the other two can work on something else, search for something to help us go faster, or ask a partner for help.
Getting distracted	Task initiation, time management, attention	Move away, set a time limit, or use positive self-talk.

FIGURE 3.7. The BSP for a long-term makerspace project. Created by Roger Reynolds at Jack Callaghan Public School in Kawartha Lakes, Ontario, Canada.

---

[2] Dawn Mattiussi, Stephanie Chislett, and Roger Reynolds teach at Jack Callaghan Public School in Kawartha Lakes, Ontario. Used with permission.

(Swanson, 1990; Torgesen, 1977), though they tend to benefit especially when taught adaptable, resourceful responses (e.g., Wong, Butler, Ficzere, & Kuperis, 1996). Second, the teachers commented that they had never seen such a polite and optimistic group of grade 7 and 8 students; it sure is satisfying to have your experiences validated and your ideas taken seriously. In addition, learning new skills feels good, especially when they allow you to bring your ideas to life.

So, reimagine your daily life in a bold, student-centred, 21st-century classroom. Where once you moved from student to student, continuously providing information and guidance, now you begin to interrupt this daily activity to ask your class, "How will this be hard for us?" and to discuss the strategies necessary for success. This is a small but mighty interruption, a flip of the script, and a radical departure from routine teaching—so radical, in fact, that we wonder if using the BSP isn't a little like a science fiction scene in which the hero rips a portal through time and space. When you stop the everyday grind for a moment to guide your class into a metacognitive conversation, you lead them to a different dimension to explore a rarely used aspect of their cognitive ability. It is like walking our students forward though the grey matter in their own brains, past simple reactions and academic ability, toward the most reflective, adaptive, and strategic structures.

From day to day, we can pop in and out of this "portal" with our students to explore math challenges, writing difficulties, or social problems. When doing larger projects, however, in which students learn and practice new skills over a longer period of time, we can step through, build a fort, stick a flag in it, and plan to come back. Using a BSP throughout these longer projects can be like creating a metacognitive basecamp: a place designed *with* children around the demands of a shared classroom task, assembled from a ramshackle collection of common tricks and strategies, and cemented by a meaningful shared experience. Built over weeks, this place becomes a comfortable, beloved, and complex structure that students will not soon forget. "Did you know this was here?" we might ask. "This place called 'metacognition' has been here all along. It's yours, and you can come back whenever you like!" It is a wondrous thing to discover.

> ### How to Facilitate the Barriers and Strategies Protocol (BSP):
> *Organic and Free Flowing*
>
> The *big idea* here is that the BSP doesn't have to be a big, disruptive, formal "thing." In this section, you'll learn more about how to do the following:
>
> - Use a "pocket-sized" BSP whenever and wherever you might need it for on-the-fly problem solving.
> - Engage in the BSP as a truly open-ended and curious form of inquiry with students.
> - Use the BSP to discover something new about your learners.

After using the BSP a few times, you might find yourself turning to it more casually and organically. These may be unplanned-for moments—perhaps right in the middle of a classroom activity, out on the playground, or in the middle of a museum while on a field trip—when you realize that your instructions have missed the mark or your students are off track. *Something* is going wrong. What begins as just a little whiff of a problem can intensify into something rather unpleasant, and like a bad smell, you might not know exactly what is causing it. Instead of jumping to a quick diagnosis, a teacher equipped with the BSP can step back, refocus, and say, "Stop. Talk to me. Let's understand what is going wrong here . . ." This process is pocket sized and universal enough to use for almost any tricky "on the go" moment.

For example, put yourself into the shoes of grade 4 teacher, Janet Rhude, who was halfway through a literacy period when she started to notice that something wasn't working. Students had been divided into groups with a page of text, and Janet had asked them to split it into sections and take turns reading aloud. The text was not too hard or too long for her students, yet almost none of them had started the activity. A few students were rocking back in their chairs. One was looking fed up, and another had put on her headphones. Scanning her class, Janet might have made a number of quick assumptions. Are they just low energy, and do they need encouragement? Or are they struggling to manage their time and perhaps need a 10-minute deadline? If neither of these approaches worked, she might have started moving from group to group, dividing up the text and assigning roles for the students.

Janet, however, took a different approach. She took a step back, and a deep breath, and watched her class for 8 seconds straight. After spending this calm, focused eternity trying to understand what was really going on, she stopped her students and initiated the BSP pictured in Figure 3.8. She discovered that, in fact, the students were not low energy, and they did not need a deadline. Rather, they were having trouble dividing up the text because they had strong feelings, both positive and negative, about different sections. Janet was surprised and delighted by their deep responses to the text, and this became a point of further conversation. In the meantime, they

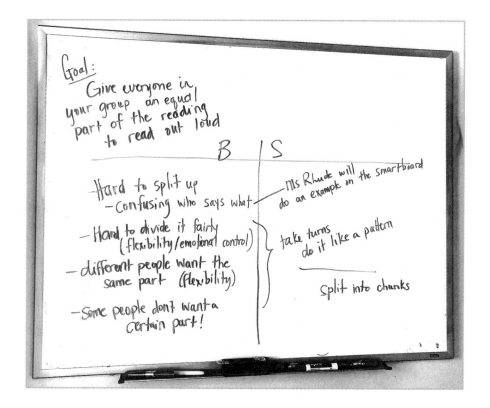

FIGURE 3.8. A Barriers and Strategies Protocol (BSP) conducted midway through a reading assignment. Created by Janet Rhude at Scott Young Public School in Lindsay, Ontario, Canada. Used with permission.

correctly diagnosed the issue as one of flexibility and emotional control and worked out a way to divide it up that was acceptable to everyone.

Consider a few days in the life of Victoria Young, an educational assistant who specializes in challenging behavior and autism spectrum disorder. On Day 1, after receiving word that the schedule had changed and her grade 4 students would have to attend French class during the last period of the day, Victoria hosted a quick BSP to set them up for success. The class brainstormed barriers, divided them up, and tasked small teams of students to tackle each one. On Day 2, Victoria was helping a mixed group of students from grades 1 through 3 to deal with some of the frustrations they were feeling while playing tag. In response to the vexing annoyance of the person tagged denying it happened, the students quickly agreed to try three things: first, to take a deep breath and count to three; second, to try using self-talk by saying, "This is no big deal"; and third, to simply move on and try tagging another person. She found she could much more confidently send this capable group out to recess. Later that same week, Victoria dropped in on a classroom and found a grade 1 group struggling to share a set of whiteboards and markers. There weren't enough to go around, and after describing how frustrated they felt, the students worked with Victoria to make a list of good strategies for sharing, getting along, and getting their work done (see Figure 3.9). Students realized that they sometimes preferred drawing their ideas on scrap paper and that they could also can arrange to use a whiteboard after another student had finished. These obvious-seeming ideas were reinvented and applied by the grade 1 students with a great deal of

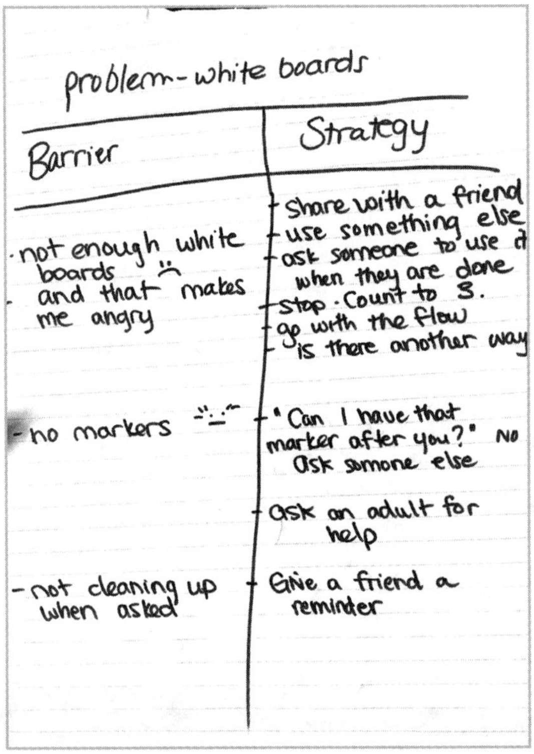

FIGURE 3.9. A Barriers and Strategies Protocol (BSP) conducted to problem-solve the sharing of materials. Created by Victoria Young at King Albert Public School in Lindsay, Ontario, Canada. Used with permission.

pride and enthusiasm. Victoria reflected that, while the conversation was hilarious in its simplicity, it seemed to work because the students did not have a problem sharing the whiteboards again.

Our final example of how quick, easy, and powerful the BSP can be comes from Julie Kuiken in grade 8.[3] It was the end of the day, and Julie's students were packing up their books for an unusually heavy night of homework. With a science test planned for the following day, the students were a little nervous and Julie needed an efficient way to help them manage. In a 5-minute BSP, she realized why they were so stressed. A few students had incomplete review notes, one was having trouble accessing the online materials, and still others weren't sure if their answers to the practice questions were correct. Before long, her class had swapped strategies and notes, made plans to copy the answers to the practice questions, and fixed the technology problems. How might these students have managed otherwise? They may have used avoidance, lowered their expectations, or externalized their frustrated feelings with anger or tears. The BSP can be a healthy and merciful support for an overloaded teenager.

With so much to get done in a day, it is always tempting to jump to a quick conclusion about the source of student problems. The task is too hard, you might assume. The game is too intense. The groups are too large. And without the help of our students to appreciate the problem in an accurate and nuanced way, we might execute one of a few big, clunky, blunt-force strategies: quickly reducing our expectations, removing parts of an activity, or providing solutions that we were hoping our students would work out independently. There is a simple genius to embracing the limitations of our own judgment and trusting students enough to ask *them* what is going on. We hope you'll let the BSP help you out at these moments; it is a compact little strategy that can be used to be more sensitive, precise, and supportive throughout your day.

How to Facilitate the Barriers and Strategies Protocol (BSP): *Working with a "Stressed" Class*

The *big idea* here is that you can use strategies and tactics to ease a more stressed group of students into group problem-solving conversations. In this section, you'll learn more about how to do the following:

- Model a mindset of self-understanding and compassion.
- Keep your barriers and strategies conversations short and snappy.
- Persist for 10 full attempts before becoming discouraged.
- Recruit as much support as you can from your colleagues and administrators.

Not to give our ages away, but when we (the authors) were growing up, stress was not a word we heard very often. If we did, it pertained to a disorder suffered by adults, not children. Over the past 30 to 40ish years, however, the effect of stress has infiltrated our communities, the word has entered our daily vocabulary, and even very young children are now sometimes described as "stressed."

Though it sometimes feels scary or hard, we can actually benefit from the stress arising from everyday challenges. As our heart rate and blood pressure increase, and our bloodstream fills with epinephrine, norepinephrine, and cortisol, we may feel energized for learning and performance.

---

[3] Julie Kuiken teaches at Central Senior Public School in Lindsay, Ontario, Canada. Used with permission.

For you, about to give a presentation at a staff meeting, and for your students, about to do a test, this is a feeling worth getting used to. This is the stress that is associated with risk taking, learning, and growth, and with any luck every single one of us will experience it on and off throughout life. Managing this stress is necessary for success in a wide variety of jobs and careers, during parenting, while enjoying relationships, and in order to stay healthy. As teachers, therefore, our job is not to minimize all stress but rather to teach students how to recognize it, embrace it, and manage it properly. Using the BSP, we have the opportunity to prepare our students with resilient, can-do habits; the confidence to involve others in problem-solving; and a familiarity with the kinds of strategies that work for them. We can rally our students to go boldly toward challenge with the firm belief that "We can do hard things!"

Stressed students come in many forms, and occasionally they come in groups. At some point, you may wind up teaching a class that is notoriously stressed. One that has "history." This is the class that everyone talks about in the staff room, the one that wasn't allowed to go on the yearly canoe trip, and the one that absolutely *has* to have the same shatterproof substitute teacher every time. This class may include a few highly stressed students who act out and make others feel unsafe, or they may just have a generally challenging dynamic. And while these students would probably benefit the most from additional strategies, self-regulated learning, and team problem solving, they may also be the ones who have the most difficulty accepting help. They will be tough nuts to crack; when conducting a BSP with a group like this, we can pretty much promise that it won't work on the first or even second try. But stay the course; this is the bold, life- and world-changing work you may have dreamed of doing in university or college. It's the "Oh Captain, my Captain" type stuff. It may take a while for a stressed group to trust one another enough to open up, talk about their challenges, and collaborate on solutions, but there are tricks that make it easier. We have several pieces of advice for initiating a BSP ritual with a stressed class:

1. *Model the mindset.* Always start the conversation by modeling self-understanding, self-acceptance, and self-compassion. So, before you ask your students what is challenging for them, share with them what might be challenging for *you* about the task. Saying things like "Organization is tricky for me. You've all seen the state of my desk by the end of the day!" might go a long way toward establishing trust, reducing stigma, and showing students that even successful people struggle sometimes.

2. *Keep it short and sweet.* Your class will probably feel quite vulnerable and out of their comfort zone the first few times you conduct the BSP. Don't leave them in this position for too long, or you stand more chance of losing their cooperation. In fact, you might want to reassure them by setting a 5-minute timer and stopping the conversation promptly when it dings.

3. *Try for a 2 + 2.* The first few times, make it your goal to model the mindset, and then work with students to discover only two barriers and two strategies. This will provide more structure, keep the conversation short, and allow everyone (including you) to feel a sense of accomplishment in a short time. When you feel they are ready, you can bump it to 3 + 3, and so on.

4. *Stay the course.* If your class has difficulty the first two or three times you attempt the BSP, don't give up. We recommend budgeting for 10 short and sweet attempts. Until you have finished all 10 attempts, try not to evaluate your success or make any conclusions. The approach will need time to work. If you can suspend your judgment and resist quitting, you might be surprised at what you can achieve.

Our colleague Irena Farkov is a grade 4 French immersion teacher at Ventura Park Public School in Thornhill, Ontario. Though she doesn't work with an especially stressed group, she adapted the BSP in a way that we think might be calming and reassuring for students. For her first five attempts, Irena asked students to write down their barriers on little squares of paper. She quickly gathered these papers in a collection box and read them out anonymouavsly. In this way, students could take their first cautious steps without really risking anything at all. While we think it is important for students to trust one another and believe in their overall ability enough to "own" their challenges, this seems like a move in the right direction. With this approach, Irena filled the room with real student voice and classmates began to understand that to struggle is normal. Soon, her students began to open up and Irena no longer needed to use anonymity as a scaffold.

Speaking of shatterproof substitute teachers, consider Miya Bradburn's story about a day she spent covering a grade 4 class in the Trillium Lakelands District School Board in Ontario. Miya sent us the note, below, to describe her experience using the BSP.[4] Her description is special because it acknowledges a supportive principal, Jamie Stone, also from the Trillium Lakelands Board, and shares the many feelings and responses experienced by both herself and her students throughout the process.

"I had a supply day booked in a class that was, by all accounts from admin and staff, going to be tricky. The regular teacher had been away for 4 days, and the group had been taught by four different teachers. The principal started our day with a community circle to discuss the barriers to learning that might come up. We then discussed strategies to handle the barriers. First block went so well! I was finding myself very present and intentional in all my words and actions and used EF language as much as I could. After first recess I could sense some upset energy, so I did another circle, this time on my own, to talk about barriers to success in Block 2 due to what happened at recess. Block 2 went pretty well! [For the] final block, they came in and seemed okay after recess, so I asked them about this and they said it went a lot better than first recess. I don't usually get compliments from students about my teaching, but today in Block 3 they said I really listened to them. They were, for the most part, really self-controlled, attentive, and on task, and this is what they told me they had been struggling with. All this to say that I had direct and immediate proof that what I felt was a practical approach *actually really was*! I almost kept waiting for the other shoe to drop and for the wheels to fall off, but wouldn't you know? Those shoes stayed on."

Miya's story illustrates so many important points. First, when working with a stressed group of students, the hands-on support of an administrator who really understands what is going on can make a world of difference. Jamie Stone didn't just pop his head in to say hello. He showed up, proved to Miya that it was okay to be bold and ambitious and compassionate in her approach with the students, and helped to shoulder the responsibility for pulling it off. Without this engagement, a teacher might simply close the classroom door, do everything possible to keep the kids quiet all day, and hope to avoid an embarrassing incident. Because of Jamie and Miya's leadership, the students seemed to have a much more connected and enjoyable day.

---

[4] Miya Bradburn teaches in Lindsay, Ontario, Canada. Jamie Stone is the principal at Mariposa Elementary School in Oakwood, Ontario, Canada. Used with permission.

What was it that made the day so much better for Miya's students? Notice that she didn't mention devising any earth-shatteringly brilliant and brand-new strategies. We think that, most of the time, the strategies mentioned during the BSP are rather ordinary. In fact, they may be the type of strategies that Miya would have otherwise asked students to use, over and over again, probably to little effect. "Take a deep breath!" she might have suggested. "Find a better place in the classroom to work!" or "Take the time to get your materials organized before you begin!" The thing is, there are plenty of strategies like this floating around in classrooms. The real challenge is to redirect the prevailing and steady little forces surrounding students so they can start moving in a positive direction and actually make *use* of a strategy. Using the BSP, we change the tone in the classroom in a way that makes children feel more powerful, capable, and ready to act.

Another thing we know for sure is that it is very comforting, connecting, and empowering to be heard. Particularly during times of stress, it means a lot to have your perspective considered, your difficulties fully understood, and your ideas for solutions appreciated. This is true for both adults and children. After working in school administration for many years, Carol (author) reflects that when parents took the time to offer thanks, it was often because they were shown the simple courtesy of attention. "I felt listened to," they'd say. From the desks in Miya's Block 3 math class, attentive listening allowed children to explain the argument at recess, explore how it was making them feel and act, and plan the best way to proceed. Miya became so much better informed about her students, and we wonder how this increased sensitivity may have affected her decisions, responses, and expressions as she interacted with them all day long. Regardless, when children trust us enough to share these kinds of thoughts and experiences, we should consider it an opportunity. Through the BSP, we enter a space where truth and sharing, a sense of mattering, and deep understanding makes genuine relationships possible—and relationships are the foundation upon which all other learning is built. We're not suggesting this will be easy, but finding connection with a stressed class is incredibly rewarding. With some patience, an extra cup of coffee, and especially with the help of a supportive colleague or principal, it is a 3- or 4- or even 6-week goal worth striving for.

How EF Literacy
Can Improve Observation

HOW WE TEND TO OBSERVE

In the following discussion, we will describe the ways that your knowledge of EF can support a more accurate and useful process of classroom observation. We will also characterize the ways that a teacher's careful observation of EFs can benefit students. By paying attention to the EF demands and subsequent self-regulation demonstrated by students, an EF-literate teacher can stir self-awareness and energize a more active process of EF development.

Have you ever seen someone clap two old-school chalkboard erasers together? We'll begin Chapter 4 with this classic bit of prewhiteboard mischief. As you remember the huge, lingering cloud of dust this created, turn your attention to what may *hang in the air* between yourself and your students. In this chapter, we will talk about the constant, quiet, invisible network of information zipping around your classroom from moment to moment as you watch and listen to your students. We'll suggest that even though observation burns a lot of teacher energy, it often operates without much notice or manipulation. We'll also describe the ways that observation works from both a teacher's and a student's perspective and argue that it is a highly active force in a classroom. Finally, we'll propose that with just a little bit of awareness and intention, EF literacy can help teachers reclaim the process of observation and use it to steer and encourage student performance.

Let's slow down for a moment to think about exactly what is going on when we observe. Imagine you're at your desk. It's about 2:00 p.m. on a typical Monday, and you're encircled by three students who are blocking most of your view. You can hear a repetitive tapping noise, and someone is laughing loudly. The classroom door bangs shut, and you realize that a whole group of desks is empty. Why? Meanwhile, over the shoulder of the student directly in front of you are four students who look very productive but who have arranged a heap of papers onto the head of another who may or may not be sleeping. This is an ordinary moment at school—a good moment—but one that illustrates the barrage of irresistible stimuli that capture our attention. In rapid succession, we are supportive, irritated, curious, concerned, delighted, and, against our better judgment, slightly amused. The point is that while we are capable of planning to actively observe something specific, it's not surprising that we occasionally go for long periods simply chasing the sights and sounds in our midst. With upward of 6 hours of contact time per day taking place in a variety of loud and active contexts, it's easy to succumb to sensory overload. This is most acute for rookie teachers or visiting parents, who are easily distracted and overwhelmed by every little movement, sight, and sound in the room and struggle to appreciate the complexity of what is going on around them (Wolff, Jarodzka, van den Bogert, & Boshuizen, 2016). The next time you're in a classroom, notice how you observe. Are you choosing where you focus your attention, or are just trying to keep up? This may be different from morning to afternoon, Monday to Friday, or bright and early in September to the day after your sister's wedding in May.

As much as we *gather* information in a subjective and disorderly way, we also tend to *interpret* it that way too. Have you ever observed the same group of students as a colleague, asked her what she noticed, and realized you each picked up on completely different things? Or, if you were focused on the same events, that your interpretation was different? This can be particularly noticeable after a scuffle on the playground, when almost every observer has a different understanding of the events that took place. There are several reasons for this. First, like it or not, we all carry unconscious biases. To some extent, the way we interpret the actions of our students will be influenced by our previous experiences with them and our own sensitivities. Goodwin (1994) coined the term "professional vision" to describe the specialized way professionals observe and accurately interpret phenomena of interest to them. For teachers, professional vision becomes more and more precise and insightful as knowledge of students, subject matter, and pedagogy grows (Kramarski & Michalsky, 2009).

Our interpretations are also influenced by our teaching experience, skills, and knowledge. For a specific subject like mathematics, the deeper our knowledge of mathematical principles, the more noticeable our student's mathematical thinking and action will be (Kersting, Givvin, Sotelo, & Stigler, 2010). Similarly, having more experience with children and knowing more about special education and child behavior enables us to clearly see and more accurately interpret a diverse range of unexpected student behaviors (Michalsky & Schechter, 2013; Perry, Phillips, & Hutchinson, 2006). With a knowledge of EFs, for example, we may observe a student repetitively tapping her pencil and suspect that she is creating stimulation to support better attention. Or we may recognize that two students are talking during math class to support emotional regulation and goal-directed persistence. This sharper vision is very beneficial, because a more accurate appraisal of student behavior enables a more attentive response and fosters closer relationships with and among students (Perry et al., 2008; Shivers, Levenson, & Tan, 2017; Yenawine, 2013). Conversely, without adequate pedagogical knowledge, student behavior can seem a little overwhelming and stressful. In response to the very same pencil tapper, a teacher with less professional vision may feel more stressed and change their approach. Research tells us that teachers tend to respond to stress by boosting structure, reducing expectations, and tightening up control (Klusmann, Kunter, Trautwein, Ludtke, & Baumert, 2008; Muller, Gorrow, & Fiala, 2011; Yong & Yue, 2007).

So, what teachers see when they look at students is highly variable. Let us now explore how observation is translated and understood on the *receiving* end. You might not realize that the little point of focus you bounce from person to person and event to event around the room is quite an important presence for your students. The National Scientific Council on the Developing Child (2004) tells us that from birth, children are wired to seek the attention they require to meet their social and emotional needs. Furthermore, we know that over the years each piece of valuable attention your students have received has made a real impression on them. These deeply satisfying experiences teach subtle lessons about what is important and what is valuable (Berland et al., 2016).

For example, imagine standing at the front of the room watching your students write an assignment. One is changing the assignment a little to demonstrate independence and free thinking, one is about to ask you for clarification to demonstrate obedience and respect, one is looking through a thesaurus to demonstrate originality and creative energy, and another is disagreeing with the thrust of the assignment to demonstrate critical and bold thinking. There might also be a student who is thinking, "Why is she *watching* me?" and feeling a little worried that your gaze is disapproving. The manner in which each of these students operates is based on their own assumption about what is valued in the process of learning and thinking. This means that not only are your observations subjective and guided by your own professional knowledge but also they will be interpreted in an almost infinite range of ways by the diverse group of students who populate your classroom. These forces of observation are strong, but surprisingly disorderly.

How can we bring more order and purpose to our observation? This will be described in vivid detail throughout the following discussion and in the subsequent "how to" sections. Essentially, we believe that by using a more mindful and intentional process, teachers can interrupt habitual practices and leverage the great many observational forces already at work. We also believe that by understanding student behavior according to a knowledge of EFs, we can appreciate it in a more scientific and coherent way. Teachers have always been masters of giving "the look." With a little finesse, we can use this quiet superpower more efficiently to support and guide the students we teach.

SLOWING DOWN AND TUNING IN
TO STUDENT PERFORMANCE WITH AN EF LENS

When you look at your students, what do you see? Their behavior may not match what you were expecting, especially if that behavior takes the form of an eccentric and personal little strategy to support their EFs and self-regulated learning. In fact, some of their best strategies could *cost* them brownie points. To function as teachers of creative, independent, and strategic thinkers, we need to get comfortable with observing the unexpected—to see it, strive to understand it, and make very clear the fact that we value it. The old-fashioned greeting "How do you *do*?" has never been more appropriate or more considerate. Looking around the room, we should wonder, "And how do *you* do? And *you*? And what about *you*?" Our style of observation should convey a genuine curiosity and delight at how our students "do" their learning.

As our familiarity with students' EF grows, we will be more able to appreciate the diversity and complexity in their approach. For example, to an EF-literate teacher, a student who responds to a writing prompt by seeking conversation with friends and teachers may look like a student trying to support his attention or emotional regulation, instead of one who has chosen to ignore the instructions. Or, we may interpret a student calling out in the middle of a lesson as, yes, a little inconsiderate, but also as one who is trying desperately to share something before it is lost from his working memory. "Try jotting down that idea," we might respond, "and remember that when you call out you make it difficult for others to pay attention." After learning about the impact of EFs on performance, you may feel as though you are looking at students through a new lens and noticing things about them you've never seen before.

When we can actually *see* all of the little ways our students' EFs affect their learning, and also notice when they are attempting strategies to work around these challenges, we have new options and choices for teaching. The simplest change we can make is to allow students the time, space, and encouragement they need to do this work. Instead of shushing those unexpected prewriting conversations, we can notice and support them. By creating this safe space, we can set the stage for even more supportive and positive relationships in our classrooms.

Consider the interesting situation we encountered while leading a workshop for a group of educators. After assigning a task, and giving participants a few minutes to get started, we began to observe our way around the room. While many tables were filling in the assigned worksheet with their responses, one group had skipped it entirely and was instead engaged in an energetic debate, scribbling notes and small diagrams for each other as they tried to explain their ideas. We loved to see their passion, but as we approached their table, it was like a dark cloud filled the room. These experienced educators assumed we were displeased with their decision to stray from the instructions, and they responded to our observation with a bit of defensiveness and a "cold shoulder." Their negative reaction stirred negative feelings from us, and we were suddenly on our way down a rather unfriendly and unproductive path.

This was a pivotal point in the workshop; thank goodness we figured it out quickly enough to salvage a teachable moment. We stopped the group to call attention to the negative spiral taking place among us and suggested that the problem was both our unclear role and our values as observers, as well as the fact that people tend to assume the worst. Operating based on their own memories as schoolchildren or perhaps their own experiences as teachers being supervised and evaluated, our participants assumed we were watching for compliance and rule following. They thought we were cross, disappointed, and exasperated, when in fact we were delighted by the way they were managing a high level of attention and persistence to the task. "We are really interested in how you learn," we reassured them. "We are so excited by your initiative and can't wait to hear about what you're thinking." It was as if the sun had come out. We learned that in order to preserve a trusting, cooperative, and supportive relationship, we needed to make our intentions, feelings, and observations 100% clear.

If the teachers at our workshop respond this way, how might students respond? For arguments' sake, let's say these teachers were experienced, capable, strong, and powerful. While it may not be entirely true, let's also say they were secure and happy adults with extensive social safety nets, a pocketful of money, a cell phone, and a teachers' union to back them up. And in actual fact, these teachers had to sit through only a few hours of our workshop before heading out the door with the option to never see us again. Now, imagine how a similar confrontation might feel for students, who attend school day after day for years, may arrive discouraged from other negative experiences, and often already believe we won't like them, won't help them, and are "out to get them." This is a well-known phenomenon. "Stereotype threat" is the general fear of being observed or judged according to a certain stereotype. Often, people who belong to stereotyped groups feel this way, including people of color, people with disabilities, people from low socioeconomic backgrounds, women, minority groups, the elderly, and many others. Someone with stereotype threat may quickly assume the worst. Imagine how quickly the situation could escalate if the student felt particularly isolated, prejudged, disrespected, or misunderstood. Reflecting on how a relatively secure and skilled group of adults responded to the ambiguous messages they received from our observation is a telling reminder of just how students may struggle to cope with something similar at school. It only takes one look to get off on the wrong foot.

So, how do we fix it? How can we observe students in a way that makes them feel respected, appreciated, and encouraged? Margaret Forster and Geoff Masters (1996) speak of a process called "spotlighting," through which specific outcomes can be targeted for special attention in one's observation. Traditionally, this practice is done by deciding to focus on certain curricular goals, such as the use of punctuation. For example, a teacher might say, "Today I'm looking out for capital letters and periods." It is a simple step that can reduce cognitive demands for teachers and make observation a little calmer. This approach is perfect for an EF-literate teacher; we love the idea of using it to transform the many confusing and zig-zagging lines of observation into one steady, warm spotlight that is focused on *process*. Throughout the day, and particularly when students are struggling, we can focus a spotlight on the unique ways our students manage EF barriers or create strategies to meet the challenges we place before them. "I can't wait to see how you manage this task. I'm interested in your strategies!" we might say. Spotlighting brings order to observation for teachers, and reassurance, confidence, and power to students. The more you can make your observation of strategy visible, the more you can make it clear that you like your students' ingenuity and individuality. For this reason, we recommend you observe as conspicuously, noisily, and overtly as possible, making sure your students know right away that you are regarding them with respect.

Any time we find ourselves watching students, it makes sense to clearly declare what we are looking for. By saying things like "I'm very interested to see how you'll do this . . ." or "I can't wait to see the kinds of strategies you use . . ." or "I'm watching to see all of the different ways you're going to manage . . ." you can nip negative assumptions in the bud and project the kind of curiosity, interest, and delight that will grow their initiative. It won't take long for your students to understand that their teacher appreciates the fiery determination and invention that lies beneath their ultimate success.

THE NEED TO BE SEEN AND APPRECIATED

Shortly, we will describe a crafty and efficient method of observation for EF-literate teachers and provide you with more practical classroom examples than you ever dreamed possible. First, however, let us share an inspiring story that is a little closer to home. We would like to explore the naturally occurring form of process-focused observation that can be found in the attention paid by a calm and doting grandparent. While we appreciate that not every grandparent is the same, we believe there is a set of qualities you will be able to recognize. By making this connection, we hope to place process-based observation deeply into the context of being *human* and suggest that it is an essential ingredient in the healthy development of children. Much like a naturally occurring nutrient, we can analyze it, understand its principal components, and synthesize it for use in our classrooms.

First, consider how a grandparent lavishes a child with attention. Often, they can't see their grandchildren every day, so by the time a family gathering rolls around they are dying of curiosity and captivated by every little detail. "What have you got there?" they might ask, or "Show us how you do that!" Meanwhile, children have spent the week desperately seeking attention by any means possible. You may know how it feels to try to read the paper, talk on the phone, or check an email while a child begs for more attention: "Hey! Look! Look at this! Are you watching? Watch! Look! Hey! Hey! Look! Watch this! Watch me!" Or, perhaps you've had the remarkable experience of having a very young child command your attention by taking your face in both hands. When you have more than one child, the demands become more intense as they jockey, jostle, and compete for either your approval or simply your most extreme reaction. Grandparents really are the perfect fit for their grandchildren.

We would like to introduce you to one particular grandparent whose unique style of engagement with his grandchildren provides an interesting example of the power of warm, attentive, process-based observation. Place yourself near the front door of Bill's house and imagine him getting ready to take his 4-year-old grandson, Adam, out for a walk. They have put on light jackets, packed a snack, and are talking happily about visiting the park as the boy struggles to put on his shoes. Placing each shoe carefully in the right position on the floor, Adam begins to receive the benefit of Bill's noisy, attentive observation. "Alright ladies and gentlemen, what will Adam do now?" Adam looks up, massively delighted, not only by his grandfather's attention but also by the silly suggestion that an imaginary crowd is watching too. Bill continues, "First, he puts the shoes in the right place!" and as Adam squishes his foot inside the shoe without first loosening the Velcro strap he begins to whine with frustration. Bill remarks, "The foot doesn't fit in the shoe, ladies and gentlemen. What will Adam do now? I can't wait to see . . ." Hearing this, Adam looks up with a worried expression, and then smiles mischievously as he turns his attention quickly to the strap on the shoe. "I know! I know how to do it!" and before he even has time to say "Look!" his grandfather chimes in "This is very exciting, ladies and gentlemen. He decides to open the strap! And now his foot fits in! How did he know how to *do* that?" Throughout this process, Bill doesn't waver in his attention. While Mom and Dad are hurriedly checking phones and performing one last multitask, Grandpa Bill sits solidly beside Adam, seemingly immune to the hustle and bustle around him.

Some readers will think this story is marvelous, and some will question our sanity. How in the world can a classroom teacher carry on like a grandparent? No matter how possible it is to do "calm, doting observation" in your context, there are a couple of interesting things to notice from Bill's example. First, Bill did not lay one finger on Adam's shoe. While a busy parent might have reached down to flip open the strap, Bill didn't budge. With a level of response inhibition borne out of maturity, wisdom, and perhaps the fact that he didn't feel like bending down, Bill made space and time for Adam to do this little job on his own. In turn, Adam responded to this with excitement and determination, perhaps because Bill's approach conveyed confidence and interest in his ability. During their walk, Adam then continued to seek Bill's doting appreciation with demonstrations of walking backward, saving a worm trapped on the sidewalk, rolling down a hill, and fixing a swing that was turned inside out. Of course, it would have been much easier for Bill to simply rush in for a quick "save": When faced with a whiny, worried, or frustrated child, jumping in is often the simplest fix. If Bill had taken this approach, however, we wonder if Adam would have been quite as resourceful when his zipper got stuck 2 minutes later, or whether he would have quickly given up and called for help. In classrooms, while we can't wait for students to figure everything out on their own, you might like to have a go at inviting student initiative and creativity with comments like "I'm watching . . ." or "You're the expert . . ." or by loudly reflecting, "What will they do?" It's a balancing act. As a teacher you have to know when it makes sense to step in, and when you have the time and energy to support your class in more self-directed problem solving.

Second, Bill did not divide his attention at all. Watching him with his grandchildren was like watching someone meditate: Not only did he focus his awareness exclusively on Adam, but also he projected a clear and calm emotional state. We're not asking you to sit solidly and calmly beside each and every student all day long, but we wonder if you could take one more breath of observation before jumping to action. In that time, you might decide that instead of bending over to point out a mistake or wipe up a spill, you can simply invite your students to self-regulate and do some problem solving on their own. The more you do it, the more confident and skilled your students will become.

Generally, our discussions about observation and attention in school are grounded in the fact that they drive performance. It is also important to remember that dedicated attention is part of a loving and appreciative relationship, which is essential to both school success and children's ability to thrive. So, what should you do about those "attention-seeking" behaviors? While we don't advocate rudeness, we think it's always important to ask the question *why?* Why are children whining, acting out, and unwilling to take risks? What might happen if we treated those behaviors as a cry for more connection rather than attention? We know our readers teach in a range of varied contexts and that everyone does the best they can—we leave the story of Grandpa Bill in your hands. Even if it's just for one afternoon, we hope it inspires you to try an even slower, more attentive, more adoring approach with your class.

How to Observe Process, Strategy, and EFs: *Early Days*

The *big idea* here is that observation focused on process and strategy will help you to get to know students in a meaningful way. In this section, you'll learn more about how to do the following:

- Pause, when you feel like intervening, to slow down, take one extra breath, and tell your students that you are watching and "can't wait to see" what they do.
- Be a noisy and conspicuous observer.

Do you believe in love at first sight? Apparently 60% of people have experienced it, including Prince Harry who swears he felt it the first time he met Meghan Markle (Naumann, 2004). Psychologists believe it results from a subconscious search for positive emotions—we study strangers for loveable qualities and quickly form positive connections when we find them. Setting aside *romantic* love for a moment, we would like to suggest that you can achieve a similarly fast, positive, and fulfilling bond with students by paying special attention to their problem-solving strategies, coping methods, and spirit of resilience. During the early days of your work with any group of students, you can use observation to very quickly seek out and "fall in love" with all of the best things they have to offer.

As teachers, we spend a lot of time preparing for our first magic moments with students in September: We want to set a positive tone, earn trust, and establish a good working relationship. The one thing we can't control, however, is the children. They will arrive in all their glorious diversity, never failing to surprise us with their personalities, ideas, and energy. Our performance in such unpredictable circumstances relies on our ability to quickly find common ground and form a team, but this can be challenging. For example, imagine the tricky first day Laurie (author) once had in grade 2. Upon arrival, her students found a puzzle, a bin of materials for making bead bracelets, and a coloring page: calming activities that might have allowed everyone to socialize comfortably. Before long, however, Butter Dumpling the teddy bear hamster had charmed his way out of his cage. Overwhelmed by the excitement of it all, and acting totally out of character, he bit a student quite hard on the finger and drew blood. Another student, suffering from a rare condition, caught sight of this, experienced a sudden drop in blood pressure, turned green, and flopped dramatically onto the beanbag chair with fluttering eyelids. Simultaneously, a student entered the hallway to have a snack and accidentally pinwheeled cherry yogurt from a floppy plastic yogurt tube all over several other students, the lockers, the floor, and himself. This was not the type of morning Laurie had envisioned, and not really the kind of situation to make a person fall in love.

What a messy, stressful moment! Students urgently needed support both inside and outside of the classroom. As the only adult in the room, it was very tempting for Laurie to wade in, take over, and try to fix both problems at once. After sorting out the ailing students, she might have entered the hall and said, "Freeze! Listen carefully—I'm going to tell you exactly what to do . . . Kevin, go and get some paper towels. Maya, move those jackets . . ." She then might have given students 5 minutes' worth of specific instructions for exactly what to do to contain the mess. When Kevin returned from the washroom with paper towels, she might have said, "No, give them to me," and started working on the students' clothes herself while continuously reminding the student with his foot in a puddle of yogurt to stay absolutely and completely still. This sounds intense, but how many times have you been in a similarly stressful situation? Most experienced teachers have a few hair-raising stories.

What actually happened was a little different. Of course, the first step was to get first aid to the ailing students. Then, newly fascinated by the power of attentive observation, and perhaps because the whole situation was overwhelming and she needed help, Laurie took a step back. Instead of rolling up her sleeves and taking over, she rallied the problem-solving skills of her class using attentive and noisy observation. Standing in the doorway with a good view of both situations, she got everyone's attention and said, "There is a lot going on right now. Kathy is not feeling well, and Ryan's yogurt is all over the place in the hall. What will you do? How will you respond? I can't wait to stand right here and watch how you all manage!" There was some urgency in her voice and a genuine flush in her cheeks. This was a real situation and the students could tell. What she was really telling them was "I want you to show me your best qualities. This is a great opportunity. Show me your character, and let's start building a relationship based on respect!"

Many different things began to happen. First, and this is important to keep in mind, not all of the students responded well. In fact, out in the hall, one fellow took a few steps back, ran, and slid, surfer style, though the slick of yogurt; these were normal grade 2 kids, and they were eager to impress each other on the first day of school. However, when Laurie repeated, "Oh, this is complicated. What will you do?" certain students really seemed to wake up and take charge. Calista said, "Oh, I know! I'll get some paper towel. You move those books, okay Maya?" This inspired Ryan, who seemed happy to help Maya, which gave Arden and Stella the bright idea to scoop up the yogurt spill with a dustpan. By providing an opportunity for leadership among the students, Laurie made space for a positive, productive tone to catch on among the other students.

Standing back to observe this, a teacher might spend a moment with her eyes wide in surprise and her hand on her heart. She might mouth the word "Wow!" to her students and nod encouragingly. Not only did *Laurie* have a chance to experience and express positive feelings about her students, but also *they* had a chance to experience and express positive feelings about *each other.* Of course, there was a bit of unpredicted chaos—there always is. Instead of heavy control and frustration, however, there was a lot of back slapping, many thanks, and several expressions of satisfaction. And after it was all over, the story about the first day of school was that it was indeed a biiiit of a disaster, but also that it was fun and that the kids left feeling good. "You know what, Ms. Faith?" asked the yogurt surfer. "I think we are going to make a great team."

How to Observe Process, Strategy, and EFs: *Time Strapped*

The *big idea* here is that you can use EF-focused observation to help shift your students into gear. In this section, you'll learn more about how to do the following:

- Spend time to save time! Invest 5 minutes in an upfront 3 + 3 BSP conversation to clarify what strategic behaviors you'll be observing.
- Avoid getting overly involved in work that is your students' responsibility.

You barely have time to take attendance, never mind sitting back to observe. If you consider your situation "time strapped," we're willing to bet you're operating at full steam, using all four limbs, eyes and ears fully deployed, and perhaps occasionally also holding items in your mouth or tucking pens into your hairdo. Below, we'll paint a picture of what extreme time pressure can look like with the understanding that it happens to the best of us. In doing so, we'll describe why time-strapped teachers sometimes abandon the awesome power of attentive observation and suggest a way to get that power back.

Ask yourself: Does the prospect of slowing down a little, taking a breath, and adding *anything* to your already very tight 45-minute period drive you a little crazy? If so, you're not alone. Though we paddle into position in August, fresh from summer, amped with energy, and ready to rip, many teachers spend September to June surfing a wave of overwhelming pressure. As the students roll in and the work heats up, things steadily become more intense, and if we're not careful, we can wind up miles off course. In the madness, we may surrender all planning and proactive measures, and instead focus on navigating the never-ending torrent of immediate needs. For example, when your students struggle to manage the EF demands of their work and seem off track or unfocused, you may circle the room to remind each of them to "get going," feed next steps, or slowly remove parts of the assignment so they stand a chance of finishing on time. You may offer corrections, encouragements, and expressions of disappointment in a steady stream, responding again and again to the same problems. It feels as if, if we stop, a giant wave will surge, crash over our heads, and utterly swamp us.

With all of this going on, we know you have no time to waste and no extra pairs of hands to do more. We will not recommend you layer something else on top, but rather that you put your foot down, clear 5 minutes, and know that we fully support you in *stopping the insanity.* You can safely dismount the wild ride for a moment, take a breath, get steady, and paddle into a much tamer and more productive current.

How? We suggest that you clear 5 sweet little minutes to do a 3 + 3 BSP (see Chapter 3).[1] After providing instructions for the day's work, grab a marker and urge your class, "Three things that

---

[1] Remember, the BSP was introduced in Chapter 3. It is a semistructured teaching protocol. Essentially, it asks teachers to gather students to discuss "What are your/our barriers to this work?" and then "What strategies can we use to be more successful?"

will stand in our way and three strategies! Go!" Don't let the conversation go longer than 5 minutes. In fact, your discussion might include some finger snapping or a timer. You may say, "Come on, everyone, what will it be? This is supposed to be a quick conversation. Who has an idea?" Then, when you're finished, tell your students you'll be watching to see them using the strategies discussed: "I'm watching. Let's see how many people use the tricks we've talked about." This is the moment you take back some control and switch from surfer to spectator. You should observe heavily, attentively, conspicuously, and without lifting a finger, knowing each student has a small handful of practical strategies to try right away.

Imagine if, with this 5-minute conversation at the beginning of class, you could drastically improve your students' ability to manage. What if the four students who might otherwise have done nothing actually get started, and what if the rest of the students do roughly twice as much as they would have otherwise? If your 5-minute investment makes the remaining 40 minutes twice as effective, you've reclaimed 20 minutes! For example, let's say you have just had a BSP conversation regarding your fifth graders' problem-solving work in math stations. During the BSP, everyone agreed that emotional control and goal-directed persistence would be challenged as they attempted to share materials and not give up on the independent activities too quickly. The strategies they created were to "rock–paper–scissors" for first choice of materials upon arrival at each station and then to read instructions out loud twice before deciding the activity was too confusing. After the teacher says, "Okay. Go! We only have 30 minutes left. I'm watching to see you use these specific strategies," the students will know exactly what to do. The teacher's main priority will be, not to wade in and help 30 students at once, but to slow down, stand back, and appreciate what they are doing on their own. We're not predicting miracles—new challenges may benefit from another 5-minute BSP the following day—but as the students head back to their desks to get started, they'll know exactly which three achievable behaviors you're looking for.

How can you afford the time? First, we would like to suggest that nothing you do as a teacher could waste more time than an unfocused group of students. They win hands down. It doesn't matter that you're behind with the science project, that the speeches are not quite ready for assembly, or that the math test is *this Friday*. For the most part, your students will proceed as usual—they will miss your instructions, get into disagreements, stress over every detail, and lose their materials. As far as time-wasting goes, your indulgence of 5 minutes to get your students on track is a drop in the ocean. If it can move the needle on their ability to use strategies that will support their EFs, it will provide everyone with a smoother and more successful experience and will definitely be worth the time.

How to Observe Process, Strategy, and EFs: *Highly Structured*

The big idea here is that you can observe students' use of EFs, process, and strategy in structured ways throughout your day. In this section, you'll learn more about how to do the following:

- Use a structured observational technique such as a running record, an anecdotal record, or event sampling to spend more time gathering data before jumping to conclusions.

- Establish an "observation post" or posture and use it regularly as a cue that you are observing.

Do you remember when iPhone launched "live" photos? Having spent a day photographing loved ones, you might recall later discovering that your device had captured not simply one moment but also the two fascinating seconds before and after. What a difference this made! For example, you could see that your sister's smile came after a glance at her dog and was followed by an eye roll, or that your child drank hot chocolate just after a little shove from his brother and just before the liquid sloshed onto his shirt. The richness of these 3-second videos reminds us that an awful lot of information can be captured in a few extra seconds. Similarly, stretching classroom observation just a little allows us to stitch together rich contexts, motivations, and emotions. It lets us connect the dots on adaptive student behavior that may otherwise seem random. And, over time, it creates a welcoming stage on which students can perform such feats. How long does your attention rest on any one student before your memory "clicks" and you move on? Let's talk about two approaches to stretch and structure your observation.

First, let's discuss a handful of highly structured approaches that might help you unravel the mystery of an unusually tricky student. These will be useful when you're feeling out of ideas and patience, or temped to say, "I know exactly what's going on with that kid" or "I've seen this kind of thing a thousand times before." When you hear yourself making comments like these, ask yourself if your stance of *frustrated already knowing* may actually be sucking the life out of your ability to observe. Are you watching for one second before jumping to conclusions? Maybe two if you're feeling generous? In these situations, your ability to observe may be crushed under the massive weight of your experience and what you think you already know. Below, we will share a few techniques to help you revive your observation and continue learning. They will function to, momentarily, pause your instinct to interpret and instead encourage you to linger a while in a more deliberate process of gathering information. Taking a closer look at a frustrating student may provide insight on underlying EF challenges or compensatory strategies, increase your understanding and compassion, and expand your ability to provide timely and tailored support.

Running Records

You may be familiar with running records as a mode of reading assessment, but they can also be used to objectively observe and understand student *behavior*. To make a behavioral running record, choose a target student, decide how long your observation will be, and then begin making notes about what you see the student doing. You should pay attention to the students' physical movements, their social interactions, their facial expressions, and the activities they seem to be attending to. This won't be easy. Your mind will be in "efficiency" mode, and you may feel tempted to make a quick assessment about what is happening. For example, in the first moments of your observation of a student who never seems to complete any work, you may see the student wandering around the room and assume they aren't interested in the activity. Or you might assume the work you've assigned is too hard. Sticking to a mostly descriptive running record of what you see the student doing before drawing too many conclusions, however, may reveal surprising information. Looking back over your notes later, you may discover that the student was much more confused about the basic instructions for the assignment than you realized. As an EF-literate teacher, you may begin to suspect that specific EF challenges are at play. Look at our example in Figure 4.1. As Katrina (the teacher) documented C.J.'s behavior, she began to notice his frustration, his confusion, and a seeming desire to participate. Could C.J. be experiencing a working memory or

Running Record		
Student name(s): *C.J.*		
Age: *13*		
Location: *Rose School homeroom classroom*		
Date and Time: *Monday, October 5, 2020, 10:45–10:55*		
Observer: *Katrina*		
Type of Development Observed: *C.J. rarely hands in classroom assignments.*		
Event	**Time**	**Notes or Comments**
Lags behind as group moves to back table. Group starts work without him.	*10:45*	*Didn't notice the transition? Attention?*
Arrives at table and looks frustrated. Rolls eyes at (other student). Listens to conversation briefly and then leaves to find pencil.	*10:47*	*Doesn't seem to know what to do. Not sure if he caught the instructions.*
Returns to group for instruction. Pokes (other student) with pencil. Asks, "What are we supposed to do?"	*10:48*	*May need more reiteration of instructions before starting his work.*
Gets up and asks to go to the washroom.	*10:49*	*Avoidance. Looks embarrassed.*
Returns, sits at own desk, and stares at workbook; sighs loudly.	*10:55*	*Did he manage to get enough information to start? Is it the actual starting?*
Significant Points	**Next Steps**	
C.J. is quite skilled at avoidance and is trying a number of approaches to not start the task. C.J. is starting to act out in frustration. C.J. wants to participate. C.J. is struggling to pay attention.	*Ask C.J. if he's having a hard time understanding instructions? Should I slow down with instructions? Would writing down the instructions help?* *Would repeating the instructions be helpful?*	

FIGURE 4.1. How a teacher might fill in a running record.

attention challenge while trying to capture the details of classroom instructions? These are the kinds of significant points and targeted next steps you may arrive at when you review the text you have created, either alone or with a colleague.

The period of time over which this observation is conducted will depend on the resources you have available and the extent of the problem you're attempting to understand. In only 5 to 10 minutes, you may be surprised at the amount of information you can gather. In truth, we rarely slow down enough to watch individuals for even this length of time. Or you may decide to conduct a few 5-minute observations to really understand what is going on. On the other hand, if you have an especially tricky student and you feel you are starting to hit a wall, you may want to consider finding time for a longer observation and running record. By recruiting the support of a colleague or administrator, you can gather a 20- to 40-minute running record and gain even deeper insight. While this will require some organization and planning, it may completely transform your ability to understand and respond to a struggling student. It may be one last thing to try before referring this student for a more resource-intensive intervention (such as an educational assistant or other specialist). The information you gather will be useful in either case. See Figure 4.1 for a simple example of the kinds of comments to include in a short running record and Figure 4.2 for a clean copy to use in your classroom.

Anecdotal Records

Collect written observations about a specific child. You don't need to follow a schedule; when something happens that you think is interesting, simply write the date and jot down a few key words, a quote, or the essence of the situation. You may wish to share the recording process among several teachers, and you may wish to focus your attention on certain EFs or other growth areas that are specified in an IEP. Much like with your running record, you should focus on gathering objective and descriptive information that can be analyzed later. Then you can work with a colleague or on your own to extract significant points and plan appropriate next steps from your anecdotal record.

Event Sampling

Once you start to notice a pattern of behavior, you may wish to confirm it with event sampling. Using this method, you simply keep a tally of how often the target behavior occurs over time. It is especially useful to work with a colleague who can observe a specific student during certain lessons or periods of the day while you are engaged with other students. You may, for example, like to compare the number of times a behavior occurs during a math lesson versus during a writing lesson. Keeping track of the time and place during which the event sampling occurred is essential.

We realize the abovementioned approaches require an added investment of time and planning. A slightly less involved method of adding structure to your observation is to adopt a cueing system. Each time you plan to observe how students are managing EFs or use strategy, you can retreat to the same "observation post," hold a notepad, or assume an over-the-top "I'm watching" gesture. Will you lean on the same bookcase, retreat to your desk, or just stand where you are? Is your gesture one of hands on hips? Or hand to chin? Or is it a slow, meaningful putting on of glasses? Routine times of the day, such as transitions or daily bell work, provide a good opportunity to get started with observation cueing. The first few times you try it, you might nudge students with a simple, "I'm watching. I want to see what you do," or "I'm watching how you manage this." On your first attempt, you may hear a defiant "I don't care!" or a groan or two. Over time, however, if you force your attention toward the adaptive, clever, creative, and positive actions taking place, and acknowledge them with little smiles, nods, eyebrow lifts, and chuckles, most students won't be able to resist the opportunity to shine. You may hear them comment, "Guys! She's watching!" as they jump to action. Over time, this bit of theater will set a familiar stage for students, and you can expand your system into less routine times of the day, such as math problem solving, creative writing, or even times when you are out of the classroom, such as field trips. Of course, this approach pairs beautifully with feedback, and we will cover this topic extensively in Chapter 6. In a pinch, all the follow-up you need is to say, "I always learn something interesting when I watch you work." You may realize that, in sometimes big and sometimes small ways, this comment tends to be true.

Running Record		
Student name(s):		
Age:		
Location:		
Date and Time:		
Observer:		
Type of Development Observed:		
Event	**Time**	**Notes or Comments**
Significant Points	**Next Steps**	

FIGURE 4.2. A blank running record.

How to Observe Process, Strategy, and EFs:
Organic and Free Flowing

The big idea here is that there are easy ways to make casual observations more effective. In this section, you'll learn more about how to do the following:

- Use a tracking tool such as a class list or seating chart to jot your daily observations.
- Notice who you tend to observe and who sometimes falls under your radar. Adjust and pay more attention to the students in your blind spot.

Picture the most organic and free-flowing woman of all: *Jane Goodall.* Jane eschewed more formal research methods in favor of long, slow observation, so she had to spend a lot of time camped out in the dry, prickly grass of the Gombe National Park in Tanzania. Quietly watching, she collected clipboards full of notes about a family of chimpanzees. She watched "Fifi" and "David Greybeard," among others, for hours, days, months, and even years, trying to understand their behavior. In your more free-flowing and organic moments, or perhaps when your students are acting like primates, you might consider adopting her approach. By taking the time to study and record what she saw, Jane began to appreciate qualities in her subjects that you, in your classroom, might understand more fully in your students: unique personalities and emotions, as well as adaptive approaches to solving problems.

Following the publication of one of her books, Jane was criticized for plagiarism. "I don't think anybody who knows me would accuse me of deliberate plagiarism," she responded, and explained that disorganized note taking was to blame (Taylor, 2014). In her enthusiasm, Jane had not made careful-enough records of *who did what* as she conducted research for her books. She was so immersed in her learning that these details escaped her—organic and free flowing indeed! This type of problem may be the hallmark of a teacher who is deeply and organically involved with students on a daily basis, so let's consider a few ways to tame and organize the process of observational note making. Figure 4.3 provides three ideas from least to most restrictive to organize your collection of anecdotal observations. This is not rocket science, but if you're not a kindergarten teacher, you may not be familiar with approaches like these.

The first image in Figure 4.3 is a class seating chart. This tool can be rendered in quick-and-dirty black marker as often as your seating arrangement changes. We recommend you copy yourself a big pile on convenient-sized paper, making the image large enough to jot notes inside each student "desk." Obviously, this approach is challenging if you are using a flexible seating plan. Regardless, if you like the idea of writing observations in boxes, there are many options. Some teachers create a template like this, but cluster the squares into other useful categories, including reading group, project group, or in groups that represent different levels of support required. As notes are added throughout the day, this tool provides a good visual map of where a teacher's attention has been paid. Over several days, interesting patterns may emerge and you might, for example, notice that you rarely attend to the students in the back row.

The second image in Figure 4.3 is a wonderfully adaptive and simple tool. When expanded, it fits onto a regular notebook-sized page. Notice that, on this version, the first five students are shaded. This can support your ability to quickly scan and find a student on the page, especially if you cluster students by group. If your class is larger than about 24 students, you might have to break this chart across two pages or make smaller charts for observing subgroups of your class on different days. Whatever you choose, this tool starts out empty each morning except for the student

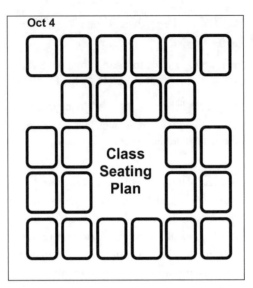

Date: *Oct 4*	SR	CS	MI	JM	IR	KI	RR	SL	RI	PI
Sketching math problem	✓		✓		✓		✓			
Hands behind back in line				✓						
"Let's try both" in groupwork				✓	✓					
Doing a 5-sec exhale	✓			✓						
Working at the quiet desk							✓			
...									✓	

Date: *Oct 4*	Sketching math problem	Hands behind back in line	"Lets' try both" in groupwork	...
Josh	✓✓ with partner		✓✓✓	
Rosa		✓✓	needs help with this	
Amara	✓	struggling	✓	
Ebo	✓	✓	✓	
Lemar			✓	

FIGURE 4.3. Three different daily strategy trackers. The class seating plan would be expanded to full page, so observations could be written inside seats. The "handwritten" contents of these forms are different every day, added as teachers observe unique strategy use and add it to their tracker. Dotted lines indicate the form continues.

initials across the top. As the day progresses and you notice a student using a strategy, you can jot it in the list on the left and check off which student you observed using it. This will provide the perfect opportunity to look around the room to see if other students are using that strategy. Or, if possible, you can remark upon the strategy you have observed so that other students will consider using it. For example, you might say, "Oh, Sam is sketching the math problem. I'm going to jot that on my strategy list." Following this comment, you may notice that Maya, Michael, and Reyhan quickly attempt the strategy as well. As you check off these names on the list, you might remark, "Four students are using the sketching strategy," which will probably encourage a few more. The beauty of this list is that it is open-ended. You can add as many strategies as you see fit throughout the day.

The third image in Figure 4.3 may be more suitable for larger classes. Students' names run from top to bottom, so more of them can fit on a page. This limits the strategies you notice to only four or five, however, as they must fit across the top of the page. This format allows for larger checkboxes that can accommodate short written notes, or multiple checks to indicate the number of times any one strategy was observed. Because this form allows you to focus on a few specific strategies, it might be suitable after a BSP (Chapter 3) conversation has been conducted and specific strategies have been agreed on. Or it can be useful for observing one specific subject, such as during a math class or when writing in a journal, at which time students may naturally tend toward using a handful of key strategies.

The great thing about collecting anecdotal notes about humans is that we can also feed them back as a source of information about how to optimize performance. The data collected on all three of these forms would support a great closing reflection at the end of a session of work, allowing a teacher to provide rich overall feedback. We might say, for example, "Would you like to know the most popular strategy of the day?" or "I observed someone using a strategy I have never seen before. Do you want to know what it is?" or "On the way out to recess, I will show you my notes and you can see how strategic you were today." Imagine if Dr. Goodall could have done this for the chimps: "Fifi, you're using the longer stick, and you seem to be getting twice as many ants out of the anthill!" How might Fifi have responded, and what would David Greybeard think? Both chimps would probably have grunted, looked around nonchalantly, and then taken off into the trees in search of a longer stick. There really are so many parallels to our human context.

How to Observe Process, Strategy, and EFs: *Working with a "Stressed" Class*

The big idea here is that you can really improve the way observation feels to a stressed student. In this section, you'll learn more about how to do the following:

- "Prime" your students with a quick, positive comment to establish the fact that you're ready to observe and appreciate the very best in them.
- Share your EF literacy with your colleagues so your students are observed through a more consistent lens.

Your presence, attention, and observation may be very difficult for a stressed student. For myriad reasons, they may jump to the conclusion that you don't like them, won't make them feel good about themselves, or aren't interested in helping them. We may reflect, "I haven't even said a word and this student has already shut down" or "She took one look at me and decided I was the enemy." When the slightest look triggers negativity, it can be tempting to give up, avoid engaging, or take it personally. In this section we will address the issue of not only observing stressed students but also, more broadly, how to simply *be* with these students in a way that is comfortable, respectful, and effective. In preparing this advice, we draw from our knowledge of EF and self-regulated learning, the wisdom of practicing teachers and principals, and also from a few practices advocated by trauma-sensitive educators.[2] We'll make two very specific recommendations, both of which relate to your role as an EF-literate teacher who sees and appreciates process. Prepare yourself for a slightly lengthy explanation of each; observation is subtle, and the practical shifts we are proposing are a little counterintuitive. These fairly simple ideas require some background.

First, we suggest that when you head into the orbit of a stressed student, either to observe or engage, you should begin by "priming the pump." If you know how old-fashioned hand pumps work, feel free to skip the rest of this paragraph. For others, the following mini-lesson will get you up to speed. Basically, there is a handle on the outside of the pump, and inside there are pistons and valves that pull water up through a line from the ground. The important thing about these pumps is that in order to pull water up, the piston and valve chamber as well as the line to the ground need to be filled with water. If it's dry, the suction you create by pumping has nothing to grab onto. You can work the handle as fast as you like, for as long as you like, and all you'll get is a sore arm. To fix this, you need to "prime" the pump by pouring water into the top until the system is brimming and full.

Similarly, many of our students arrive primed and ready to connect and learn. They are topped up with positive past experiences at school, solid learning skills, healthy home lives, and a sense of confidence. When we approach these students with a smile, a connection can easily be made and only a slight effort is needed to get their positive participation flowing. Other students, however, arrive in our classrooms quite empty and hollow, and instead of being ready to connect and learn, they may be preoccupied by fear and distrust. These are the students who need to be filled up before we try to tap into their potential as learners.

How to best "prime" these students? You should assume that any message, expression, or gesture that is not overtly positive may be received as a negative. Experts in trauma-informed practices suggest that stressed students require ongoing and deliberate support to feel connected, protected, and respected (Hummer, Dollard, Robst, & Armstrong, 2010). As EF-literate teachers, therefore, we are just what the doctor ordered. Our challenge lies in quickly establishing the fact that we are ready to observe and appreciate the best in them, that we understand and appreciate the diverse ways each student manages, copes, and solves problems. Table 4.1 includes several types of priming comments that may help your students understand how you're "seeing" them. Don't delay: Deliver these messages as soon as your students venture round the schoolyard gate or appear in your classroom doorway. Yes, they *do* seem a little heavy handed and obvious. They might feel conspicuous and clunky the first time you try them, but as with many new approaches, we suggest you commit to using them 10 times before deciding they don't work. For children who

---

[2] Our insight on trauma-informed classrooms owes a lot to the work of the Trauma and Learning Policy Initiative at *http://traumasensitiveschools.org*.

TABLE 4.1. What to Say to "Prime" Stressed Students for Learning

After saying "hello," these kinds of statements meet student needs for . . .			
Connection	Protection/safety	Respect	Skill/competence
I'm so glad you're here. I missed you yesterday.	We have everything we need today.	We really needed your perspective yesterday. Glad you're back.	You're going to like our topic today. I bet you'll be good at it.
I always feel happy when I see you.	Here you are. My team! My people!	I was thinking about what you said yesterday.	I was thinking of you when I wrote today's plans. I can't wait to see what you do.
It is really not the same without you.	We are all going to take care of each other today.	I was trying to use your strategy this morning.	We're doing X today. Mr. Y said it's totally your thing.
You're so important to me. I'm glad you're here.	We're all safe here.	Thank goodness you're here. Nobody else knows your trick for . . .	We're starting a new topic. Not naming any names, but I suspect a few of you are going to really excel.
You're just in time! It was feeling *wrong* without you here.	It's going to be a great day in our cozy classroom.	You figure things out in a way I would never have thought of.	
Ms. X was telling me how much she liked what you did yesterday!	We're all going to support you today.	I really like the way you think about things. I really like watching you work!	I really like to watch you problem-solve.
I'm so glad you're here. I need your help!	We don't have to do this perfectly. I'm interested in seeing how you explore and problem-solve.		

automatically assume the worst, these messages will help to replace negative thoughts, begin to fill an achy void, and make it more likely for connection and learning to take place.

Our second piece of advice is to let go of the idea that you will be *the* turnaround teacher. Often, the more educators discover about the stress and disparity among their learners, the more single minded they are in their desire to help. Unfortunately, it often takes years of slow and steady nurturing and the attention of a number of teachers before any impact is made on a stressed student. We make this suggestion not only to set you on a realistic course and help you prevent burnout but also because it may cause you to take actions that will be more effective.

In a practical sense, this might mean that you proceed quite differently. For example, consider the approach used by a community of EF-literate teachers at King Albert School.[3] Their EF work started in a typical way: A handful of really keen teachers began teaching children about EFs, talking to them about barriers and strategies, and observing their performance through an EF lens. They felt gratified by their work; the approach felt appropriate, fair, efficient, and most of their students were responding in positive ways. At this point, they might have simply closed their doors and basked in this feeling of accomplishment and satisfaction. They noticed, however, that their students sometimes needed support outside of the classroom. They recalled students' emotional outbursts in the hallway, inflexibility in the playground, and inattention while under the supervision of a gym teacher.

With the support of a wise principal, a small group of interested teachers designed a feasible

[3] Dean Burk, Victoria Young, and Christine Alldred teach at King Albert School in Lindsay, Ontario, Canada. Used with permission.

strategy to build a basic level of EF literacy among all students *and staff.* They wanted, at the very least, for their students to feel as though they were being observed and understood through a similar lens throughout their school day. Their first move was to host monthly assemblies at which the principal himself read and discussed EF-oriented storybooks and presented recognition awards to children demonstrating growth in strategy use. They also created a schoolwide behavior management approach. Using several centrally located rings of small, laminated cards with the names of 11 EFs and their definitions (like a key ring), any staff member supervising a common space like the yard, the hallway, or the main office could support a student in crisis. Without requiring too much expertise, the EF cards could simply be presented to a stressed-out student. The child could then point to the EF they were struggling with, effectively translating their experience for the adults (and sometimes students) present. The teachers told us that using these EF cards helped to pivot the situation toward a more tangible, practical focus.

In this way, these teachers built a community of understanding observers and supporters for their students. Using a handful of staff meetings, a few hallway chats, and a shared commitment to serving their stressed students, they found a way to extend their program across their whole school staff. Their ideas may need some adjustment to suit your context, but their example reminds us of what can be done when we put our heads together. There is always a way to support the learning and growth of a team of colleagues.

Working with stressed students is a challenge, but we suspect you're the type of teacher that even the toughest students often grow to love. In fact, due to your dedication and hard work, your students may start to panic at the end of the year when they think about leaving you. While this sure is flattering, we'd like to suggest that you could aim even higher. The greatest gift you can give your stressed students is not one remarkable year but the continuity of a number of years nestled within a whole community that truly sees and respects them.

CHAPTER 5

How EF Literacy
Can Improve Feedback

HOW WE TYPICALLY GIVE FEEDBACK

Teachers talk with students all day. By 4:30, or 6:30, or whenever staff meetings, homework club, and play practice are over, we may be a little dehydrated and feel as if our *lungs are tired*. We may savor a perfectly quiet trip home, dive straight into sweatpants, and truly appreciate a few peaceful moments before the evening's activities begin. And while the armchair teaching experts at home think our days would be a breeze if we "just let the kids do silent reading!" the fact is that all of that talking is absolutely necessary. Giving effective feedback is the big kahuna of high-yield classroom practices. In a well-respected meta-analysis of more than 100 factors influencing achievement at school, effective feedback earned a top five ranking, right alongside direct instruction and students' prior cognitive ability (Hattie & Timperley, 2007). It is for this reason that understanding and refining feedback is such a central goal of this book. You will see that by becoming EF literate (Chapters 1 and 2), learning to use the BSP (Chapter 3), and learning to observe process (Chapter 4), you have vastly expanded the quality of feedback you are able to give. This feedback will allow students to learn about the obstacles they face and the most effective strategies to use, and to further develop their EF.

In this chapter, we will discuss the powerful psychological forces at work within your day-to-day feedback approaches. This will be a realistic and practical discussion that acknowledges your need for external motivation and short-term control, and suggests fresh approaches for longer-term, intrinsic motivation. To be clear, this chapter's discussion of feedback will handle the *formative* verbal and written exchanges that occur during learning to help steer and improve performance, leaving the *summative* assessment conducted at the end of a task for Chapter 6.

How do classroom teachers tend to give feedback? This is a tricky question to answer. We are isolated from the daily practices of our colleagues by closed classroom doors, and we tend to mis-estimate our own habits. On top of that, researchers are rarely welcomed to study teachers' enacted classroom approaches because their presence seems so evaluative. Turns out, few teachers are excited to have a random person perched in the corner, writing down everything they do. Anecdotally, we all know that feedback comes in many forms. Sometimes we conduct long follow-ups with individual students, and sometimes we roar though lineups with quick "Yup! Good! Keep going! Check the second paragraph!" encouragements. Occasionally, we sharply correct, express displeasure, or lavish students with praise. Or have you ever seen a teacher who can communicate almost anything by varying the speed, pitch, and tone of the word "shhh"? Some teachers achieve "written" feedback through several checks on a rubric, while others compose a paragraph of personal and thoughtful comments. These may represent different teachers and different classrooms, but more likely they describe the various feedback practices that each of us conduct every day; each has its place within a dynamic and effective approach.

Over the years, researchers have been able to determine a few general feedback types. One very clear and straightforward contribution is Tunstall and Gipps's (1996) "spectrum" of feedback (see Table 5.1). While this is from an older study, we feel the typology remains the best of its kind. After making detailed observations of primary-aged classrooms, Tunstall and Gipps proposed four distinct types of feedback teachers gave when talking to students about their work and learning. See if these types sound familiar: Feedback that punishes or rewards they call Type 1, feedback that communicates a teacher's feelings in the form of judgment they called Type 2, feedback that is corrective or notices and names a student's process they called Type 3, and feedback involving a back-and-forth discussion of specific aspects of process they called Type 4. As you can imagine, we are most intrigued by Types 3 and 4, because these are the types in which organization, time management, or other EF processes can be noticed and discussed. We are also grateful to have clear, straightforward categories for feedback that is punishing/rewarding or judging (Types 1 and 2) because these types are used often and have a variety of specific advantages and disadvantages.

As Tunstall and Gipps sorted through their observations, they realized that their four types could be further grouped into that which was *evaluative* or *descriptive*. This was probably an exciting moment, because much is known about the markedly different impacts of evaluative and descriptive feedback; look in the final column of Table 5.1 for a breakdown of the differences. Basically, research tells us that after our *evaluative* comments, students may do exactly what we want them to do but may also wind up feeling guarded, nervous, or eager to avoid mistakes in the future. While this may sound okay, they may also begin to suspect we are simply watching for winners and losers, and they may respond by hiding errors, faking expertise, and avoiding things that are hard. Even if we have made a positive judgment about their performance, they may respond by fearfully guarding and protecting this status, afraid to take any risk that might endanger it. This is the basis of extrinsic motivation, which is powerful and necessary but seriously limited.

Meanwhile, our *descriptive* messages may cause students to feel competent, independent, and clear about what is expected. In response, they may be keen to engage in more of the thinking, strategy, and process that we noticed, named, and wanted to discuss. Descriptive feedback may begin to convince them that their struggling, striving, strategies, and yes, mistakes too, are not only acceptable but also fascinating and important parts of their learning. This is the basis of intrinsic motivation, which is truly fulfilling and causes students to persist longer and conquer more challenges than those who are only extrinsically motivated (Pintrich & Garcia, 1991). The important thing to remember is that there is no such thing as throwaway feedback. For better or for worse, the words we say to children have slow and steady effects that build up over time.

TABLE 5.1. A Typology of Feedback According to Tunstall and Gipps

	Description	Examples	Impact
Evaluative			
Type A: *Rewarding and punishing*	Simple rewards and punishments.	Stickers, treats, or special privileges and recognition. Or exclusion, removal of privileges, destruction of work, or ignoring.	Shapes performance quickly. Students focus on doing better than others or appearing to succeed with little effort. Students have greater failure avoidance and feel embarrassed when things aren't easy for them.
Type B: *Judging*	Expressions of general approval or disapproval.	Body language, voice modulations, or comparisons or comments that express negative/ positive feelings or disapproval/ approval.	
Descriptive			
Type C: *Noticing and naming, correcting*	Factual observations from teacher to student about the small steps evident in students' work, or the small steps necessary to improve specific work.	Noticing and naming process steps. Providing models of success or giving specific practice. Naming errors in work or restating criteria. Information flows from teacher to student.	Shapes performance slowly. Students focus on learning, mastering, and demonstrating a willingness to try. Students have greater failure tolerance and are more willing to expend effort, use strategy, and work through a process.
Type D: *Discussing*	Reflective and strategic conversations among teacher and learners about what has to be and will be done on work. Often facilitated with groups of students.	Discussing processes, strategies, challenges, or ways to improve. Often conducted in group settings with teacher taking role of facilitator.	

Note. This table summarizes the literature review and original research presented by Tunstall and Gipps (1996) in their article "Teacher Feedback to Young Children in Formative Assessment: A Typology." The **bolded categories** "rewarding and punishing," "judging," etc., were added to provide a more straightforward reference point for teachers. Used with permission.

To be clear, nobody gives only evaluative or only descriptive feedback. In fact, we often mix several types together in one utterance, the flavors blending like a fine wine. So, when you say, "Great job, Group 2. So smart! You made a chart in the margin. Look at your punctuation in the second paragraph," why not imagine a sophisticated feedback "sommelier" standing in your classroom, interpreting the individual components:

"Now *this* feedback has a typical balance of evaluative [Great job. So smart!] and descriptive [You made a chart in the margin. Look at your punctuation in the second paragraph]. Notice it opens with a rather heavy, toasty note of judgment [So smart!] but finishes with a bright, crisp dash of notice and name [You made a chart in the margin] and corrective [Look at your punctuation in the second paragraph]."

Or imagine you said, "Naz, let's sit down and talk about your next steps. I have no idea what you've been doing, but that can go straight in the bin." The sommelier might swirl, sip, and comment:

"Now this feedback is very fruit forward. It opens with a structured, citrusy note of descriptive discussion [Let's sit down and talk about your next steps], which is then almost overwhelmed by a rather gritty and acidic pop of evaluative punishing [Your work can go in the bin]."

Think of the ways your own feedback includes a blend of different effects. Some of our comments will quickly shape students' performance and bring them in line with our rules and expectations, while others will stimulate deep feelings of satisfaction and engagement. While this is normal, it's important to remember that the benefits from our descriptive comments can be overpowered if combined with too many of the evaluative ones (Bennett & Kell, 1989). Thus, while our feedback habits are often well aged and stable—comfortable habits that work to keep our classrooms running smoothly—it's worth questioning whether they achieve quite the most effective balance of immediate satisfaction and aftertaste.

DESCRIPTIVE FEEDBACK, GROWTH MINDSET, AND THE PROBLEM WITH "EFFORT"

If Table 5.1 seems familiar, it's because it relates to a field of motivation research also referred to by Carol Dweck in her book *Mindset* (2006). In it, she considered all of the studies on descriptive and evaluative feedback, both hers and others, and coined a couple of useful buzzwords to capture the frame of mind resulting from each: a "growth mindset" and a "fixed mindset." Most teachers discovered Dweck and the idea of growth mindset though her TED Talks, but if you haven't already, we highly recommend actually reading her book. Dweck earned her PhD in 1972 and has continued to think about motivation ever since. She has a knack for explaining things simply and brings a giant range of life experience and insight to the topic; her examples will take you deeper into the theory than you thought possible. In fact, you may find yourself reading a page, destroying it with dog-ears and margin scribbling, and then requiring several moments of wide-eyed contemplation. It's a tasty, inspiring, game-changing book.

Something very interesting occurred, however, as teachers began to read and interpret Dweck's message. She initially referred a lot to "effort," talking about how commenting on this could support a growth mindset. So, she told teachers, don't dwell on students' fixed qualities like intelligence; highlight their effort instead. Before long, however, she realized this had become a problem and began to correct the pesky phenomenon of "false growth mindset." Turns out many people wound up trying to support a growth mindset in children by simply encouraging them to try harder; Dweck's "effort" was assumed to mean something more like *intensity*. But have you ever struggled to do something really challenging, such as, say, learning to drive a standard transmission car or taking care of a newborn baby, and had someone suggest you ought to just try harder? In both cases, like many of our students, you were probably white knuckled with effort and intensity already. What you might actually have appreciated was some clear, specific feedback on effective strategies: "You wrapped the baby snugly and she seemed to calm down," or "The engine is revving high—now is the time to shift to second gear." Turns out, being a "Yet! Yet! Yet!" cheerleader isn't very effective when the only prescription is more effort. Instead, Dweck clarified that our feedback should focus on specific elements of process so students can connect their strategies to their outcomes. This is welcome news to EF-literate teachers, who are already so tuned in to and ready to comment on the components of process. Carol Dweck, you had us at hello.

To simplify this idea of focusing more on strategy than effort, think of a child trying to push a very heavy rock. While one growth mindset teacher might stand beside the child chanting encouragements, with reminders to exert more effort, another might encourage the child to stop for a moment. This second teacher might say, "Let's consider what might be standing in your way," and guide the child in a little "walk" around the problem. On this walk around the rock, the student and teacher together might notice that several smaller stones were resting in the way of the larger one. In the same way, a classroom teacher might engage a student in a discussion about helpful strategies for writing an essay or completing math problems and find that a little trick (such as drawing a picture, making a list, or clarifying instructions) was all that was necessary to accomplish the primary task. Thus, the way to move the larger stone was not with more sweaty intensity, or "effort," but with a strategic approach whereby obstacles were identified and removed. Perhaps you'll be dazzled by Laurie's Sharpie rendering of this difference in Figure 5.1.

Day by day, interaction by interaction, our feedback nudges students toward these different mindsets. Our specific comments and conversations about aspects of strategy may leave our students feeling growth oriented, seeking out larger and larger rocks to push, confident that they can manage almost any challenge as long as they identify and remove obstacles. Meanwhile, evaluative comments may support fixed mindsets, causing students to focus more on how we will rank their ability and judge their finished products. They may find a way to avoid pushing the first rock, and then head off in search of smaller and less daunting challenges at which they are sure to succeed. For these students, classroom opportunities to get better, learn, or improve may only be embarrassing reminders of their inadequacy. This may affect them in one class or subject more than others and can be either triggered or soothed by daily experiences.

Just one of the treats in *Mindset* is Dweck's (2006) comparison of a more "growth"-oriented mindset to the "exuberant" learning of babies:

> Infants stretch their skills daily. Not just ordinary skills, but the most difficult tasks of a lifetime, like learning to walk and talk. They never decide it's too hard or not worth the effort. Babies don't worry about making mistakes or humiliating themselves. They walk, they fall, they get up. They just barge forward. (p. 16)

Can you imagine a baby with a fixed mindset? Picture a 9-month-old utterly embarrassed by his inability to put a spoonful of mashed bananas in his mouth. He might refuse spoons permanently and commit instead to a lifelong diet of Cheerio handfuls, satisfied that anyone observing his eat-

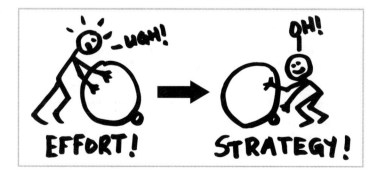

FIGURE 5.1. A sketch illustrating the change from focusing on effort to focusing on strategy.

ing would always find him *perfectly* skilled. How much more successful would our students be if they greeted challenge with an infant's can-do exuberance, totally at peace with their messy process steps, knowing their efforts were completely typical, important, and valued by others?

You may be realizing that a decent-sized portion of your daily feedback tends to be evaluative. You may also notice that it works pretty well, in terms of disciplining and controlling student performance. What's more, your class may seem a little addicted to it. They may be dying to know *not* where their errors are, what you appreciate about their process, or what their next step is but whether you think their work is good, deserving of an A grade, and furthermore, whether you think it is *better* than that of their classmates in some way. Good grief, even their parents ask us, "So just where does Amy place in comparison to the rest of the class?" Your students may have developed a taste for the rewards of evaluative feedback and gotten comfy in their fixed mindset. They may be a "handful of Cheerios" kind of group, and while this is something you'll want to balance out, it's not all that unusual or shocking. Our advice is to let it go . . . for now. Give yourself a break—make a cup of tea (yes, another one) and take the night off. A better plan is to begin the day tomorrow well rested, feeling accomplished for having done some professional reading, and focus simply on using your EF literacy and sharp professional vision to introduce just a little more descriptive feedback.

A REALISTIC LOOK AT EXTRINSIC MOTIVATION

When researchers and experts suggest that you reduce your punitive/rewarding and judgmental (Types 1 and 2) feedback and replace it with descriptive (Types 3 and 4) feedback, you may think, "Okay, sure. Whatever." This is a realistic teaching book, and we realize you've probably been given this advice before. Whether or not you are vocal about it, admit it to yourself, or are even aware of it, this advice likely hit your radar with a bit of a dull thump and fell to the floor, where you stepped politely over it. The fact is, you may be a great teacher with years of fabulous results under your belt who uses Types 1 and 2 feedback regularly. You may roll your eyes and tell us that in fact *these approaches often seem to work like a charm.* For example, you may spend a lot of money on stickers and rewards that your students delight in. When choosing among them, your students may hop from one foot to the other, barely able to contain their excitement. Then perhaps they run back to their desks to complete another "perfect page" of spelling, math, or handwriting. "They love them. I love them. So, what's the harm?" And who can deny that there's a very special little moment of connection shared when a reward or a piece of positive judgment is delivered. "Oh, Kai, look at how nicely you've done your work. Why don't you hand out the snacks and go to recess early?" "Honestly, if it ain't broke don't fix it," you might think. "There are too many other things to worry about." Even negatively judgmental and punitive feedback seem to serve a purpose—we use it to create order in our classrooms, calm the students, and get things done. "Listen, if I don't command the power in my room, one of my students will be only too happy to take control—and that doesn't feel safe for anyone." Types 1 and 2 feedback are not some mythical naughty teaching behavior that nobody ever uses. They are approaches that actually solve classroom problems. We use them, you use them, everyone uses them because we care deeply about our work, want our classrooms to run smoothly, and want to help students feel calm, safe, and successful. Of course, when we remove the treats, praise, and grades, the motivation stops (DeLong & Winter, 2002), but overall, for a teacher in a busy classroom, it's a pretty good deal.

In fact, hoping students will act based on intrinsic motivation alone might be a disaster! Trained to use only intrinsic motivation, our students might complain about revision by saying, "But miss, I don't *enjoy* doing that . . ." or "I didn't study for my exam because the French Revolution is not *interesting* to me." In fact, many experts now believe our feedback should be a combination of both intrinsic and extrinsic motivation (Cerasoli, Nicklin, & Ford, 2014). They say that while intrinsic motivation predicts *quality* of performance, extrinsic motivation predicts the *quantity*. In many ways, our efforts to leverage extrinsic motivation gets our students through the door and keeps them in the room so we can do the deeper and more powerful work of promoting intrinsic motivation.

THE BSP[1] AND INTRINSIC MOTIVATION

Have you ever scrolled past an online video of an animal doing something that looked playful or curious? Think of cows romping around in a field, a deer rolling and splashing in a mudpuddle, or a crow sliding down a snowy rooftop. If this doesn't sound familiar, Google it! These phenomena exist. In all cases, you may wonder if there is an external reason for the behavior. You might suspect that the cow has an itch, or that the deer is trying to unearth a food source, or that the crow is trained and will earn a small reward. In fact, just as extrinsic motivation exists in both animals and humans, so does intrinsic motivation, and it is a wondrous thing. Intrinsic motivation feels good. It is the state of being personally invested and interested in learning and doesn't rely on rewards. In general, people (and animals) who are intrinsically motivated choose to do challenging tasks and can remain focused. They take pride in their work and enjoy doing it. It is associated with high academic outcomes, independence, and the ability to understand, monitor, and direct one's own learning (see, for example, Patall, 2013). As you can imagine, an intrinsically motivated citizen, be it a student, employee, spouse, or parent, is a highly productive and valuable asset to society. Intrinsically motivated animals, on the other hand, can be cute or annoying, depending on whether their project involves romping around in a far-off field or digging up your lawn.

Regardless, intrinsic motivation is an old idea that you've likely heard about a million times. To many teachers, however, it is a rare, random occurrence. We may see it in a child who joins our classroom after a few years of homeschooling, or during the handful of times that our projects perfectly suit our students' interests, but as a mental state it often seems impossible to *cause*. Will it somehow grow naturally, like a fungus, in the vacuum left by stickers and other incentives? Like growth mindset, there is a disconnect between how much we like the idea of intrinsic motivation and how much we actually know about fostering it. Also, like growth mindset, we may find ourselves trying to prompt intrinsic motivation in our students by simply suggesting or recommending it. "Have a growth mindset! Have intrinsic motivation!"

In fact, lo and behold, much is known about the conditions in which intrinsic motivation develops. There are four key factors, and we love to describe them because almost all of them can be directly stimulated using our nifty little back-and-forth, group feedback practice called the Barriers and Strategies Protocol (BSP). According to Deci and Ryan (2000), they are as follows:

---

[1] This chapter includes reference to the Barriers and Strategies Protocol (BSP), which was introduced in Chapter 3. It is a semistructured teaching protocol. Essentially, it asks teachers to gather students to discuss "What are your/our barriers to this work?" and then "What strategies can we use to be more successful?"

- Autonomy: The ability to make choices based on one's own free will.
- Relatedness or belonging: A sense of connection, caring, and interaction with others.
- Competence: A sense of mastery and control.
- Meaning: A sense that learning has purpose and is meaningful.

We are not the only team trying to find clever ways to incorporate these factors. A program called Responsive Classroom, for example, weaves these factors across a whole bunch of different instructional approaches and activities; they have good results (Rimm-Kaufman, Fan, Chiu, & You, 2007). In contrast, our BSP is just one practice. It is a very carefully designed and compact approach that can be learned in 5 minutes and used to improve your instructional conversations. It can be pocket sized and quick, or unfurled to occupy a whole period of discussion, but you will see that in all its forms it encompasses the factors for intrinsic motivation. Table 5.2 breaks down exactly how it achieves each of the key conditions for motivation.

Thus, the BSP quickly sets the stage for an intrinsically motivating feedback encounter of the descriptive, growth-oriented type (#4) characterized by Tunstall and Gipps (1996). Instead of moving from student to student conducting speedy semiprivate interactions, we tap into the social

TABLE 5.2. How the BSP Addresses the Four Key Conditions for Intrinsic Motivation

Construct	Instructional goal	How the BSP addresses it
Relatedness/ belonging	Help individuals feel as though they matter and are valued in a supportive learning community. Emphasize common goals and shared ideas.	When a challenge is set, students are gathered in a group to discuss it. The experience of problem solving, students' barriers, and their strategies are derivatized and shared. Students get to know each other as problem solvers, sometimes acting as experts for one another, sometimes receiving support. Through this process, teachers and students learn information that may have previously been kept hidden about themselves and each other as learners.
Competence	Help students see challenge as a way to improve ability and skill. Create a structured way for students to attempt challenges, use strategies, and try again when they fail. Reinforce strategy use and reflection though process-based feedback.	Within a short, structured, routine conversation, a T-chart is made in which students list their barriers and work together to devise matching strategies. This coupling of barriers and strategies reinforces a strategic habit.
Autonomy	Share decision-making power and support students' choice in how they practice and demonstrate their ideas and skills.	The opportunity to develop strategies positions students as experts. Teachers then encourage students to choose and use an appropriate strategy and watch attentively as they attempt it.
Meaning	Help students connect instructional concepts to their personal interests, values, goals, and dreams.	Whether students are EF literate or not, having a structured, shared opportunity to explore and understand one's own personal barriers and strategies is inherently meaningful.

power of belonging by working with the whole classroom community at once. We make time for a more student-driven discussion of barriers and strategies and provide the opportunity for students to choose and use the strategies *they* like. As we saw in Chapter 3, the BSP is handy because you don't need to overhaul your whole classroom to start using it. Rather, it is one straightforward practice that you can establish in any context. After a few uses, you may notice it spreading seeds of intrinsic motivation throughout your classroom. You'll be better informed about processes and strategies taking place among your students so you'll be more able to notice and name them. From one small tweak, a mighty change will begin to occur.

Mighty though it may be, don't expect intrinsic motivation to grow overnight. The funny thing is, it *does* grow like a fungus—slowly, steadily, and quietly. We're not talking about the mess that springs up between your patio stones. Instead, imagine the famed white truffle, valued at upward of US $3,000 per kilogram, or even better, the rare yartsa gunbu, which grow on dead Himalayan ghost moth caterpillars and are valued at a whopping $50K each. Like yartsa gunbu, intrinsic motivation is worth the time and effort. It's potent and powerful, even millennials think it is cool, and the demand for it has skyrocketed in the past decade.

How to Conduct Powerful Feedback: *Early Days*

The *big idea* here is that getting to know students should be all about discovering (and feeding back) the processes and strategies they use to operate. In this section, you'll learn more about how to do the following:

- Create a culture of strategy talk in your classroom.
- Share the EF-based feedback you give to your students with their parents using a homework book, notes on an assignment, or one of many online platforms.
- Create classroom systems and routines for delivering process-oriented feedback.

While sitting in the dirt, chipping away at wheels and trying to spark up fires, perhaps the ancient cave teachers gave their students rudimentary feedback: "Ugh. Hey, kid. I see you. You're doing neat stuff." Nowadays, searching Google for "ways to give feedback" yields 223 million hits. In hundreds of different spoken dialects, you can find examples of verbal feedback delivered in whispers, shouts, acronyms, rhymes, raps, songs, community circles, huddles, or using the magic of traditional Indian Kathputli puppets. Some teachers dabble in sign language, while others make up gestures or use specific facial expressions. These messages may be delivered hourly, daily, or during special meetings that sometimes include peers, parents, or principals. Written feedback, meanwhile, is given on paper, adhesive notes, charts, diagrams, journals, or cards, using comments, callouts, stamps, stickers, or a variety of symbols. Sometimes we digitally record feedback using fancy apps. One teacher we know uses a whiteboard marker to scribble feedback right on students' desks, while another uses washables to jot friendly comments up and down their arms! There is no shortage of feedback approaches in our modern times, but the basic message has remained the same: You are cool, kid. I see you doing important stuff.

What *has* come a long way is our ability to notice, understand, and accurately name the kinds of processes our students are using to pursue their goals—even during the earliest of days and in the most basic of interactions. Imagine, for example, it is the first day of school and you're walking by a crowd of third graders in the hall. Before you even enter the classroom, you can begin to guide and shape your students' performance with feedback. If you say, "Boys and girls! You're so noisy!" they will probably be noisy again tomorrow. If you say, "You really stick together!" you might see more of that sticking together at recess. If you say, "Everyone in grade 3 seems to be friends with each other!" you might find that the group continues to grow. Most teachers know how this works. For better or worse, when you notice and mention something, especially to a group, they can't seem to resist leaning in and doing more of it.

Research tells us that students actually spend a lot of time ruminating about unclear or vague feedback, and this distracts them from their work. Researchers suspect that the provision of more "elaborative" feedback that connects success or failure to specific process steps or strategies would ease this rumination so students could quickly process it, understand it, and get back down to business (Baadte & Kurenbach, 2017). As EF-literate teachers, we can use the language of EF to achieve this specificity. Indeed, as soon as you meet your students you can start noticing and naming the little strategies they use. We have learned much from Paula Barrow, a primary teacher we know who gives great EF-oriented feedback.[2] Walking around a full table of children jostling to share a bin of markers and finish a worksheet, she might say, "I notice that four students have used their task initiation to get started right away." In Table 5.3 we imagine a few other pieces of feedback that Paula might deliver to a group of students using her EF lens and compare it to what a teacher might say otherwise. Notice that, without an EF lens, typical responses often include reduced expectations, solutions for problems, or expressions of judgment.

The process-based feedback we have imagined for Paula's class names a whole range of stellar performance. We know, however, that in real life students aren't always quite so picture perfect. In this very class there might have been a bit of pushing between two of the more squished kids, a few students might have been making careless errors, and one student might have been stalling and wasting time. The struggle is real—in fact, another teacher might have walked in, picked up on it, and wondered aloud whether the kids were off to a rough start. Meanwhile—and this is the fun part—Ms. Barrow could have barged ahead with her process-based feedback, observing positive and effective strategies regardless of how prevalent they actually were. Even better, in a pinch, she could have used her imagination and "observed" Jonny or Janet X, the invisible student who *was* doing the right things, filling her students' ears with feedback about target behaviors that weren't quite happening yet. Saying, "I see someone who is making a great choice" or "Someone just took a moment to get organized" or "I see someone who is paying close attention" can have a surprisingly effective impact on a group of students who need clear guidance and motivation to make good choices, get organized, and pay attention. Regardless, by searching for even the tiniest little whiff of effective process and commenting on it, we cultivate good ideas among our students. In response to the EF-based feedback we imagined in Table 5.3, the students sitting in Paula's classroom might have straightened up, paid closer attention to their pages and the clock, and made extra space for the elbows of their seatmates.

This careful process of cultivating performance is much like conducting a science experiment. If you ever took any upper-level biology, you might remember using a petri dish full of agar jelly to grow cultures of bacteria. Agar is a nutrient-rich material, and about a week after you run a dirty swab across it, a whole bunch of different bacteria will start to bloom. You'll see a variety of desir-

---

[2] Paula Barrow teaches at Fenelon Township Public School in Cameron, Ontario, Canada. Used with permission.

TABLE 5.3. Two Different Feedback Types

Challenge	EF-based feedback	Other feedback
Students jostling for space at a table with limited space.	I just saw someone use response inhibition! Their elbow was bumped. They just said, "No problem," and moved over a bit.	Boys, please move to the table by the window. Boys. Boys? Come on. That seat really isn't working today. Maybe you can try it again tomorrow.
Students trying to write stories and getting stuck.	I see someone rereading her story to plan what comes next. She's planning and prioritizing!	Okay. Let's see what you've got. Okay, so what would the bird do? Would he fly away? I think so.
Students managing materials for a project.	I see a student who has organized her papers in three piles. I don't think she'll lose any of them.	Before you do anything else, Jack, please get those papers organized.
Students stalling and not getting things done on time.	Someone just looked at the clock. I think he is managing the time he has left before recess.	Okay, guys. Just a reminder! You only have 10 minutes left to finish your stories!
Students making careless errors.	I see someone reading his story to make sure he didn't mix up what he was thinking. That's a big help to his working memory!	I see a mistake in the second line, and are you sure you want to put that question mark there?
Students distracted by others while working.	Devon and Jason noticed the front table was getting too full, so they decided to move. That's metacognition!	Remember, if you can't get that done in class, you'll have to take it for homework.
Students arriving or becoming upset.	I see someone taking a minute to relax, take a deep breath, and practice emotional control.	If you can't behave properly, you won't be able to join us at the assembly later.
Students failing to proofread properly.	I see someone who is using sustained attention to check work carefully. She points to each word with her pencil.	Read this out loud. Did you do that? Does it make sense to you?
Students getting frustrated or stopped by lost materials or changes to routine.	Peyton couldn't find her book, so she's just using loose paper. She doesn't mind doing something different today. That is so flexible!	Peyton, honey, if your book isn't in your backpack and you've searched the classroom, I can't help you. Find some scrap paper.
Students losing momentum and failing to finish their work.	This group is working together to make this work more fun. They are using goal-directed persistence to get it all done today.	Let's go, guys. I don't know why I'm seeing so many people fooling around because only two of you are finished.

Note. "EF based" refers to the kind of feedback that may be possible in a classroom with an EF-literate teacher and students. "Other" refers to classrooms without this emphasis.

able and undesirable specimens in different colors and patterns—very much like the many different behaviors you see in your classroom. In the science lab, a researcher will look at this mixed-up culture under a microscope, choose one target specimen, carefully pick up a tiny smudge of *only the target specimen* with a cotton swab, and carefully swipe the separated single sample onto a fresh dish. In about a week: voila! With any luck, the little smear will have replicated, and the researcher will have a dish full of that one special specimen. Do you see the similarity? We watch our students carefully, notice a few really productive, effective processes, and emphasize those things with highly specific feedback. We need to watch closely and be quite precise about what we notice—a good background in EFs helps with this. We also need to have an open enough mind to recognize the really unusual (but valuable) specimens in the diverse cultures we begin with.

Of course, there are other ways to give good notice and name feedback. Paula, for example, has evolved to using EF "cards" on which the names of different EFs are featured (see Figure 5.2). When students are caught using an effective process or strategy to support EFs, they receive a little laminated card to acknowledge their achievement. Below, Paula reflects on her choice to use a token. You will see how cautiously she applies externally rewarding elements like tokens and competition, blending them artfully with intrinsically motivating elements like her attention, recognition of process, and a sense of community.

"Noticing and naming is powerful, but sometimes my kiddos need something tangible. I like to go stealth and set a card quietly in front of a child so as not to disturb, but to let them know

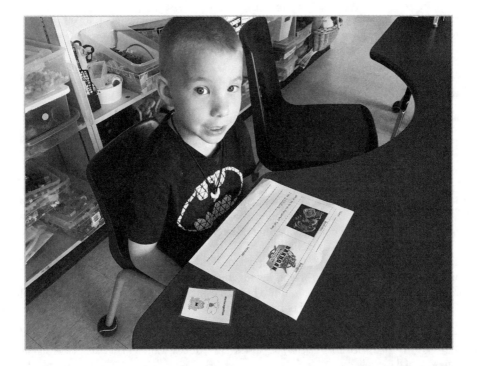

FIGURE 5.2. Earning a "ticket" for metacognition in early primary. This photo features the formidable Eli Watson from Paula Barrow's SK/1 class at Fenelon Township Public School in Cameron, Ontario, Canada. Used with permission.

that I am noticing. I watch them sit up a little straighter and a silent smile spread across their face. Then I sit back and watch even more effort going into their work. Budget wise, I do not let the kids keep these tickets. They get a friend to take their picture holding the ticket or a video snippet, which is uploaded to the parent communication tool called Seesaw. Parents and children get feedback, and parents learn about EFs with their child. It gives parents the same language to use at home and hopefully inspires them to notice and name EFs in another setting. I am considering black-and-white paper copies to keep. . . . I think I will ask my students today! I thought about placing them on my bulletin board for showing off with student names, but I can't bring myself to make it a competition at this young age."

As we reflect on Paula's choice, we admire the design of this temporary, quiet, visible token. Because it is a silent acknowledgment, this feedback can be given while students are deep in a train of thought without interruption. Silent though it may be, this feedback is highly visible, not only to students, but also to their parents and whomever else peeks into their Seesaw account. Most importantly, these tokens won't be accumulated, counted, and compared among students. The brief feeling of excitement and pride won't be followed by an ominous worry that "oh no, other students are getting these too, and maybe they'll have more than me!" Similarly, these tokens won't be piled up, crumpled, lost, and start to lose their value in the back corner of a desk. The choice not to give takeaway tokens or post tokens to a bulletin board is probably a good one—though we love that she's asking her students what they think, and we wonder what they'll say. Regardless, we truly appreciate this powerful, yet highly sensitive and child-friendly approach.

> ### How to Conduct Powerful Feedback:
> *Time Strapped*
>
>
>
> The big idea here is that there are many everyday routines that can be modified slightly to deliver powerful feedback. In this section, you'll learn more about how to do the following:
>
> - Get students involved in giving "shout out" EF feedback to one another.
> - Use exit slips for self-reflection on EF strategy use.
> - Do a quick BSP with strategies that will provide a basic script for what to say as you provide high-quality feedback.

Perhaps you cycle through 120 different students every week as an instructor of art, French, or Spanish. Maybe you're a homeroom teacher who runs three different reading groups plus an enriched project, all while providing accommodations for students with special needs. Or, who knows, maybe your principal has you teaching something completely unfamiliar and you're feeling stretched. All of these examples, and many more besides, would place you squarely into the category of a time-strapped teacher. Regardless of what you're doing that makes you strapped for time, we recognize that whatever EF-based feedback approach we try to sell you needs to be quick and seamless. Below are a couple of suggestions that might work.

First, we know several middle school teachers who maintain "shout-out" routines, through which students themselves are encouraged to notice and name each other's performance. They set up a bulletin board with several EF categories, often simply printing out a set of EF posters and using sticky notes to add student observations about effective process.[3] This is efficient because a single setup can last all year; you simply create a bulletin board to collect strategies and run with it for as long as you like. And while using EF categories adds coherence, you certainly don't have to set your display up this way. In Sallie Byer's classroom, shout-outs are added on a random collection of sticky notes and colored paper, written casually and quickly.[4] The strategies noted on Sallie's board regarding goal-directed persistence include the following:

- "Sit away from other people to do independent work."
- "Email teacher for extended time when life has surprise problems."
- "Take the lead with growth mindset (possibly by encouraging classmates?)."
- "Make time after school or at lunch to work on projects."
- "Ask lots of questions so I know exactly what has to be done."
- "Edit and revise repeatedly to make sure there are no mistakes."
- "Ask for extra work to improve in a class."

To solicit these ideas, Sallie might have stopped the class midway to see if anyone had noticed an effective strategy: "Any shout-outs on how to do this?" In response, students might have said things like "Jo is using an app to make notes"; "Reema is putting her research in colored folders"; or "We're reading these questions to each other and it's helping." This conversation could also take place during a transition, while students were gathering their books and materials or tidying up equipment. "You have 5 minutes to tidy up and get going to your next class. I'm writing down shout-outs. Call them out. What were our innovative approaches today?"

As the bank of "shout-out" ideas grows, it can be used in different ways. Considering the breadth of strategies collected in Sallie's classroom, she might consider responding to off-task students by having them tell her one strategy they plan to use to get their work done. If they aren't sure, she could ask them to refer to the chart and choose a certain EF to focus on. Or she could ask the whole class to jot down the strategies they plan to use at the top of whatever assignment they're working on. If Sallie wanted to spend a few extra moments creating small "exit slips," she could have students attach one to their daily work before leaving, declaring the strategy they used, rating how successful it was, and writing down what might have worked better. Figure 5.3 provides a simple model of how this could look. Again, this is a premade tool that could be created in September, copied hundreds of times, and kept piled up and ready for use all year long.

No matter how busy you are, you should consider hosting a modified version of the BSP. This will give you the raw material you need to provide high-quality, EF-oriented feedback. Consider these two options: a rolling BSP or a lightening round BSP. To do a *rolling* BSP, teachers designate certain pages in a flip-chart pad for certain subjects, EFs, or even classroom routines. On the math page, for example, all kinds of different barriers and strategies can be added throughout the year for quick reference. Then, on a particularly busy day, the chart can simply be opened up for students and teachers to refer to. As students make use of the noted strategy ideas, their teachers can use the chart like a script to provide high-quality, EF-based feedback.

---

[3] Oh, yes. We know those sticky notes will lose their stick and flutter maddeningly to the ground. For a lasting effect, and your own sanity, we suggest you reinforce them with a little piece of tape.

[4] Sallie Byer teaches at Central Senior School in Lindsay, Ontario, Canada. Used with permission.

The strategy I used today . . .	
It worked . . . (circle one)	very well | well | poorly | very poorly
So, my next strategy will be . . .	

FIGURE 5.3. Exit slip for quick feedback/formative assessment of process.

The other option is to do a *lightening round* BSP. This can take place in a snappy 3-minute back-and-forth. In a hurried tone, you can say, "Okay. 3 + 3 BSP! Before you start, tell me three barriers and three strategies. Go!" If you do this regularly enough, your students will become fluent and efficient and may only take a few minutes to articulate the obvious stumbling blocks and appropriate strategies. By quickly generating a few agreed-upon strategies, you will be able to vocalize very specific and useful group feedback throughout the work period.

How to Conduct Powerful Feedback:
Highly Structured

The big idea here is that you can revamp traditional feedback systems to deliver EF-focused feedback. In this section, you'll learn more about how to do the following:

- Create a rubric that incorporates the EF strategy targets.
- Use EF rubrics during longer projects.
- Use a scoring system on an EF or strategy rubric.

Let's imagine a typical day; some of your students are off track, and some are tackling EF challenges using innovative strategies. One is diagramming a math problem, another is using a supportive technology, while another needs your help to organize folders of notes and materials on the computer. It would be nice to have a record of these processes because, first, it will be report card *gold* (see Chapter 6). Second, collecting data and information on your students' ability to manage their EFs will also provide immediate benefits. Right away, you can feed it back to them for motivation and direction. There are many convenient ways to collect this information—we'll present one for daily use, one for yearly use, and one for special projects. Hopefully, you can modify, change, and spin these off into as many other variations as you need.

First, however, you need to do some planning. Most teachers we know who provide structured feedback on EF strategy use base their observation and comments on strategies that have already been discussed among the class within a BSP (see Chapter 3). Following a conversation like this, your students will have a good idea of the kinds of strategies that might work, and you will be much more likely to witness the kinds of clever approaches you're hoping to record.

A daily writing task, such as journaling or creative writing, is a perfect opportunity to give structured EF-based feedback. Consider Figure 5.4, on which a grade 4 teacher we know listed academic goals *as well as the EF strategies her class had discussed and planned to use.* In this case, students were working in pairs to learn how to craft proper expository paragraphs. Right away, the teacher conducted a BSP. She then transferred the strategies to this sheet to use while observing students at work. Walking around the room as they worked on their paragraphs, she could easily record what she saw. When students managed an academic or EF skill independently, this was tracked with a "3." If a reminder was given, the teacher tracked a "2" (with reminder). If students required one-on-one reteaching, the teacher tracked a "1."

As this data was gathered, the teacher conspicuously *narrated* her note making. In this way, the daily tracking page became like a lyric sheet for daily feedback, reminding both students and their teacher to focus on the five agreed-upon strategies. For example, regarding a student who was stuck, the teacher said, "Just a reminder to choose and use a strategy. I'm watching to see you choose independently," and tracked a small "2" on the chart (reminder). When the student required further assistance, the teacher said, "Let's practice rereading the examples together" or "Let's reread each sentence together," and tracked a small "1" on the chart next to these strategies (required 1:1 help). This approach is particularly effective if students know the goal is to move toward independent use of these strategies. We've seen this done in many ways, but the simplest is to tell students exactly what a 1, 2, and 3 mean. Over the course of one period, you may track a "1," and then a "2," and finally a "3," indicating the progression of a student from one-on-one support to a reminder and finally to the independent use of a strategy. In this example, students knew they had met their goals when they heard the teacher say, "You're using positive partner talk indepen-

Academic skills	SR	CS	MI	JM	IR	KI	RR	SL	RI	PI
• Use three transition words.										
• Use a clear topic sentence.										
• Use three supporting sentences.										
• Use effective collaboration.										
• EF strategies										
• Restate what your partner said. (Attention)										
• Say, "Okay. What's next?" (Planning)										
• Reread the examples. (Goal-directed persistence)										
• Reread each sentence. (Attention)										
• Use positive partner talk. (Emotional regulation)										

FIGURE 5.4. Feedback chart with academic and EF targets. This chart has been abbreviated at the right-most column to save space. It can be produced in landscape format to include all student initials. Or it can be produced with a smaller number of students to facilitate feedback that is focused on specific groups each day. Teachers may use the following code to enter data: 1 = one-on-one support, 2 = with reminder, and 3 = independently.

dently. I'm tracking that." Many of them took an interest in how their independence seemed to be growing, asking to see the teacher's records of their 1's, 2's, and 3's.

Structured feedback can be provided regarding yearly goals as well. Early in a school year, general classroom behavior can be discussed and agreed upon according to EF categories. In fact, this is a nice way to introduce the idea of EFs because it provides students with clear, grounded examples they can relate to. Consider Figure 5.5, in which a team of grade 7/8 teachers and students at Montcrest School in Toronto, Ontario, engaged students in a more general discussion of the barriers they might face in class and the strategies they could use to be successful. Notice that they chose to focus on only a handful of EFs that seemed most relevant to their context. Once co-created, this chart was copied for each student and placed in the teachers' assessment binders. It provided a useful ongoing record for the teachers to return to over the course of the term. As the teachers gathered simple ✓ or ✗ data, they conferenced with students about their progress. Even though the indictors under each EF were quite general, the teachers often circled back with students who were struggling to ask, "I've noticed you're not demonstrating these attention strategies. Do we need a more specific strategy?" In this way, the teachers' feedback was specific, process oriented, and based on targets that were well understood by everyone.

The final example of a highly structured feedback approach we'll provide refers to a very specific, monthlong project taking place in a grade 2 classroom. For this project, students were matched up with two classmates they were not used to working with and were asked to use a kit of wooden materials to build a creative structure. In previous years, this project had been rife with student fighting and disorganization. It required a seemingly never-ending amount of class time,

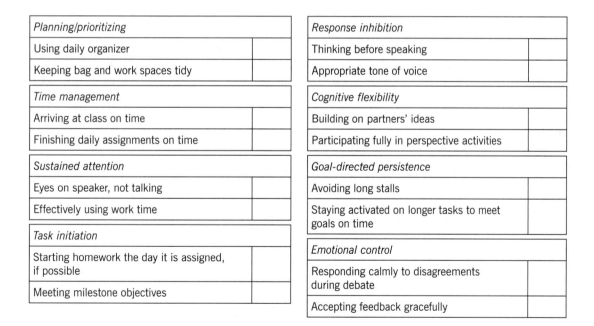

FIGURE 5.5. A chart of Term 1, grade 7/8 behavior expectations. Created by senior teaching staff and students at Montcrest School, Toronto, Ontario, Canada. Used with permission. This chart has been abbreviated at the right-most column to save space. It can be produced in landscape format to include all student initials. Or it can be produced with a smaller number of students to facilitate feedback that is focused on specific groups each day.

and students only made reasonable progress when attended by an adult who would feed them specific next steps. Moving constantly from group to group, the teachers felt as though *they* were slowly building all eight creative structures. How is this teaching them anything, they wondered? Regardless, the teachers felt the project had potential and they were committed to making it work.

The first step toward making their students more independent was to devote a full period to a discussion of BSP. After describing the task, they explained that its purpose was not only to apply a handful of science principles but also to build key 21st-century skills (goal setting, listening, speaking, turn taking, and resolving conflicts). As the students explored the kinds of things that could go wrong, and the kinds of steps they could take to be strategic and successful, the teachers created a chart of behaviors to "look for" and "avoid" (Figure 5.6). The chart had been created based on the students' own ideas, so they were familiar with the expectations. This class happened to be EF literate, but you could easily create a chart of behaviors to look for and avoid without connecting them to EFs.

This chart was used in an interesting way. Every building day, each group of students was given a fresh copy of the sheet to place in clear view at their workstation. It then became a landing pad for teacher feedback. Circulating the room as usual, teachers were no longer pulling up a chair, rolling up their sleeves, and trying to make the students' design ideas work for them. Nor were they taking students into the corridor to talk through their disagreements or help them "cool off." How did they spend all of this saved time? They were glancing at the chart and making comments such as "I see you playing the blame game. Can you choose a 'look-for' strategy?" As this comment was made, the teacher placed a little check next to "playing the blame game" on the rubric. "I'm watching to see how you use our strategies," they added. A few moments of calm, focused observation after these comments often yielded a rather awkward, sarcastic, or lame attempt at using a strategy. This was the moment of truth, at which the students stood at a fork in the road between old, ineffective, but comfortable habits and new, possibly more effective, but frighteningly unfamiliar and risky ones. In much the same way that you might coach a child to let go of training wheels on a bike, the teachers at this moment needed to be fully present and jump on the least

Skill	Look for Level 3	Avoid Level 2	Comment
Goal setting (organization)	"First . . . second . . . third . . ." Plan who does what. Check in as you go.	Doing before talking. Making huge goals.	
Listening actively (inhibition)	Look at speaker and nod your understanding. "So, I heard you say . . ."	Just waiting and not really listening. Finishing the speaker's idea.	
Speaking (attention)	Wait for readiness. Use eye contact and clear voice.	Bossy tone. Negative body language.	
Turn taking (flexibility)	Explore and try your partner's ideas.	"Closing or slamming the door" on an idea.	
Resolving conflicts (emotional regulation)	"Can I explain that again?" "I'm not sure if that will work because . . ."	Ignoring or avoiding. Playing the blame game.	

FIGURE 5.6. A daily tracking sheet for groupwork.

sign of willingness, positivity, and courage. The moment the teachers saw a student trying a new strategy, they checked it off on the rubric right away. "You just explored your partners' idea! I'm tracking that," the teacher might have commented, and an upward spiral would begin: Even the most awkward use of strategy started to untangle the students' problems, they felt more successful, they realized that using the strategies worked, and they began to use them with more conviction and ease. They were off! At the end of this unit, the students were proud of their accomplishments. They all felt as though their EFs had grown. They also made reference to the way certain strategies had helped them to get to know new people and form satisfying new relationships.

We know there is nothing particularly groundbreaking about the recording sheets we have suggested. In fact, you could easily upgrade them with apps like Plickers, Padlet, or Google Jamboard. In our experience, the kind of feedback that helps children build EFs isn't necessarily fancy. It simply helps them to understand how, when, and why they are successful, and teaches them to think for themselves and to be strategic. Anything you add beyond that might add convenience, allow for faster communication, or impress the heck out of parents, but it will only ever be the cherry on top.

How to Conduct Powerful Feedback:
Highly Structured Project Work

The *big idea* here is that to succeed at highly structured projects, students need ongoing feedback to support their management of complex processes and EF demands. In this section, you'll learn more about how to do the following:

- Use your support of EF and process skills to persevere when the going gets rough.

- Use a variety of conversations, rubrics, tracking sheets, daily written reports, and personal journals to steer your students' performance.

Teachers who are perceived to be highly structured by their peers often have a good laugh at the idea that it comes easily to them. We hear this in workshops—after being outed by colleagues, they will say, "You think I'm *naturally* structured? You have no idea how hard I've worked on it! This is not my natural state!" They tell us that their structured approach to teaching was something that evolved over time, in response to all kinds of emergencies, missed opportunities, and mess ups. As the demands of their work evolved and changed, things got tougher and they realized they needed a proper, structured plan in order to manage. They tell us, "For goodness sake, I organize myself in this way because I would have drowned in chaos otherwise." If you're one of these "structured" types, the following discussion may be right up your alley.

It may be counterintuitive, but we've noticed that students working on the least structured academic units often require the most carefully planned systems of ongoing feedback. To cultivate 21st-century learning, for example, we may offer students complex projects with authentic, open-ended problems. To facilitate these projects, we need to step back and allow students the time and space to wrestle with tricky problems, but it takes finesse to counterbalance this freedom with appropriate support and discipline. In fact, many of us dread student-centered projects because the idea of giving a class more responsibility *and even less guidance* seems completely absurd—like jumping straight off a cliff. How can teachers build in students the EFs they will need to manage such open-ended projects?

In business management, control in an open-ended thinking environment is called a "constraint" and is considered very important. When the goal is to balance innovation with some stabilizing coherence and focus, expert managers talk about using *enabling constraints* (Davis & Sumara, 2006). This doesn't have to be complicated, but it usually requires some planning to set up. Enabling constraints force children to exert executive control, even in creative and open-ended environments, because they funnel activity through specific, safe, agreed-upon channels. This is very much like creating boundaries for a game of hide and seek or designating one specific room for your kid's wild and crazy sleepover party. The trick is to design constraints that feel comfortable and don't intrude on the target activity. Cue the BSP, and let us enter the busy grades 6, 7, and 8 makerspace classrooms of Roger Reynolds and Dawn Mattiussi.[5] We think their adaptation of the BSP and subsequent feedback process provide just the right level of constraint.

Makerspace? If this context sounds unfamiliar, we encourage you to translate the following example to something more familiar; Dawn and Roger's insights apply equally to many different teaching situations. You might imagine an art room, a typical primary classroom, or a middle school math class. In Kawartha Lakes, however, our makerspace teachers are in their preferred habitat: surrounded by glue guns, saws, drills, electrodes, and computers. For the first time they are allowing their students to progress through several projects at different rates. They have pulled their students out of lockstep because they feel that following a specific timeline is limiting creativity and innovation. So, while they all started at the same time making roller coasters, each group will then work through three other projects (robots, mobility devices, and disaster-proof houses) at their own pace. Although their students now have even more freedom, Dawn and Roger are faced with an additional challenge in the logistics of providing EF support and control. They want to design a structured feedback process to stay ahead of the chaos.

At the beginning of this unit, Dawn and Roger sat their students down to conduct several big BSP conversations. They wanted to zoom in on a few important skills for makerspace, including getting started quickly, using positive self-talk, and being open minded to different ideas. They described these goals to their classes, and then asked them what EF barriers might stand in their way and what strategies they might use to be successful. You can see what their students came up with in Figure 5.7. Based on these conversations, Dawn and Roger were able to circulate around the room giving feedback. They might have said, "I see that you're procrastinating. Which of our strategies do you plan to try?"; "I see you're breathing to control your frustration"; or "This group is listing pros and cons of a new idea!" The students knew what types of strategies they could use to be successful, and the teachers knew exactly what kind of performance to notice and name with their feedback. The straightforward expectations added a sense of predictability and calm for both students and teachers. And to their delight, the students knew that as long as they demonstrated the agreed-upon strategies, most of the creative decisions would be up to them. This is an example of "enabling constraints": The students knew that if they used the agreed-upon strategies, they would remain on track and be allowed the autonomy they wanted to make creative decisions.

As certain groups finished more quickly than others and moved on, however, Dawn and Roger realized it would no longer be practical to host one big BSP conversation. Students were at very different points in their work, and the conversation seemed too general to be useful. At this point, they thought carefully and designed a new structure for their feedback—they started to experi-

---

[5] Roger Reynolds and Dawn Mattiussi teach at Jack Callaghan Public School in Kawartha Lakes, Ontario, Canada. Used with permission.

Goal
Stop procrastinating and begin
tasks immediately

Barriers
Talking and socializing
Not knowing how to begin
Social media/other distractions
Not wanting to work

Strategies
Move away from distractions
Ask friends or teachers
how to start
Shut off devices
Use a reward system when
work is finished

Goal
To use positive self-talk when
encountering difficult situations

Barriers
Not knowing triggers
Too upset to care
Being angry at certain people
Feeling sad

Strategies
Ask for help (parent, teacher,
peers, counselor)
Breathe
Listen to relaxation music
Give yourself space and time
before working through
problem
No sad music—only happy,
uplifting music

Goal
Be more open-minded to
receiving new ideas and using
new strategies

Barriers
Unwilling to implement
group members' ideas
Arguing
Some students take control
all the time

Strategies
Consider pros and cons
Consider how you can
implement new ideas
Remain positive and look for
the value in new ideas
Assign roles to all group members
Change roles often

FIGURE 5.7. Using the BSP to troubleshoot makerspace skills. Reproduced from posters created by Dawn Mattiussi, Roger Reynolds, and their students at Jack Callaghan Public School in Kawartha Lakes, Ontario, Canada. Used with permission.

ment with daily BSP *journals.* Before and after each session of work, they provided their maker design teams with several prompts (below) and gave them 5 minutes to collaborate and respond in writing. These moments of wide-awake, metacognitive thinking would not have happened otherwise. Without this opportunity, Dawn and Roger knew that many of their students would head into the classroom with unclear plans and make the same types of mistakes over and over again.

Journal Prompts to Be Answered Before the Day's Work

1. "As a group, identify your goals for today."
2. "As a group, identify barriers and strategies to achieving your goals."

Journal Prompts to Be Answered After the Day's Work

1. "Individually reflect on your group's progress toward achieving your goal. What worked and didn't work?"
2. "As a group, decide on your goals for tomorrow."

The resulting journals became something the teachers could easily collect, read, and respond to. When desired, they could gather the class to share an especially insightful entry, or to ask for help strategizing on a particularly challenging barrier. If a group was not performing as desired, Dawn and Roger could note this in their response to the students' writing, commenting, "You didn't make much progress today. What went wrong? What will you try next?" Or if students devised strategy ideas that were vague, they could ask for more specificity. This approach allowed for a high level of personalized structure for each student without taking too much class time or overcommitting the teachers. Imagine how Dawn and Roger could have provided feedback on the following student journal. They may have asked for a more specific plan for avoiding distraction, or to hear more detail about how time was conserved.

> "Goal: Our goal today is to have a reliable button that works perfectly. Two things that are going well are our board for melody and the buttons on our board. We have been paying attention to our work, we have conserved time reasonably well, and we were able to change our plan when we needed to. A barrier that we are having trouble with is a few distractions. We will overcome that barrier by focusing more on our work and less on other people."

There are many ways to share feedback, but delivering it while maintaining our students' sense of freedom and creativity takes finesse. Like architects, we can plan structures that provide support and safety, that fit the ecology of the context, and that provide the least obstructed views for the students who dwell inside. During one term's worth of maker activities, Roger and Dawn explored several different feedback structures and were able to foster their students' metacognition as well as big, broad transdisciplinary EF skills. When we are comfortable with the basic setup of EF-literate teaching, the adaptations we make are only limited by our courage and creativity.

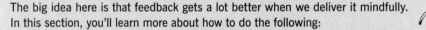

How to Conduct Powerful Feedback:
Organic and Free Flowing

The big idea here is that feedback gets a lot better when we deliver it mindfully. In this section, you'll learn more about how to do the following:

- Breathe deeply before delivering feedback. As you inhale, think, "Why . . ." and as you exhale, think " . . . are they doing that?"
- Respond to children based on your EF literacy rather than on a habitual reaction.
- Notice and name the EF barriers or strategies at play in your students' performance.

A student is behaving unexpectedly. Instead of finishing a math test, for example, he is creating a dusty, black scribble on his desk with a pencil. Your feedback may be so organic and free flowing that it emerges before you even have time to think: "Ten minutes left," you might say, or "Start with the ones you know." Or you might remark, "You've got this—almost done!" or "Underline the important words." Alternatively, you might simply walk closer to the student, say his name, point to the next step, or gesture toward the clock. Each of these pieces of verbal or nonverbal feedback supports a different EF. Did you notice? First was time management and then prioritization, emotional control, working memory, attention, and finally organization. What's your style? Do you tend to give *time* reminders? Are you a reliable source of *emotional support*? Or do you give a wide variety of different responses? How often do you think you hit the mark, and how often do you miss? For example, have you ever given a time reminder to a student who was actually frustrated and overwhelmed and in desperate need of emotional support? Depending on the student, this can cause a giant meltdown.

Whether we realize it or not, classrooms are overflowing with EF challenges and teachers are walking dispensaries of EF remedies. But ask yourself if you often dispense the same type of "medicine." Stuck on a question? Check the time. Disagreeing with your group mates? Check the time. Don't know how to finish your essay? Check the time again—you only have 10 minutes left! We spend a lot of valuable time offering these corrections, so improving their accuracy would be worthwhile. We believe the fix lies in better everyday diagnosis and that this begins with better everyday observation.

Take a deep breath: in for two seconds and out for three. Even if you count fast, this is all the time you need to organically, naturally, and easily improve the quality of your feedback. The trick is, while you're breathing in, to think, "Why . . ." and as you're breathing out, to think, " . . . are they doing that?" Then, glance at your EF posters and change up your feedback. What *if* the problem was related to organization? Or could it be related to task initiation? Should emotional control be considered? When your students are behaving unexpectedly, slow down, take a breath, watch carefully, and consider interpreting the situation through an EF filter.

Teacher Janet Rhude describes the way her EF lens and a few seconds of extra observation changed her perception and dictated a different feedback approach.[6] After weeks of frustration with her grade 4 class, she made a discovery:

> "In my daily math warm-up, I always assign a problem that all students can solve. I noticed that the weakest students, the ones who most needed review or to build skills before beginning the next unit, avoided the task at all costs. It was so frustrating because I was trying so hard to encourage them, but they didn't seem to want to even try . . . so I changed my teaching. Under the problem, I gave steps: First draw the problem, second write the information you know, and third write the information you want to find. Now they had a way to get started. Over time they started getting to work and trying."

Janet had been focused on pumping her students up to feel confident, but emotional support wasn't what they needed. When she took a deep breath and asked herself, "Why are they doing that?" she realized that her students actually needed scaffolding to prioritize and get started on the task.

How to Conduct Powerful Feedback:
Working with a "Stressed" Class

The big idea here is that there are strategies and tactics that make delivering powerful feedback to stressed students less tricky. In this section, you'll learn more about how to do the following:

- Convey feedback in less confrontational ways, such as a back-and-forth journal response, an exit slip, or a written chart of observed strategy.
- Gently infuse your teaching and classroom feedback with an emphasis on process.
- Convince your students that you really are interested in their strategy use and process steps.

---

[6] Janet Rhude teaches at Scott Young Public School in Lindsay, Ontario, Canada. Used with permission.

Quite a number of students are stressed about their performance at school. Some are highly capable, but perfectionist. Some have lagging academic skills and spend their days hiding behind disruption and distraction. Still others come to school hungry, tired, and discouraged from challenges at home. Teenagers, meanwhile, can go entire school years seeming to be irritated by every little thing. Add in a fire drill and a fight in the parking lot, and you might be tempted to scratch "feedback" right off your list of daily tasks. If you've ever experienced these feelings yourself, you know that getting "advice" at the wrong moment can be extremely grating. Our goal is to offer you ways to support stressed students that are genuinely helpful, without poking the bear or becoming yet another annoyance. It may only take a little tweak to make feedback work in a stressed environment.

Stressed students have 99 problems, and you shouldn't be one of them. How can you become part of the solution? First, there are many ways to reduce the emotional intensity of feedback. You might try using a daily feedback journal, asking students to respond privately to prompts such as "What strategy did you use today?"; "Did it work?"; or "What might you do differently?" This will allow you to respond in a quiet and nonconfrontational way with congratulations, requests for more information, or gentle nudges to try something new. Similarly, private exit slips can be a good way to start with a stressed group, helping you get the ball rolling by gathering data on "Most helpful strategy used today" or even "What strategy didn't work for me today?"

With younger students, who are sometimes so sensitive that even the *slightest* attention causes embarrassment and sets them off, you might try using nonverbal feedback. We know early years teachers who use hand signals, small tokens, little cards, or small symbols that get jotted on work. No matter what you choose, this approach works particularly well if your students are EF literate. Instead of giving a generic "good job" type token or card, you can give one that more specifically identifies effective performance. You might like to create a set of laminated EF cards as Paula Barrow did. Remember Paula, from Fenelon Township Public School in Cameron, Ontario? We discussed her cards in the "Early Days" section. She makes several copies of each little EF card and then simply and quietly places them before a student who she feels is using a strategy to support a certain EF. For example, when she saw a student independently looking at the clock while completing daily work, she placed a "time management" card discreetly at his desk. Paula remembers the day on which one of her students mimicked her discretion and sensitivity when sliding a response inhibition card (a little stop sign) toward a friend who was playing a little too roughly in an activity center. "The behavior stopped immediately without adult intervention," she told us, "and nobody got defensive or argumentative."

Another key feedback approach for stressed students is to help them appreciate their own progress. This can be accomplished by collecting a simple form of performance data over time in a visual format such as a tally chart or graph. For example, you might consider making a bar graph to display the number of times you observe a student independently using a calming strategy. Over the course of one week, you can check in with this student several times, letting them see the way their performance is slowly improving. For our most dysregulated students, negative thoughts often dominate the inner monologue and your visual feedback may come as a pleasant surprise. In fact, for some students a visual representation almost *gamifies* their strategy use, creating a colorful pattern that can be irresistible to try to build upon and extend. In any event, with a visual representation, you can cut through days that might be muddled full of frustration, self-doubt, and stress with a clear and encouraging indication of growth and improvement.

These visual tools solve another problem for a stressed student. By cutting down on the amount of verbal rhetoric, they may help us work around what amounts to a total system shutdown. Imagine how our highly stressed students may respond to the sound of a well-meaning teacher trying to explain the implications of their performance. As the sounds of "nagging" or "judgment" start to trickle in, do some of our students close up like space-aged transforming robots, all senses mechanically shuttered and sealed? They might not even be in control of this reaction—it might begin like an inevitable, automatic protective response. As the barrier begins to form, both you and the student might realize the imminent failure of all verbal communication. "I'm sorry! I'm losing you! I feel too much humiliation to hear you!" the student, in a perfect world, might shout from across the void. "I know! And I have no idea how to talk to you without sounding negative and exasperated!" you might holler back. "Forget talking! Just *look* at this!" you might say, as you throw the charts like a lifeline. Students like these, despite their uncontrolled emotional response to our intervention, often truly do want and appreciate help. By sharing the raw data we gather using charts, graphs, or lists, we allow them to process and interpret the data themselves, with a boosted sense of competence and autonomy. Most importantly, by letting go of the traditional verbal approach, we reduce the temptation to steer away from tricky students with feedback; they need it just as much as the others. With a little finesse, we can ensure that feedback to stressed students is delivered, received, and processed.

It is worth remembering that solving problems in the more communal space created by the BSP can, in itself, be calming. Instead of always relying on an *adult* teacher with whom they may have little in common, students can draw inspiration and feedback from one another. This contrast is particularly stark in communities in which there may be historical, cultural, or racial conflict between students and their teachers or the very institution of school. We're not saying a teacher–student connection is a lost cause. There are plenty of teachers who manage to overcome these challenges and enjoy rich, respectful relationships with their students. For a vulnerable learner, however, diversified feedback systems may provide a needed boost.

We may have a hard time convincing our most stressed students that we truly value their process steps. As we know, without correction, many students have a fixed sense of what is cool. They want us to think they execute brilliant performance with little effort because they are . . . geniuses! You may be aware that one of the highest accolades among your students, when considering a successful peer, is the observation that "she doesn't even have to *try* . . ." A friend of ours, the parent of a grade 4 girl, was lamenting this challenge. Trying to coach his stressed-out daughter through a big homework project, he realized she was absolutely process averse. He explained, "She is very uncomfortable just experimenting and trusting the value in the process without concern for the outcome." In fact, many adults leave school feeling the same way and struggle with a sense of inadequacy for the rest of their lives. Particularly for someone who is already stressed out, it takes a lot of courage to let people see your messy, behind-the-scenes, "I'm not done yet, hang on!" process steps. What can we do in school to help students avoid this fear? The key seems to be, again and again, to pull back the curtain, focus our attention on all of the muddled and imperfect developments hiding back there, and reassure students that what we see is interesting, useful, and often delightful.

CHAPTER 6

How EF Literacy
Can Improve Summative Assessment

THE ENDURING IMPORTANCE
OF SUMMATIVE EVALUATION IN AN EF-ORIENTED CONTEXT

In this chapter, we complete our very practical tour of EF-literate teaching with a discussion of summative assessment. If you recall, we have moved from building EF literacy in Chapter 2 to applying it to a whole-class pedagogy in Chapter 3, bringing an EF lens to our observation of student performance in Chapter 4, and using a feedback approach that acknowledges and cultivates EF-based strategy and process in Chapter 5. We'll now describe how tests, evaluations, and reporting can be improved using an EF lens. Before providing practical guidance, however, we will tackle some of the issues surrounding summative assessment with a particular emphasis on those most relevant to an EF-literate teacher. What is the role of strategy assessment alongside test scores, and how does it fit into a report card?

It may surprise you that we wish to begin with a defense of *academic* summative assessment. How does a deep focus on daily process square with cool and objective academic summative evaluation? As teachers and students focused on EFs, should we even concern ourselves with final tests and data? Our answer is an emphatic yes—being focused on day-to-day details doesn't mean that overall performance data no longer counts. Rather, having information upon which to set long-term goals is essential to our sense of "discrepancy"—the distance between where we are now and where we want to be next (Bandura & Locke, 2003). Imagine, for example, a long-distance swimmer churning through miles of water with singular focus on shoulder rotation, breathing patterns, and stroke rate. Similarly, in our classrooms, we (teachers *and* students) may feel as though we're utterly preoccupied by the little daily strategies we use to improve performance. Our knowledge of EFs allows us to look beyond academic achievement to the adaptive transdisciplinary skills used to get there: Kevin designs strategies for managing time, Joey creates tricks for noticing details in her writing, and Mae works with Reema to organize large projects. Pull, breathe, kick, glide—we know that by optimizing these processes, we can finish the race with "personal best" results. Just like long-distance swimmers, however, we need to look up every so often to sight the next marker, assess our position, and make overall adjustments. This is the role of academic summative assessment, and it applies just as much to an EF-focused learner as to anyone else. It is so important to "look up" from the hypnotic routines of our daily grind to determine whether our approaches are moving us in the right direction. Are we actually improving reading and math scores?

The fact is, teachers who collect and use student data to make decisions make better modifications and changes to the way they teach. Without this information, they are prone to making faulty decisions according to unreliable gut feelings and bias (Schildkamp, Lai, & Earl, 2013). As teachers, we must be cautious not to assume we know what is happening as a result of our teaching. There are many frames of mind that may lead us in this direction, but our two favorites are the bright-eyed, "My approach is way beyond tests," *super-innovator* perspective and the strong and steady, "I've been doing this for 20 years," *trust me* perspective. For teachers with the *super-innovator* perspective, who may begin their teaching units with a single sweeping arm across the tables of tradition, the idea of testing and assessment may seem too reductive and standardized. "How can we gather standardized data on an educational experience that has become so applied, individualized, and creative?" they may wonder. We would respond that when school is a playful, diverse rumpus room of creativity, it is even more important to pause occasionally to take a breath, look around, and gather a few sober facts about student achievement. Safety first, right? Conditions of authentic mystery, challenge, and change can be thrilling, but they provide even more reason to double-check our assumptions.

It is all too easy to assume that, when teaching feels good for us or seems fun for students, it is productive. Even if your students are peacefully lost in their own creative thoughts, applying fabulous learning strategies, and knee-deep in papier mâché, you may be missing key benchmarks for your grade level. This is a giant problem for students, because academic targets that seem hard to achieve in a grade 3 classroom may be almost impossible to remediate in grade 5, especially when caregivers don't have the resources needed for extra support at home. Getting and staying lost for a whole school year can be a real disaster. The hard data we gather from good overall assessment supplements our assumptions and helps us make appropriate, even *lifesaving*, instructional decisions. When delivered in individual classrooms, and even when conducted by whole schools or school boards, summative evaluation is how we ensure that each of our students will leave our care with the literacies required to graduate school safe and sound. This is not an either/or situation; we don't have to give up on creativity or our process focus to fulfill our civic and moral duties toward our students.

Academic summative assessment is just as important for very experienced teachers who have, over time, steadily honed and perfected their knowledge of both children and teaching. These are the teachers who might say, "Trust me, I've learned a few tricks in my 10 or even 20 years in the classroom." They not only have amazing lesson plans and materials but also often seem to intuitively understand the processes and strategies students use. Regardless, the first time these veterans teach a class of students who have been bussed in from a neighboring community, they may miss the mark. Blinded by their superb materials, confidence, flawless discipline, and immaculate organization, these teachers may miss deeper academic problems. Is the tried and true approach allowing these particular students to master key writing, math, and reading objectives as usual? To call back our swimming metaphor, even for a very experienced swimmer, unfamiliar waters can be surprising. The greatest of the great are strong, steady, prepared, and still self-aware and flexible enough to change course when necessary.

GATHERING AND REPORTING DATA THAT TELL A TRUE STORY

Oh, reporting. First you collect a pile of summative data—you give tests, do reading assessments, and review quiz scores—and then you spend a ton of time sorting it into report cards to send home with students. Still recovering from this process, you enter the third leg of the triathlon in which you navigate parent responses. They show up at your classroom door, find you outside the school, or send you an email to ask, "So, what's the story?" They might say, "I saw the report, but tell me what's *really* going on." When you ask if they have any specific questions about the report, they usually don't: "Just tell us what you think." It is as though those 2 weeks you spent trying to do your daily teaching from underneath piles of tests, class lists, and crashing computer servers never happened.

Parents often want more information than our reports contain, and we can't really blame them. Scores, numbers, thresholds, and benchmarks can only tell us so much. Parents want context, implications, conclusions, and a clue about what they should be doing in response to the report. Pat on the back? Grounded? Less media time? Tutoring? They may also probe to understand how vigorously they should take these actions, at the worst of times demanding a ranking. "Do we need a 1-week consequence, or should we pull him right out of all extracurriculars?" Parents are desperate for next steps and control.

Report card comments about EFs may address this need by providing information about aspects of performance that can be deliberately improved. As you begin the heavy work of gathering academic data, you may begin to notice interesting patterns: Larisa started paying better attention and has gone up a whole reading level; Shaw's math result isn't high, but he really improved his organization and his progress is awesome; and even though Zach is really bright, his planning skills for essay writing seem to be regressing. Equipped as you are with not only the academic scores but also a day-to-day knowledge of the EFs through which these achievements were won, you will understand the *stories* behind your students' learning.

There is actually a whole method of assessment called "Learning Stories," and the science behind it is illuminating. It was first developed in New Zealand in 2001, and has since been used around the world (Carr, 2001). Using this approach, teachers work with children to collaboratively "describe," "discuss," "document," and "decide upon" how to interpret their learning. In this way, the teacher can avoid making assumptions and instead respects the unique personal, physical, and cultural context of each child. Like all process-oriented approaches, it aims to make the daily operation of learning "visible" and thus knowable and reproducible (Project Zero & Reggio Children, 2011). It also promotes children's capacity for self-reflection and self-education (Liljestrand & Hammarberg, 2017; Schulz, 2013).

We realize that by advocating "story-based" or "narrative-based" assessment, we risk running seriously afoul of busy teachers. We are not talking about writing the next great novel about each and every one of your students. We are also not talking about spending hours making an adorable scrapbook to celebrate how cute and lovely they are. The meaning we seek is a simple remedy for summative assessment that often strips away important context and veers toward *meaninglessness.* Imagine, for example, the information you would want and need if *you* were being assessed. If an adult received an email from a superior categorically indicating poor performance, odds are they would immediately try to add contextualizing information to the record. "June is a slow month for sales throughout the whole company," they might say. "My team was down two members, and I was experimenting with a new analytic platform. My results were actually quite good, given those factors." Similarly, imagine how our students with disabilities, challenging home lives, cultural differences, unusual approaches, or just a *mind of their own* might feel when faced with categorical assessment. Indulging students, parents, other teachers, and ourselves in contextual information when weighing summative academic data is hardly an indulgence at all. In fact, for a student with any conceivable investment in his or her progress and result, it may be the only option that is not outright infuriating and absurd.

To further illustrate how ordinary this idea is, let's return to the long-distance swimming metaphor. As a swimming coach, instead of simply telling our athletes, "Your time was 23:30 minutes!" we can say, "Your time was 23:30 minutes! The water was choppy, and you were swimming about two degrees off course for the first 10 minutes." The summative evaluation will be even more useful if the swimmer is encouraged to participate. She might add, "Yeah, and my goggles were foggy!" Which summative assessment is going to yield better learning and future performance for both swimmer *and coach,* do you think? In response to the second type of summative assessment, the swimmer will enter her next race thinking about staying on track, and the coach may realize that foggy goggles are a bigger problem than she had realized. What if half of the swim team has faulty goggles? By involving your students in a more contextualized process of interpreting their performance, everyone learns so much more.

Dr. Amy Fast, a principal at McMinnville High School in McMinnville, Oregon, recently tweeted that "one of the saddest and most ironic practices in school is how hard we try to measure how students are doing . . . and how rarely we ever ask them" (@fastcrayon). We couldn't agree more. Inside the body and mind of many students at school sits a distinctly *unlicensed* driver, quietly holding deep and valuable insight about their learning. This wisdom may far exceed what teachers and other experts have access to. When asked, for example, "Why do you think you did so well on our novel study?" a student will not say, "I answered all 14 questions correctly," as their test result would indicate. Rather, he might say, "First of all, I love cats and I read about them all of the time. Some words in this book were difficult for me, but I actually knew a lot of them already." While our actions based on our test result might have been to give the student more challenging reading material, our actions based on our conversation might have been to find more books at approximately the same level. In addition, while we wouldn't necessarily have time to scour the library for other cat books, we might make mention of cats in the afternoon math lesson. Either way, involving a student in summative assessment allows us to provide more timely and tailored follow-up. It is so easy to get it wrong and miss opportunity when we make unilateral assumptions and rely solely on test scores.

Our students are complex in ways we can scarcely predict. Just when you think you've understood them, you realize there is even more to learn. Consider the unique and personal learning approach of Joelle, a grade 8 student.[1] When asked to recall a list of random pictures, she succeeded with flying colors. It would have been easy to assume that this type of task came naturally

---

[1] Joelle Inguagiato is a student from Menlo Park, California. Used with permission.

to her. When asked how she did it, however, she told us, "I put them into categories. So, I put the chair and tree together because they are both made of wood. I put the pencil and the books together because they are school supplies." We thought we understood Joelle's approach, but then she said, "I put the iPhone and the brush together." This surprised us. Was she wrong to group these items? According to our schema, a brush and an iPhone do not belong in the same category. Based on this, it would have been easy for us to assume that her strategy was flawed. When we continued talking to her, however, we discovered that these items went together as *stuff from my mother's purse.* From this interaction, we realized that memorization wasn't *easy* for Joelle but that she quite naturally and imaginatively used a strategy to accomplish the task. Regardless of whether a student succeeds or fails, there will almost certainly be much more going on than our summative assessments can tell us. Research shows that when students struggle, they often struggle in many overlapping ways that change as our demands and their context evolves (Aitken, Martinussen, Childs, & Tannock, 2017). Much like looking into a kaleidoscope, looking at our students at one point in time may present a very different picture from what we see only a moment later.

The stories of our learning are personal and special. Through them, we make meaning of seemingly random events and learn lessons for the future. When you think of your own proudest accomplishment, the tale that accompanies it might be one of your favorites to tell. In the next section, we'll talk briefly about how to balance information about EFs and strategy use with academic data on report cards, and then we'll provide you with five different practical examples of how to make your summative assessment more meaningful and powerful.

BALANCING ACADEMIC AND EF GOALS
IN SUMMATIVE ASSESSMENT

If you're reading this book from back to front, you may now be dabbling with a few new teaching tricks: EF literacy, close observation, barriers and strategies conversations, and process-oriented feedback. In this case, we won't be surprised if you have accumulated quite a bit of information regarding your students' use of strategy. You may have collected anecdotal notes on how they managed a group project. You may have a chart on which you have kept track of specific organizational strategies used during math class. Or you may have a week-by-week record of attention, flexibility, and emotional control shown during lessons. Alongside your math scores, reading levels, and project rubrics, any information you have managed to gather about your students' EF strategy use will be very useful and important come report card time.

Many jurisdictions have finally begun to emphasize the teaching of "soft" skills related to EF, process, and 21st-century learning skills. It is about time! At school, EF often explains more than half of all variation in academic performance (Visu-Petra et al., 2011). Recent guidance from the Center for Curriculum Redesign suggests that teachers should focus as much on "soft" skills, those related to collaboration, communication, and self-regulated learning, as on foundational knowledge such as mathematics, literacy, and science (Bialik & Fadel, 2015).

So, the shift toward reporting this learning has begun, albeit slowly and inconsistently. For example, you may have a whole page of tick boxes devoted to learning strategies. Or you may find EF indicators such as "organization" woven among character-based indicators such as "responsibility." Many report cards have empty text boxes in which anecdotal comments must be entered. When filling in these boxes, teachers are often encouraged to describe their learners in terms of their accomplishments and next steps. Armed with actual observations, information, and data about how your students have accomplished their learning, you may *finally* feel prepared to fill in those boxes. An EF-literate teacher with a lot of notes on process and EF strategy can have a field day. Can you imagine writing comments that balance academic and EF strategy reporting like this?

- Johan can add, subtract, multiply, and divide whole numbers. He prefers to use a highlighting strategy to focus his attention on each detail in written questions when applying these skills to problem solving.
- Michael has made solid progress on his time management skills this term, which has supported his ability to plan and complete a three-part essay. He said, "I discovered that if I chunked my time and wrote down how long I worked on each section, it helped me complete my essay on time."
- Mae uses written notes to help organize and prioritize the ideas she presents during debate. With this preparation, she presents clear and well-reasoned arguments with confidence.

In Figures 6.1–6.3, we present the report cards from just a handful of English-speaking places—Toronto, London, and New York—and highlight the ways they facilitate summative reporting about EF strategy use. It is important to note that each of these report cards also includes space for anecdotal comments, so a teacher using any of these templates could include as much information about EF strategy use as desired. In the Toronto District School Board, teachers use a provincewide (Ontario) report card, and a rating of "Learning Skills and Work Habits" occupies the whole first page. On the NYC Department of Education report, a similar section sits at the bottom and is called "Academic and Personal Behaviors/Teacher." In London, the report cards are not as standardized, but one designed by a typical state (public) school includes a rating system for assessing independence, engagement, and behavior. In all cases, references to EFs were easy to find, either explicitly or implicitly. Take a look; when we found a connection to an EF, we highlighted it and described our connection in brackets. If you look hard, you'll probably find a connection we missed. You may also notice that we weren't able to find a reference to working memory on any of these report cards. We wonder if there might be a way to refer to this EF in parent-friendly language. It might sound something like "Can manage complex tasks with multiple demands."

The evolution toward tracking process and EFs in report cards is important for several reasons. First, a report card is a formal and important document, and our choice of what to include on it sends a message about what we value. By including a comment about a student's most effective strategy alongside their academic results, we reinforce the idea that these two types of performance are equally important. While we may personally convey this message in our classrooms, we cement it as fact by making it a part of our official assessment documentation. This phenomenon has been studied and researched, and is referred to as a "backwash" effect, through which our formal, summative assessments dominate what students are oriented toward in their learning (e.g., Baartman, Bastiaens, Kirschner, & Van der Vleuten, 2006). If learning to use strategies is a part of our classroom program but those strategies don't make it onto the report card, they won't really "count" as far as students are concerned.

There are even deeper psychological reasons to include information about EF strategy use on report cards. Decades of research confirm that one of the biggest predictors of academic success is an understanding of and belief in one's own capabilities, also called self-efficacy (e.g., Bandura, 1997). How do our report cards affect this important feeling in our students? Well, for those who are highly skilled academically, reading a report card might feel pretty terrific. On report card day, a student in this situation might rip open the envelope, devour every glowing detail, share it with anyone who will listen, and think, "I am so powerful! I can do anything!" A student like this will likely begin the next term of study full of energy, determination, and self-efficacy, and in this way, the "rich" get richer. But what about students who are not as academically skilled and won't receive

Learning Skills and Work Habits	E – Excellent G – Good S – Satisfactory N – Needs Improvement
Responsibility	**Organization**
• Fulfils responsibilities and commitments within the learning environment (*goal-directed persistence*). • Completes and submits class work, homework, and assignments according to **agreed-upon timelines** (*time management*). • Takes responsibility for and **manages own behavior** (*response inhibition*).	• **Devises and follows a plan** (*planning and prioritizing*) and process for completing work and tasks. • **Establishes priorities** (planning and prioritizing) and **manages time** (*time management*) to complete tasks and achieve goals. • Identifies, gathers, evaluates, and uses information, technology and resources to complete tasks.
Independent Work	**Collaboration**
• **Fulfils responsibilities and commitments** (*goal-directed persistence*) within the learning environment. • Completes and submits class work, homework, and assignments **according to agreed-upon timelines** (*time management*). • Takes responsibility for and manages own behaviour.	• **Accepts various roles** (*flexibility*) and an equitable share of work in a group. • **Responds positively to the ideas, opinion and values of others** (*emotional control*). • Builds healthy peer-to-peer relationships through personal and media-assisted interactions. • **Works with others to resolve conflicts** (*emotional control*) and **build consensus** (*flexibility*) to achieve group goals. Shares information, resources, and thinking to solve problems and make decisions.
Initiative	**Self-Regulation**
• Looks for and **acts on new ideas and opportunities for learning** (*task initiation*). • Demonstrates the capacity for innovation and a **willingness to take risks** (*emotional control*). • Demonstrates curiosity and **interest in learning** (*attention*). • Approaches new tasks with a positive attitude. • **Recognizes and advocates appropriately for the rights of self and others** (*response inhibition*).	• **Sets own individual goals and monitors progress towards achieving them** (*goal-directed persistence, metacognition*). • **Seeks clarification** (*goal-directed persistence*) or assistance when needed. • **Assesses and reflects critically on own strengths, needs, and interests** (*metacognition*). • **Identifies learning opportunities, choices, and strategies to meet personal needs and achieve goals** (*metacognition*). • **Perseveres and makes an effort when responding to challenges** (*goal-directed persistence*).

FIGURE 6.1. Learning skills and work habits. Implicit and explicit references to executive functions in a report card from Toronto, Ontario, Canada. As of 2019, this figure appeared as the first of four pages on the Ontario provincial report card. The following two pages presented grades for each academic subject with space for teacher comments regarding strengths and next steps. The fourth page included a description of each letter grade; space for teacher, principal, and parents' signatures; and space for parent and child reflections and comments. Bolding has been added to highlight aspects related to executive functioning; parenthetical and *italicized* comments have been added by the authors. Copyright © 2014 Queen's Printer for Ontario. Reproduced with permission.

Descriptors of Learning	
Independence	
1	Works independently **using a variety of strategies to ensure full understanding** (*metacognition*). Homework is always handed in **on time** (*time management*) and goes beyond what is expected of a student at this stage. Always **fully equipped** (*planning, organization*) for lessons.
2	Works independently the majority of the time with some support occasionally. Homework is routinely handed in on time and completed to a good standard. Usually well equipped for lessons.
3	Can work independently on occasion but needs support to do so. Homework is not always handed in on time and may be late and/or lacking in effort. Sometimes does not have the correct equipment for lessons.
4	Is not yet working independently and routinely needs to be guided through tasks. Homework is often not handed in. Regularly does not have the correct equipment for lessons.
Engagement	
1	Is **fully engaged** (*attention*) with all areas of the subject; **always keen to contribute to class discussions and group work** (*attention*).
2	Engages well in most areas of the subject; often contributes to class discussions and usually makes a positive contribution to group work.
3	Is not always fully engaged with the subject and needs prompting to question and develop ideas, making limited contributions to class discussions and group work.
4	Shows little engagement with the subject; often needing to be kept on task or frequently missing key ideas as a result of not participating adequately.
Behavior	
1	Demonstrates impeccable behavior at all times. **Makes mature choices** (*response inhibition*), **consistently works hard** (*goal-directed persistence, attention*) and is a role model for others.
2	Demonstrates good behavior. Generally chooses to work hard with only occasional lapses.
3	Does not consistently demonstrate a high standard of behavior and/or is easily distracted by others. Shows the ability to make positive decisions but does not always do so.
4	Does not behave in an acceptable manner in lessons therefore progress is impeded. Behavior is a serious concern as it is often detrimental to the learning of others.

FIGURE 6.2. Implicit and explicit references to executive functions in a report card from London, United Kingdom. As of 2019, this figure appeared as the third of three pages on the report card for an 11-year-old student at a typical state school in London. It explains numerical scores that will be awarded on the first page. The first page of this report was filled with academic and independence/engagement/behavior scores for autumn, spring, and summer, and the second page held explanations of the academic scores, which were explained. It represents a typical format that is adjusted and tailored slightly from school to school. Bolding has been added to highlight aspects related to executive functioning; parenthetical and *italicized* comments have been added by the authors.

a report that satisfies their need to feel capable and competent? In this case, reading a report card might be a real drag. This student might leave the dreaded school envelope in his or her backpack for several days and share it only when asked, eventually pretending not to care about its contents. "I can't do anything," such a student might reflect, "so why even try?" Because we know about the impact of self-efficacy, we understand that a report card focused predominantly on lack of skill is a big problem. By failing to confirm any evidence of efficacy, it can further disadvantage and deplete an already "poor" student.

Academic and Personal Behaviors/Teacher	Marking Period		
Manages time (*time management*) and **consistently demonstrates effort** (*attention*) to **independently achieve goals** (*goal-directed persistence*)			
Works in an **organized** (*organization*) manner			
Persists through challenges (*goal-directed persistence*) to complete a task by **trying different strategies** (*metacognition*)			
Asks for help (goal-directed persistence) when needed			
Respects school rules and works well in the school community			

FIGURE 6.3. Implicit and explicit references to executive functions in a report card from New York City. As of 2019, this figure appeared as part of a large one-page table comprising the standard grades 3–5 of a New York City report card. Schools can either use this report or create something different with different grading methods. Bolding has been added to highlight aspects related to executive functioning; parenthetical and *italicized* comments have been added by the authors. Used with permission.

Because of this worry about self-efficacy, we may be tempted to blur and obfuscate a tough academic result. While understandable, it may not be necessary to compromise accuracy in such an important record of learning. Rather, we can worry less about reporting below-average academic performance if it is balanced with other indications of efficacy. At any academic level, every single one of our students is capable of doing really cool, innovative things. Students with learning disabilities can dazzle us with compensatory strategies, use of technology, and self-advocacy, among many other things. Students with no background in a subject can impress us with their ability to quickly form personal connections, access information using partners, and develop personal systems for staying organized. Our reports should include these types of important accomplishments, whenever possible. By including this information about EFs, process, and strategy use in report cards, we can balance information about core academic skills and ensure these documents reflect the whole picture of our students' efficacy. This is important! Recently, researchers have begun to carefully tease the feeling of self-efficacy apart from other forms of positive thinking such as "grit" or an effortful attitude. They have found that a student who thinks he or she has the skills necessary for success—self-efficacy—will far outperform one with a simple commitment to working hard (Usher, Caihong, Butz, & Rojas, 2018). This means that a report card documenting a students' specific strategy use will be much more powerful than one focused on effort. We have been talking about educating the whole child for so many years. Isn't it time that we started to *report* on the whole child?

Of course, we will also come across students who are struggling academically but not doing anything else that we find particularly innovative or impressive. These are the students who have given up on being efficacious according to socially acceptable means and may instead be pursuing nonstandard and much less helpful forms of mastery. We may find them absorbed in despairing or angry activities, at which they have achieved all-time superstar status: a first-rate absentee, bully, or prankster perhaps? There may be more than one of these students. Some years, it may seem as if this describes your whole class. In this case, we've got some bad news and we've got some good news. The bad news is you may be trying to report on students who have previously had a very discouraging time at school. They may not know their processes and strategies are delightful and important. The good news is that fixing that problem is what Chapters 1 through 5 of this book are all about. Your hard work learning from those chapters may turn the tide.

> ### How to Assess EF Strategy Use:
> ### *Early Days*
>
> The big idea here is that it is tempting to stop after you've taught students about EFs. We'll encourage you to teach students how to use their EFs. In this section, you'll learn more about how to do the following:
>
> - Ensure you have embedded EF literacy deeply into your daily pedagogy, observation, and feedback. You can't assess it if you haven't taught it!
> - Change your teaching approach. The time is now, so be bold!

"How to" or "how *not* to do," that is the question. This, the first of five practical sections on summative assessment of EF-based skills, takes a slightly new approach by focusing on what *not* to do. This may seem a bit too theoretical for a "how to" section, but let us explain. We'll describe such an exceedingly common mistake that we feel our warning will resonate with many teachers. To help you fully appreciate the scenario we're alerting you to, we'll frame our discussion in a "ghost of schoolyear future" type of story. To really evoke Dickens's *A Christmas Carol,* you may wish to imagine a sleepy version of yourself in old-timey pajamas and a long nightcap.

We'll describe a mistake that teachers often make despite the very best of intentions. Think of your own best intentions: If you've read this far, you might feel full of enthusiasm for "growth mindset" teaching. You may have risen today fresh from a good night's sleep, strode energetically across the room, and thrown open the shutters to look out at the day with a great deal of satisfaction. Life is good! Teaching is good! You might have whistled as you logged in to social media, scrolled through inspiring growth mindset postings, and clicked on a podcast discussing grit. You might have smiled as you reflected on chapters of this very book, or the big assessment conference you attended this summer in which the value of process skills was mentioned. No matter what you've learned, let's assume you plan to end your unit, term, or school year with big student improvements to things like grit, growth mindset, and EF strategy use. Further, let's imagine you also intend to emphasize them in conferences, in portfolios, or on report cards. The mistake we're referring to is often innocently committed by people just as knowledgeable and invested as are you.

The mistake is simple. It is a comfy little *partial* approach to being a growth mindset teacher that is often substituted for the deeper and more pedagogical change that we and others (Dweck, 2016) have advocated. The partial approach does not operate on your regular observation, instruction, and assessment activities. Rather, it takes place in addition to and around these things during special add-on periods and lessons. Below, we'll briefly reemphasize the value of using a fully pedagogical approach, but more importantly we'll characterize the partial approach we're troubled by. Our goal is to forewarn you; while the partial approach can be added on with only a few simple handouts in a period or two, it cuts an awful lot of corners. Much like old Ebenezer Scrooge, you might not fully appreciate where this penny pinching is leading you, and how it might affect your results. So, before you get started, let's talk about the early days of September.

Let's step into the future. Do you see yourself among all of those teachers heading off into classrooms? There are your students, there is your desk, and there is your coffee mug. The bell has rung, and your school year has begun. As a teacher, you have a few new tricks: The *future you* is well equipped and optimistic, making frequent mention of growth mindset, effort, and grit. You have designated a period to explain what growth mindset is, and if you listen carefully you may hear yourself saying, "Students, you should have a growth mindset because you can do anything you set your mind to! Effort is what counts!" During this period, based on an activity you found online, you may ask your students to write one thing they like about themselves for a display on the classroom door. Look along the back wall of your classroom—you might have set up a bulletin board that says, "Grit Is What We Got!" and tomorrow you might ask each child to write a few words about a time that he or she worked hard or showed effort. The next day, you might ask the class to sort a list of 12 phrases, including "This is too hard" and "It'll take me some time to get through this," into either growth or fixed mindset. You might even start to introduce the idea of EF, using one of the practical approaches from Chapter 1 of this book. These are powerful things to do. They will set a positive, optimistic tone and show your students that, in theory, you respect their process. All of these activities will take place before or after your academic work, requiring a special period or two. The problem is that you may not go any further—you may avoid making any substantive change to your core observation, instruction, and feedback practices. This happens for a very good reason—your habitual approaches are comfortable and familiar, and in a busy, stressful classroom that's a big advantage. When using your established pedagogy, you may feel most relaxed, in control, and well prepared. It may make you feel more lighthearted and playful, which is beneficial to your relationships with students. By naturally taking your growth mindset teaching along a path of least resistance, you reduce your stress, but you do not directly and regularly teach students how to respond to challenging situations with a strategic attitude.

What happens next? Weeks may pass and you may continue to refer to the bulletin board either a little or a lot. When your students are discouraged, you may remind them to maintain a growth mindset and you may even walk them over to the bulletin board for a refresher. They will understand that they should have a growth mindset, but your students' ability to respond to challenge with a strategic approach may remain about the same. They will not have learned when and how to apply strategic processes because, actually, they have not been taught. You may begin to feel frustrated and annoyed, and you may begin to suspect that your students' ability to use EF strategies is fixed: "Some of my kids can do it, and some just can't," you may think. This future is distinctly *not* leading toward a growth mindset and is almost certainly where you will find yourself if you don't specifically decide to do something different. This is the type of approach taken by many, *many* teachers who identify with the growth mindset movement. The partial approach relies more on lip service and cheerleading than deep, substantial *pedagogical* change.

We realize this is the first time that we've come right out and characterized something as a "mistake." We do this because there is a lot on the line. We want to draw a bright line between *pedagogical* and *partial* growth mindset approaches because they are so often muddled. We are concerned that the type of substantial change we advocate will be lumped together with other, more superficial approaches. So, to be frank, we do not advocate lip service, cheerleading, or simply whistling a new tune on an old path. Or, to follow our literary theme, we do not believe children will become more powerful simply because we've clicked our heels twice and mounted a bulletin board saying, "Growth Mindset! Growth Mindset! Growth Mindset!" We believe you need to make substantive change in your core teaching practices to foster substantive change in your students. In the end, despite your best intentions, you will either be able to write report card comments about how your students *talk about* growth mindset and *define* grit or be able to write comments about the specific and tangible strategies that they *actually use every day*.

Now step into the future of *pedagogical* growth mindset teaching. While the preceding chapters have provided a detailed description of a new, EF-literate approach, you might want a more straightforward and specific way to actually get started. Below is a glimpse of a tiny little weeklong plan that drives a dash of growth mindset deeply into your daily observation, instruction, and feedback. Though it is condensed, it may be the perfect way to get your feet wet and gather baseline information about what works and what doesn't. Also, attempting this plan will give you plenty to talk about with your grade partner, if you're lucky enough to have one willing to collaborate. Look! Here you are in a different future. Can you imagine?

1. On Monday, you define "executive functions" and describe a few key EFs. Perhaps you gather your students in front of a list of a few simple, intuitive ones, such as organization, time management, or attention. "These are the processes we use to meet our goals. Think about which one you are best at. I'm best at attention. It helps me when I listen to you speak and when I read your writing," you might say. After describing the ways you show attention to meet your goals, you may allow students to participate in the discussion.

2. On Tuesday, you bring EFs into your instruction. For example, you might say, "I'd like you to solve the following problem with a partner. Think about the barriers you will face. Which EFs do you think you will use? Which one will be hardest for you? And what strategy might you use to be successful?" You don't worry about making this conversation perfect—you simply write whatever ideas your students have on the board. Keep doing this several times every day and watch the conversations become richer.

3. On Wednesday, you start observing students' use of strategy to support their EFs. You challenge yourself to really watch and appreciate how your students operate. That's it—you just open your eyes and ears and really notice what they're doing. While you watch, you might comment, "Oh, how interesting!" or "Hmm . . . I just saw something I wasn't expecting."

4. On Thursday, you give students a typical academic task and start giving them feedback about the strategies they are using. For at least 5 minutes, you drop everything and just walk around the room noticing and naming, say, their organizational strategies. For example, you might say, "I just saw Josh pulling out his math book. He knows we have math class after recess. That's so organized!" or "I see three people making a list before they begin. Nice planning strategy!" or "Sadia just checked the time. I wonder if anyone else will use Sadia's time management strategy?"

5. On Friday, you feel ready to sit down with a colleague to discuss your progress. What approaches worked? What needs to be modified? What needs a little more discussion or teaching? With just 1 week of experience, you have a feel for a wide variety of approaches and are hungry for more information. At this point, you flip back though Chapters 1–5 to find examples of classroom practice that will be right for you and your students.

For teachers, time marches forward unrelentingly. We do not have the luxury of putting off decisions about how we will teach—before we know it, the summer, the break, or the weekend is over, and there we are again standing in front of a room full of students making decisions and changing lives. Just as quickly, it will be report card time and we will be conducting summative assessments. We hope this discussion has given you a sense of the distinct choices you have as an EF-literate teacher and where they may lead.

> ### How to Assess EF Strategy Use:
> ### *Goal Setting in the Early Days*
>
> The big idea here is that your students can get started by targeting specific EFs to work on. In this section, you'll learn more about how to do the following:
>
> - Model goal setting for your students. By mentioning an EF you struggle with and telling your students about a goal you would genuinely like to achieve, you can show them it is safe to be self-accepting, self-compassionate, and strategic.
> - Encourage your students to create their own goals by asking, "What EF do you struggle with?" and "What EF goal will you create for this term?"

After you get your feet wet, you might be interested in doing a goal-setting activity. The creation of goals falls naturally at the beginning of a cycle of summative assessment and can provide focus for both you and your class. In the same way that we work with our students to make academic targets, such as moving up a reading level or mastering certain times tables, we can also encourage them to think about the learning skills, process steps, and EFs they would like to improve upon. We'll focus our attention on teachers who have developed EF literacy in their classrooms, but much of the terminology they use can suit a generic conversation. EFs such as attention, time management, organization, and emotional control, for example, can be discussed with very little background preparation. The most important thing is to open up a conversation about what approach they would like to take to achieve their academic goals; we can then reflect on whether those approaches were effective in our summative evaluation. We have two interesting examples.

Stacey Falconer, who teaches a group of eight students (grades 4–6) with learning disabilities, begins her term by setting process-based goals.[2] But before asking a group of unfamiliar, nervous students to reveal their areas for growth, she will include them in a conversation about a goal of her own. Once she told her class that she wanted to become a better teacher by improving her time management skills: "I want to remember to give 2-minute warnings before we start something new, but it really doesn't come naturally to me. How can I manage? Does anyone have a suggestion for me?" After a discussion during which the students helped Stacey devise strategies and approaches, she noticed they were more willing to open up about their own challenges. To further ease the process of goal setting, Stacey followed her example by charting her students' ideas about "the types of goals students like us *might* have." By easing the conversation toward personal goals slowly, Stacey provided the time and safety needed to reassure any feelings of reservation, discouragement, or distrust. This modeling of self-understanding and self-compassion is a key approach that is used by many successful EF-literate teachers and is particularly important when working with students who may be stressed or defensive. We'll provide information about an even more in-depth calming trick that Stacey uses in our "how to" section relating specifically to stressed students.

Kirstyn Pepall also sets EF goals with her grade 5 class, according to a similar process.[3] After a brief introduction to EFs, her students are asked to decide in which area of EF they feel most

---

[2] Stacey Falconer teaches at Lakeshore Public School in Burlington, Ontario, Canada. Used with permission.

[3] Kirstyn Pepall teaches at Legacy Public School in Markham, Ontario, Canada. Used with permission.

challenged and to create a simple goal for improvement. For example, a typical goal for organization might be "to always put my materials neatly into my binders," a goal for response inhibition "to listen more patiently during groupwork," and a goal for time management "to use my calendar more often for homework deadlines." Then these goals are jotted on small, individual "EF Goals" sheets and posted in a quick and cheerful display.

When the goals are set and displayed, they become very useful. They can be referred to often and woven into daily conversations about learning. A teacher like Kirstyn, for example, can wander by the display and mention posted goals during teaching, perhaps grouping teams of students who are focused on similar EF goals for certain tasks. For example, when assigning an essay, she might say, "Before beginning, I'd like those students with planning and prioritizing goals to get together to discuss strategies. Please report back to me with three good ideas before starting." Or, when assigning multistep math calculations, she might ask the students with both working memory and attention goals to develop strategies and share them with the class. The working memory team might suggest that students say each step out loud or work with a partner to avoid errors. The attention-focused students might suggest strategies such as quiet workspaces, underlining questions to show a double-check has been done, or wearing headphones to block out distractions. In this way, teachers can keep students' goals front and center during teaching, ensure they are building useful strategies, and also have specific targets to reflect on when making summative assessments. Stephanie Walker also asks her students to set EF goals and described how they sometimes spontaneously refer to them.[4] Knowing one of her students was working toward better response inhibition made it extra satisfying to hear him quietly reflect, "I really didn't mean to just shout that" after finishing a task and hollering, "I'm *done!*" For Stephanie, this particular student's emerging self-awareness and self-monitoring represented huge progress. Watching students awaken to goal *striving* is so exciting.

How to Assess EF Strategy Use:
Time Strapped

The big idea here is that you can get your students to help you gather data on their EF growth. In this section, you'll learn more about how to do the following:

- Work with students at the end of a project, unit, or term to determine specific EF barriers and strategies that played a role in their success.
- Work with younger students in age-appropriate ways to gather end-of-term data regarding their learning, reflections, barriers, and strategies.

The report card deadline is a week away. Your academic assessment is finished, and your grades have been calculated and entered. Depending on how comment heavy your report cards are, you now have somewhere between 2 and 20 hours of work left. This task of crafting comments about students' learning often takes forever because we have so little substantive information to work with. Instead, we engage in an often agonizingly slow process of weaving tidbits about our program ("This term, Alexa participated in a geometry unit . . .") with chatty, subjective commentary ("She enjoyed manipulating 2-D shapes to make a patterned quilt . . .") and with vague qualifiers to explain any highs or lows in grades ("Alexa required occasional support to manage

---

[4] Stephanie Walker teaches at Scott Young Public School in Omemee, Ontario, Canada. Used with permission.

the expectations of this unit.") To complete your class list, you may be writing upward of 8,000 words that don't feel very useful, and nothing fires up writer's block and resentment like a lack of purpose. To remedy this frustrating and time-consuming situation, some teachers rely heavily on cut and paste, which further depletes the meaningfulness of the work. Others advocate slashing report templates back to checkboxes or marks-only. Who can blame them?

We think, however, that when based on tangible, personal information about process and EF-based strategy, writing report card comments can feel like time well spent. They can provide essential information about context, process, and next steps and, just like the "discussion" and "conclusion" sections of a well-written research paper, make raw data points meaningful. The challenge is that we often just don't have enough information. We sit down to write thinking we must know so much about our students, and then spend hours grinding through what ends up being a *creative* project. How is it possible not to know everything about students after so much time spent together? If we haven't been gathering information about process and strategy all along, accurate information about it often hides behind our erroneous assumptions, students' crafty excuses and compensation, and the sheer volume and intensity of what we manage in a classroom. For example, you may pick up on the fact that Adele's book report is late because of a written organizational problem, but maybe you won't. Maybe that information will be confounded by the fact that she's also noisy or messy. Or maybe you'll miss it because eight other students were late and there was just too much going on. We're suggesting that after months of FaceTime with students, what you have passively gathered about why they perform the way they do may be much skimpier than you realize. This is a well-known, normal phenomenon called "illusory superiority," and it refers to an exaggerated feeling of expertise. This is good news, actually, because it probably explains a large part of the struggle we have when writing anecdotal report card comments. We have a suggestion for how to quickly deepen them.

For this discussion of "time-strapped" teaching, we'll assume you haven't been documenting EF or process-oriented information about your students throughout the term; let's talk about how to quickly gather it up. You probably already know this, but *student self-evaluation* is a huge time saver. While, of course, rich information is gathered through longer-term observation, feedback, and documentation, in this case there's nothing wrong with doing an intense little burst of assessment right at the end of a learning cycle. To do this, you'll need a period with your students and a few focused questions. Julie Hough provided us with a good example of how this can work.[5] While she typically uses a range of both fast and slow assessment approaches, she finds that this little trick works no matter how much information she already has.

Julie was getting ready to write report card comments for grades 7/8 English language arts. During the first term, her students had focused much of their attention on a book report project, so she simply jotted two questions on the board: "What was your biggest executive functioning challenge when working on the novel study? What was your biggest executive functioning strength when working on the novel study? Give examples." It is not necessary to refer specifically to EFs in your question, of course. You could simply ask students about their biggest "challenge or barrier" and most useful "strategy." A student responded as follows:

> "My strength in my novel study is working memory. I say this because whenever I am reading my book I can remember what I read so I can apply it to my work. An example of when I used

---

[5] Julie Hough teaches at Central Senior Public School in Lindsay, Ontario, Canada. Used with permission.

working memory is when I was reading *Grown* and *The Perfect Ten*. I remembered important events to add to my summary for the novel study. I struggle with task initiation. I say this because sometimes I run out of time during the week so I get stuck doing both of the novel studies in one day. An example of when I did this was for our 15th and 16th entries. I left the two entries for one day.”[6]

Armed with a pile of student responses like these, Julie would be much more informed about her students; she would know them better as individuals and as a class. Reviewing many responses, she might notice patterns of challenge or strength, and might come up with ideas for how to improve her classroom context or instruction. If, for example, many students mentioned time management as a challenge, she might front-load a lesson dealing with time management onto her next unit of study for these students, and onto the book report unit the next time she taught it. Julie would also be much more prepared to document meaningful information on a report card. Assuming this reflection was submitted by a student with good book report results, Julie might have followed a sentence describing the academic results with a comment such as this:

"For [this student], reading, understanding, and remembering grade-level material is less of a challenge than managing time. She sometimes rushes work meant to be done throughout the week and packs it into 1 or 2 days. With better organization, planning, and time management, [this student] could get started earlier and earn even better results."

In just a few short sentences, this report card comment presents an encouraging and unique record of efficacy (strength in academic performance *and* working memory are noted), a specific record of difficulty, and an actionable recommendation for next steps. A student, future teacher, tutor, coach, or parent receiving this report would know a lot about this learner and exactly how to proceed.

Consider how Julie's task of composing personal and useful comments for every single student in her class might have been eased by the wide variety of responses she received. For example, when answering the same two questions, one of her students mentioned challenges with flexibility ("I need to see it through more than one person's view"), while another mentioned challenges with metacognition ("I make the same mistakes over and over again and don't try to make my novel study better"). The students' reflections on their strengths were just as diverse. In our experience, when you actually have the information you need, writing good summative comments on report cards isn't actually that hard. Instead of grinding them out based on foggy recollections and artful repetition, we can use them to document information that is genuinely interesting, useful, and unique. Julie comments, and we agree, that when she takes the time to collect process-based information from and with students, her report cards seem to "write themselves."

Is there any way for teachers of younger students to reap these benefits? We think so. With a little more time, and perhaps simpler vocabulary, this approach works just as well for those with basic writing skills. For prewriters, teachers can gather simple smiley and serious faces, or checks and crosses, on photos or sketches of different classroom EF challenges. For example, students can put "ratings" on a page with six small photos or sketches of different classroom challenges such as sharing (flexibility), turn taking (response inhibition), sitting on the carpet (attention), being pushed (emotional control), threading beads or cutting (goal-directed persistence), and following

---

[6] Some details changed to protect privacy.

two-step directions (working memory). Collecting these pages, a teacher can see that for Alita, goal-directed persistence feels like a big frown and response inhibition feels like a giant smile. This would provide just a little bit of information about which EFs may be more or less challenging, and it might be surprising and useful. This activity would be even more revealing if done during a one-on-one chat, in which teachers ask for further information, engage students in discussion, and isolate them from the temptation of parroting their friends' responses.

At any level, this simple approach is a big win in terms of logistics, and it might help you to get your reports done more quickly. You could easily use it as the final class for each and every unit of study you do. Even more importantly, however, is that it is itself a tremendously powerful process. Even if you accidentally leave all of the student responses you collect in the staff room and some-one shreds them by mistake, you will have created a formal, shared, structured time for summative reflection that may not otherwise happen.

How to Assess EF Strategy Use:
Highly Structured

The big idea here is that students can play a major role in assessing the growth and development of their EF skills. In this section, you'll learn more about how to do the following:

- Involve students in a self-assessment of their learning skills and strategies using your school's actual report card (or a simple chart that is similar).
- Recruit students to be your report card editors. They can adjust or add more detail to your comments about the processes and strategies they use.

If you have the luxury of starting early, a more structured approach to summative process-oriented assessment can be powerful. In this section, we'll describe Julie Hough's (grades 7/8) yearlong summative activities, including self-assessment, goal setting, frequent check-ins, and collaborative report card writing. There's a lot here, but don't be overwhelmed. This represents a year's worth of material, but it is all very simple, straightforward, and practical. In fact, her approaches are so classic that you could probably modify them all the way down to grade 1. These are approaches she used single-handedly with a full-sized class.

Do you recall seeing the front page of the Ontario report card in Figure 6.1? This page forms the basis of Julie's summative assessment process. At the beginning of the year, before starting any assessment, Julie makes sure her students really understand what those indicators mean. To do this, she copies the first page of the report, cuts the learning skills into strips, and has her students sort them into piles of "do" and "do not understand"; then they work together to rewrite the tricky ones into more student-friendly language. This would be easy to do with a wide variety of different report cards.

Then, at the beginning of school and again before each of the three report cards, Julie con-ducts a self-assessment survey with her class using each of these "learning skills" indicators. There's nothing very fancy about this; she simply takes each and every indicator exactly as it appears on the report card, provides precisely the same scoring system, and asks students to self-assess. In this way, they complete a *mock* report card. You can imagine how informative and useful this is for students at the very beginning of a school year, when they may not know exactly what Julie is looking for in their performance. Starting the year with overarching expectations clearly in mind is like beginning a race with a wide-open view of the finish line.

To her survey of report card learning skills, Julie attaches a series of reflection questions, which you will find in Figure 6.4. These questions probe students' thinking about their strongest and most challenging EFs and ask them for specific examples for each. It is important to note that Julie's students have plenty of practice with this type of reflective self-assessment, because she also incorporates it into rubrics for projects and assignments. Regardless, Julie is often surprised by what students write. The fact is, the way EF strength and weakness look to a teacher is often different than the way they feel to a student. So, for example, a student who seems to struggle with organization may reveal that time management is the source of the kerfuffle. Or what appears to be a strength in flexibility may feel to a student like a weakness in emotional regulation: "I need strategies to make sure I don't just cave in and do all of the work for the group." Much can be learned about individual students through this process, and there are also many enduring, general lessons for teachers. Never underestimate the extent to which biased and incorrect assumptions about student performance are made.

Working with her class in this way offers great benefit to Julie. She manages to supervise students through this process with only light, whole-class support, gathering learning skill levels and reflective comments that can be applied directly to her report cards. When there is a discrepancy between student and teacher perspective, Julie has time to indulge in one-on-one consultation: "I noticed you rated yourself as 'excellent' for 'self-regulation.' I'm concerned this doesn't reflect your challenges with mapping groupwork. Tell me what you were thinking?" While this allows Julie to consider the student's perspective and gather information she may not have been aware of, the students know the final decision belongs to Julie. Could you manage a process like this? When estimating how long it may take you to attempt it, you should subtract the time you might otherwise spend on your own searching for data and contemplating students' learning skills without their input. How long does that ordinarily take, do you think? Julie can conduct this process in one focused 45-minute period.

Speaking of involving students in a meaningful summative assessment process, you might be surprised at how Julie actually *writes* report cards. After several meetings with her bosses, Julie received permission to write her anecdotal comments both *to and with* her students. Let that sink in—we think it's fabulously cool and contemplated it with a good 10 minutes of "oh man, I wish I had thought of that" revelry. So, after drafting a first copy and submitting it to her admin for the usual approval, Julie makes a photocopy so students can add their edits. This serves a few purposes. First, students become more invested, as coauthors, in the process of formal reporting. They feel aligned in an important and authentic project as partners and collaborators with their teacher and principal. And this is not an empty gesture. The students often find inaccuracies, over- or underrepresentations, or omissions in Julie's description of their learning skills. She said it keeps her honest and reminds her to steer away from "edubabble." On a basic and obvious level, this process also just ensures the kids have read the darn things. Julie comments that this makes a big difference because it allows her to refer to them throughout the year, asking the students about their goals or how they feel they are progressing on certain tasks. To return to a long-distance swimming metaphor, can you imagine if a swimming coach wrote, "You were swimming to the left the whole time and it cost you 5 minutes. You need to defog your goggles and steer more to the right," and the swimmer took it home, gave it to her parents, and never looked at it? Absurd.

You will discuss two EF skills, one that you feel is a strength and one that is a challenge.

1. My biggest EF strength is _____. I show it when I

_____

_____

_____ .

2. I showed this during the year when I _____ .

_____

_____

_____

_____ .

3. Next year I will (set a goal for yourself) _____ .

_____

_____

_____ .

4. My biggest EF challenge is _____. I show it when I

_____

_____

_____ .

5. I showed this during the year when I _____ .

_____

_____

_____

_____ .

Next year I will (set a goal for yourself) _____

_____

_____

_____ .

FIGURE 6.4. Worksheet for reflection on EF skills. Created by Julie Hough at Woodville Elementary School in Woodville, Ontario, Canada. Used with permission.

Because she uses this structured process, Julie's report card comments are very specific. A sample has been included below, with the student's name and specific details changed to protect privacy. We have **bolded** aspects of the comment that resulted from student consultation. You can see how they comprise about half of the comment, in balance with other information about "Alex's" academic and social work.

"Alex, you made a very smooth and positive adjustment to life at [school name]. You continued to consistently complete all tasks thoroughly and with attention to the expectations. **I enjoyed seeing you become an independent learner who developed systems to organize large-scale projects like your sustainable city and novel study. You enjoyed the responsibility that came with having choice, and you rose to the challenge each time. I was regularly impressed with the strategies you used to keep track of work or your notes. Make sure you continue to think and work like this next year. You checked in with me throughout the day to make sure you were 'on track.' Advocating for yourself like this is very important, and you need to ensure you do it next year as well.** Your social achievements this year were strong too. You made new friends, had fun throughout the day, and developed positive relationships with peers and adults outside of your classroom. You leave others with a warm impression. Putting in the effort in a new school is important. I hope you continue to make good choices about your peer group next year so you can avoid any conflict or trouble that would prevent you from having a good experience at school. **On a learning skills survey you highlighted a number of achievements you are proud of this year, particularly being so organized and independent. You felt your hard work paid off in math, literacy, and social studies. You need to keep all of your strategies and tools in mind for next year, where you will be expected to take more ownership over the day.** I look forward to seeing the great things you'll do next."

After all this summative reporting is behind them, Julie conducts one last activity to help prepare her students for their transition to high school. At the end of the school year, Julie and her students create a summary of the most important insights about their learning. They call it a "passport" because, although it is an essential reflection experience for the students themselves, the intended audience is the following year's teacher. Though every teacher, year, and curriculum is different, Julie hopes it will remind students of their effective processes and strategies and also give the following year's teacher a little heads-up. The passport focuses on many different academic areas and project types: "Anything I think the students may encounter again," Julie told us. In Figure 6.5, you'll see two different examples of the simple, point-form notes students typically make about their strengths, challenges, and strategies. Julie conducts this activity with upward of 30 students, so she does not tweak, perfect, or otherwise change the students' responses. Accordingly, you'll notice that some students wrote more than others, and within each students' passport, the entries vary from being really on point to a little incomplete. Creating this document helps students notice patterns in their strengths, challenges, and strategies across subjects, so they can stitch together a sense of what they are like as learners. Julie told us that it also stimulates a real sense of pride and satisfaction, because students can appreciate the depth and breadth of their learning at a glance. As such, Julie sometimes adds an extra dose of this experience around midyear. Regardless, by the time this passport activity rolls around, Julie's students are pretty self-aware with plenty to share.

Julie tells us that during her first year of teaching, a more senior colleague suggested she not "waste" too much time on report cards. "They have a 5-second shelf life," she was advised. Julie,

Area (project or situation)	Info (strengths, challenges, interests)	Strategies I have for this (be specific)
General executive functioning strengths	Thinking through, taking my time	Focusing on it and not talking
General executive functioning challenges	Not always reading the last piece of information	Taking my time
Group projects	City, Playground	Splitting the work
Reading	Crossover, The Hate U Give, The Hunger Games	Making a schedule for times to read
Writing	Proof writing, using the whole paper	Not saying the same thing
Math	Problem solving, reading the question	Taking my time
Other things you need to know	I like shoes.	

Area (project or situation)	Info (strengths, challenges, interests)	Strategies I have for this (be specific)
General executive functioning strengths	Emotional control, planning tasks	Ask a teacher.
General executive functioning challenges	Organizing materials, monitoring	Use a binder.
Group projects	I'm easy going and get along with people, but I usually end up doing all the work.	Just not do work for other people or section it so I know what to do.
Reading	Fluency is a challenge for me. I like books that are about real-life problems.	Read more and find audiobooks or use Overdrive.
Writing	My writing is messy and I can't spell. I can write rough drafts quickly so I get feedback.	I use a computer and want to write more often. I want to make sure I check my work over.
Math	I know all my facts, although sometimes I forget them and just need more time. I'm not afraid to try things. I pick up on new things quickly. I find measurements and conversions hard.	I need a conversion chart—I know how to use it.
Other things you need to know	I will not be afraid to ask for a rubric. I want a binder.	

FIGURE 6.5. Sample summative "passports" created by students for next year's teacher. Some details changed to protect privacy. Created by Julie Hough at Woodville Elementary School in Woodville, Ontario, Canada. Used with permission.

being highly practical and more than a little determined, decided that if she was going to have to do them, she may as well make the process, as well as the final product, worthwhile. We like imagining the advice *she'd* give to a first-year teacher.

How to Assess EF Strategy Use:
Organic and Free Flowing

The big idea here is that in-person conversations with students are a powerful way to stimulate reflection and learning and gather assessment data. In this section, you'll learn more about how to do the following:

- Use a 10-minute one-on-one conversation to expand your understanding of a student's EF strengths and challenges.
- Provide a safe space for your students to share their fears and negative thoughts about their learning, and use this safe space to offer reassurance and a more positive interpretation of their abilities.

It's the end of a school term or year, and you're preparing to comment upon your students' process skills in report cards. You may have gathered little bits and pieces of data as part of your ongoing formative assessment, but you want to take one last look at the strategies your students have learned to use. Using a "free flowing and organic" approach, you hope to weave this final round of data gathering into your program in a way that is meaningful, personal, exploratory, and constructivist, avoiding methodology that seems mechanical. How can this be done?

We searched our community for a good example and found grade 4 teacher Charlene Chapman.[7] Like many of the summative assessors we spoke to, Charlene was eager to engage students as partners using reflection and self-assessment. Instead of asking for written reflection, however, Charlene created a schedule and recorded personal, one-on-one reflective conversations with each of her students. Each conversation took about 10 minutes, give or take, and she achieved several per day by scattering them creatively throughout her schedule. Though this was time-consuming, Charlene realized benefits for students, their parents, and for her own practice as a teacher.

Charlene used these conversations to reassure each student with a very important statement about her role as their teacher and assessor. This seemed long overdue. For years, Charlene had worried that, for those with difficulties at school, report cards had become a bit malodorous; written in private and often containing a few difficult truths, they seemed to be a kind of last word from teacher to student. After many months of trust and collaboration, it didn't make sense to deliver such important information in a one-sided, written document. *You thought your teacher liked you,* the report seemed to imply, *but wait till you see what's going into your permanent record!* While it is not common, we have probably all seen a report card that sounded a little ranting and negative. Rather, speaking to her students in person vaulted Charlene into a more healthy and professional position of caring and support. In each meeting, she softened the big black-and-white process of summative assessment with several clear, direct messages: I'm gathering information because I have enjoyed watching your progress, you are important and valued, your strengths are delightful, your challenges are understandable and okay, we can all improve performance through strategy

---

[7] Charlene Chapman teaches at Queen Victoria Public School in Lindsay, Ontario, Canada. Used with permission.

use, and I care about your long-term success. Charlene and her students came together across a table, looked each other in the eye, and negotiated new roles as assessor and the assessed—in our estimation, this shift in policy and tone was a breakthrough moment in report card diplomacy.

"Interviews allowed me to dig out the most surprising information," Charlene told us. She explained that, though she began the interviews knowing an awful lot about her students, the process often seemed to double her insight. She would begin with simple questions such as "What is your best strategy?" and "What is your biggest barrier?" It wasn't the initial question that mattered most, however, but her follow-up. Instead of having a student reply simply "My flexibility in groups has improved," Charlene used a spiral of "Why," "But, exactly how?" and "Can you tell me more?" prompts to move toward a deeper understanding of challenges and improvements. For example, a student with improved flexibility revealed that he used the strategy of asking more questions, which reduced his tendency to be controlling, allowing him to feel involved with group mates without being so overbearing. These more nuanced insights were safely recorded on an iPad video recorder placed unobtrusively on the table so they could be reviewed later, making perfect material for report cards. Charlene could share whole, full interpretations of her students' performance. Her learning about her students was profound. "I realized," she reflected, "that I should be doing these interviews earlier in the year."

Investing 10 minutes per student for interviews had another benefit. In addition to identifying students' growth in terms of strategy use, she could *triage and begin to address* any unproductive mindsets. For example, as her conversations progressed, she was struck by the persistent belief from a small handful of students that despite knowing exactly what they needed to do, they would "never be able to change." After several follow-up questions, these students all confided the same general feeling: hopelessness. "I am not really changing. I am not really growing. I am not the sort of person who will be successful." Reflecting on a hodgepodge of different types of performance, stretched out over months, struggling students simply couldn't pick out and believe in their successes. So, before the meeting was over, Charlene would roll up her sleeves and help these students sort through the jumble of experience. Together they could make a neat little pile of small but steady victories and make a plan for the growth to come. With unwavering support, she'd say, "Are you kidding? You've made really important progress this year and I'm *proud* of you." Her message was "You, too, are a changer and a grower." This is yet another example of something that is perfectly simple but may be overlooked in the rush and bother of classroom life: simply responding to a child having hopeless feelings with reassurance, confidence, and appreciation. And while there is no simple solution to the problem of hopeless mindsets, Charlene's moment of connection provided the bump she needed to continue building optimism and a sense of opportunity among her students.

Drawing upon these conversations, Charlene can write report card comments that refer deeply and specifically to individual student learning. And after all of the interviews are over, and report cards are written, Charlene thinks they make a nice tool for educating parents about the evolving function of school, teachers, and assessment. She hopes that, with this boost, parents will be more likely to reemphasize a growing and improving mindset among their children, and understand that though every problem cannot be solved in 1 year, a toolbox of strategies is steadily being accumulated. The final comments on Charlene's reports sounded like the excerpt below (names and some details have been changed to protect student identity). You may notice that while several ongoing challenges are described, the language is largely positive and encouraging.

"Learning skills are an important part of Lauren's learning. She has worked this year toward understanding herself better as a learner—her likes and dislikes, as well as her strengths and weaknesses. She has participated in classroom discussions around bettering ourselves by understanding the barriers we face and strategies we can choose to help us overcome these issues. When discussing her executive functions, Lauren said, 'I am good at planning and prioritizing. When we were building structures, I tested all of my motors first to make sure they were working.' Lauren has found it challenging to work in a group. Conflicts arise when she doesn't compromise her views. She has learned to be more flexible by asking questions, so everyone can feel involved and heard. Lauren is very comfortable and capable when leading students younger than herself. Overall, Lauren does a very good job at regulating herself when she attends school on a regular basis, but the longer her period of absence, the more she struggles. Lauren's next challenge is to develop strategies to ensure that she comes to school rested and prepared to learn."

Owing to this in-depth process, Charlene finishes her year with a healthy appreciation for her own strengths *and challenges* as an educator. More than ever, she is painfully aware of her students' leftover academic gaps, missing strategies, and discouraged mindsets. Like every teacher, she will worry over these challenges during the summer, plotting and planning for even better logistics and approaches next year. In addition, however, this process has helped Charlene tune in to some pretty encouraging victories. She knows that many students leave her classroom feeling they are growing and becoming more skilled. They report feeling proud of their accomplishments and eager to face new challenges. Also, a number of her students describe having expanded their social networks. Reflecting on this, she suspects that her approach "pulls students out of their boxes." Those who were once "pigeonholed" by lagging skills and excluded from certain classroom groupings are now more often seen, appreciated, and included by their peers. "The diversity of groups has tripled!" she reflects. Charlene also delights when the big, overall message she advances in her program, and summative assessment approach, is received. She's not trying to be right all the time, or dominate her students, or have the last word in some kind of snarky report card slam dunk. When trying to explain it, Charlene says, "I don't need to make smarter students; I need to make more strategic, self-aware, and conscientious students. I need to create lifelong learners." In a note written to her on the last day of school, one of her students nailed it: "I love that you don't just want me to be good this year; you want me to be great always."

How to Assess EF Strategy Use:
Working with a "Stressed" Class

The big idea here is that there are strategies and tactics to make self-assessment a little more manageable for stressed students. In this section, you'll learn more about how to do the following:

- Teach students to put some distance between themselves and difficult challenges, feedback, or assessments.
- Create specific, predictable times and spaces in which students can anticipate an open and honest conversation.

Stressed students are not always thrilled to engage in reflection, self-assessment, or anything requiring vulnerability, so attempting to tackle personal qualities like EFs or process skills may be even harder. How can we make it more likely that stressed students will open up and engage with us in the various forms of summative reflection and assessment we might attempt? In this section, we'll present an approach that works with younger and older students, and that connects satisfyingly to a niche of research of which you may not be aware.

First, let's dig into the science. To begin, get inside the emotions of a student who is ruminating over a challenging or disappointing result. In your world, this might translate to, say, showing up late for recess duty twice in one week and feeling that a couple of colleagues are subsequently irritated with you. Can you relate? The science tells us that if you feel bad about this, and worry about it quietly and alone, keeping it all to yourself and remaining absorbed in it, you might dwell on some rather unproductive feelings. Your troubled mind might cycle through feelings of inadequacy or frustration, or maybe even anger at the perceived reaction of your colleagues. You might call up a friend on your way home from school to vent. Conversely, however, if you find some distance from the mistake, separating it a bit from your *self* and seeing it a little more objectively, you might have an easier time. You might realize that you'd just had the kind of bad week that most people have from time to time, and that two lates aren't really that catastrophic. The difference, according to research, is *distance*. If we can take a step back and reflect on our challenges from a little bit of a distance, we can ease some of the most difficult emotions, reduce the temptation to blame, respond with more insight, and experience more closure (for review, see White, Kross, & Duckworth, 2015). It's a subtle insight, but when you're trying to engage stressed students in a moment of real, open, frank discussion about their performance, every little bit helps.

This research is hardly surprising. In fact, it seems obvious. Upon hearing it you may line it up with comments you typically make in your classroom, such as "Don't worry"; "It's no big deal"; or "Tomorrow's another day and we can try again." These are, indeed, *reassuring* comments, but if you really pay attention to the science, you notice that it recommends something just a little more specific. You would be closer to the science if you said, "Your behavior is not you"; "Yep, that's a problem, but let's step back and see it from a bit of distance"; or "Let's move away from it so we can actually see it." Do you notice the subtle difference? When helping students to create distance from challenges, we are not aiming to shrink or discount the importance of those challenges. Rather, we can confirm the importance of the challenge but encourage students to remove themselves from it. Taking this approach allows students to process the situation from a higher level, with more of a "big picture" perspective. From this position, removed from emotion, one can see a situation in its entirety.

To model this calm and objective self-reflection, Paula Barrow asked her primary class (senior kindergarten/grade 1) to help her reflect on her own teaching practices. "Just like you, I want to learn and get better every day," she told them. "I would like you to help me think of a few things I need to work on." Her students then helped her create a chart of successes and things she should change (Table 6.1), but before they started, she took a moment to confirm their trusting relationship:

"Teaching my students to be empathetic is a big thing for me, not just toward each other but toward anyone. I front-loaded this discussion by asking students to consider their comments a moment before sharing. I asked them to be reasonable and not make requests that I certainly cannot honour, like, for example, 'play all day' or 'no more writing.' I also asked them to consider my feelings. I told them that words can hurt and that we need to use metacognition and response inhibition before raising their hands."

In the list of things students suggested Paula should change were a few items that might have stung had she ruminated quietly upon them. She may have thought "Snacks? We missed snack on, like, one day!"; "Yeesh, I go to garage sales all summer and all you notice are the broken toys?"; and "Oh, man. I've really failed them if they are asking me for more stories . . ." Just like the kids, had she kept this process close and quiet, Paula might have indulged in blaming or self-doubt. Rather, while conducting her reflection in conversation with her students, she modeled an objective attitude. In response to their comment about toys, she said, "Oh. Hold on. That's a surprise but let me take a step back. Okay. Well, that is easy to fix!" While there is nothing particularly earth shattering about being calm and objective about your mistakes in front of kids, it is pretty crafty to intentionally create a space in which your real, genuine challenges will be exposed so you can model a healthy, objective response. It's even better if you can apply state-of-the-art science and intentionally use "distancing" language. To be even more direct, Paula might have explained how she was responding: "Oh! When you mentioned toys, my first feeling was a little hurt and defensive." At this, their eyes might widen; teachers' disclosures of personal feelings are often fascinating to students. She might continue, "But then I decided to put the problem down, stand back, and really get a look at it." She might have even gestured to a spot on the floor where she had "placed" the problem. This is one good way to teach even very young students to maintain their self-esteem and confidence, and to remain objective, when talking about challenges.

TABLE 6.1. Kindergarten/Grade 1 End-of-Year Feedback for Teacher

What should my teacher keep doing?	What should my teacher change?
A little bit of play	Jenga
See Saw	Snack everyday
Executive functions	More stories
Persuasive writing	Throw away broken toys
Math	Put old toys/games in storage and get different ones
Telling time	Agendas
Crafts	
Outside gym	
Keep tables where they are	
Chart paper talks (Barriers and Strategies Protocol)	
100th day of school	
Daily 5 and Daily 3	
Kinder sight words	
Day of the week/months	
Puzzles	

Note. This table is based on a chart created in Paula Barrow's senior kindergarten/grade 1 class at Queen Victoria Public School in Lindsay, Ontario, Canada. Used with permission.

Stacey Falconer, a grades 4–6 special education teacher, uses a slightly more involved method.[8] As a special ed. teacher, she spends a lot of time helping her students to understand themselves as learners and refine personal strategic approaches. Her class, therefore, is very well equipped to comment on the teaching approaches that Stacey uses to support their learning. She uses a survey called "Feedback for My Teacher" (Figure 6.6) to collect their initial responses. This tool offers three to five different examples of environmental supports for each EF, and asks students to rate the extent to which each one is provided in the classroom. These supports include accommodations to time, space, materials, and interactions, and just reading over the document is like taking a course in special education.

Imagine Stacey administering this tool with her students: About half of them retreated to a quiet place with the survey to read and contemplate, while others worked through it in a chatty, collaborative group. After about 20 minutes, the students regrouped with feedback that was, for Stacey, truly useful and often quite humbling: "I told them that I was genuinely shocked at some of my areas for growth." In a few cases, what she intended and what the students said they were receiving was completely different. For example, she thought she was providing students with adequate reminders about timing, deadlines, and transitions but realized she needed to drastically increase the dosage and frequency of this support to register any impact with students. As they watched her respond to their feedback, Stacey's students saw her progress through a series of feelings. Initially, Stacey tells us she genuinely felt bad. She was disappointed with herself, was a little mistrusting of the feedback, and felt tempted to assume her students had somehow misrepresented what she was doing. Sitting in her teachers' chair, however, mindful of modeling her very best behavior, she managed to slow down, consider the feedback more objectively, and finally use it to improve her performance. "Feedback can be hard, but it is so important," she reassured them. "I just needed a moment to take a breath and step back from what you told me. Now I can see it more clearly. I get it and I'm excited to try a new approach."

In addition to using distancing language and modeling objectivity, Stacey emphasized how *much* of her own sharing, connecting, honesty, and vulnerability it took to cultivate trust among her students. There is no faking it. "You have to be willing to take a risk," she told us, "reveal some weakness, admit to a few mistakes, and share your true feelings." From here, in Stacey's classroom, the students became more open to discussing strengths and challenges, first in private conversations and then among their peers. This is not to say that her students walk around all day in a permanent state of vulnerability—they are perfectly typical kids. Instead, Stacey dedicates specific time, sets a stage, and cues students for short, intense bursts of sharing. "It takes a lot of trust on both sides," she clarified. "We sit down on the floor together, and it may take a moment to shift gears." It is perhaps because they know she won't expect them to remain perfectly exposed that they feel comfortable sharing in the first place. When the room is calm and quiet, and everyone feels safe, Stacey can engage her students in objective discussions about their goals, their most effective strategies, and where they plan to go next.

---

[8] Stacey Falconer teaches at Lakeshore Public School in Burlington, Ontario, Canada.

Feedback for My Teacher	*How much does my teacher help my executive functions?* (a **T**on, a **L**ittle, **R**arely, almost **N**ever)

Response Inhibition

My teacher gives instructions slowly, so I can keep up.	T L R N
My teacher helps the class calmly and patiently.	T L R N
My teacher finds time to talk with me about personal things of interest.	T L R N

Working Memory

My teacher makes charts, posters, and other strategies that help me remember things.	T L R N
My teacher gives her instructions out loud and with some kind of visual.	T L R N
My teacher believes me when I tell her that I forgot.	T L R N
My teacher helps me connect new learning to things we already know.	T L R N

Sustained Attention

My teacher lets me eat a healthy snack or take a walk when I need it.	T L R N
My teacher tries to eliminate distractions.	T L R N
My teacher makes sure I know what to do before asking me to start my work.	T L R N
My teacher reminds me to get back to work if I become distracted, but she doesn't make me feel bad about it.	T L R N
My teacher posts the daily agenda, so I know what to expect.	T L R N
My teacher tries to make classes interesting and meaningful.	T L R N

Emotional Control

My teacher talks to us about emotions (both ours and others') and how to handle them.	T L R N
My teacher lets me have a break or go to a "safe, quiet spot" if I'm frustrated.	T L R N
My teacher lets me know when she's worried about me.	T L R N
My teacher has given me strategies that help me to calm down.	T L R N

Flexible Thinking

My teacher tells us when something unusual is going to happen—just gives us a quick "heads up."	T L R N
My teacher explains new situations and lets me ask questions if I'm unsure.	T L R N
When my teacher gives me a "next step," she also reminds me of the things I do well.	T L R N

(continued)

FIGURE 6.6. "Feedback for My Teacher" assessment tool. Created by Stacey Falconer at Lakeshore Public School in Burlington, Ontario, Canada, in cooperation with Laurie Faith. Used with permission.

Organization				
My teacher helps me to make systems to stay organized, like online binders, folders with colors, bins, etc.	T	L	R	N
My teacher has a place for the things I need.	T	L	R	N
My teacher helps us keep an organized classroom.	T	L	R	N
Prioritizing and Planning				
My teacher checks in on my independent work to make sure I'm not falling behind.	T	L	R	N
My teacher helps me to break jobs into chunks, so I know what parts need to be done.	T	L	R	N
My teacher makes checklists and success criteria with me, so I know what I should be learning.	T	L	R	N
Time Management				
My teacher gives me the "2-minute" warning before we finish.	T	L	R	N
My teacher helps me to remind my parents of upcoming things.	T	L	R	N
My teacher lets me have input into how I finish tasks.	T	L	R	N
Task Initiation				
My teacher is clear about what I should be doing.	T	L	R	N
My teacher makes the work "just right for me."	T	L	R	N
My teacher makes me believe in myself by letting me know *she* believes in me.	T	L	R	N
Perseverance				
My teacher lets me learn with and from other students.	T	L	R	N
My teacher gives me ideas or examples to help me keep trying.	T	L	R	N
My teacher lets me have choices in some of the things I do.	T	L	R	N
My teacher checks in with me to see how I'm doing.	T	L	R	N
My teacher makes things easier, so I can do well.	T	L	R	N
Metacognition (thinking about my thinking)				
My teacher goes over finished work with me, so I know where I went wrong and what I did well.	T	L	R	N
My teacher develops next steps with me.	T	L	R	N
My teacher doesn't just give marks; I get to help decide on my marks by thinking about what I understand.	T	L	R	N

FIGURE 6.6. *(continued)*

CHAPTER 7

How EF-Literate Teaching Supports Other Educational Priorities

In this chapter, we describe how an EF-literate approach can support your work on six other educational priorities: the achievement gap, global competencies, equity, IEPs, Universal Design for Learning, and the reduction of teacher burnout. We point out the advantage of building a basic EF literacy among your students (and colleagues) and focus heavily on the utility of the BSP.[1] To navigate this chapter, you may flip through to find the topic you're especially passionate about, read up on the issue your district is currently focused on, or tackle the whole lot. In any case, we hope it will make your EF-supportive teaching more satisfying and that it will help you find efficiencies and opportunities to "kill two birds with one stone."

A little disclaimer before we dig in. Writing this chapter was like galloping up to seven powerful tribes, wielding a peace offering and asking for a parlay. In essence, we entered the traditional lands of the achievement gap, global competencies, equity, IEPs, UDL, and healthy communities and said, "Let us summarize our interpretation of your needs and suggest the ways that we can work together." Then we sat ourselves down and began the intense process of trying to find interconnection. Hours, days, and weeks of slow, careful negotiation would pass, and when we finally rode away, we'd mumble an exhausted "Um, that went well, don't you think? That was helpful?" About an hour later, however, we'd be circling back after reading, hearing, or conversing about something new on the topic. "Nope. Not right," we'd say. "Missed something." All this to say, we've done a lot of learning, thinking, and editing, and, doggone it, we know there's very little chance that we've got it all right. Regardless, we remain dedicated to traveling outside of our small territory of EF-literate teaching to discover connections with other domains.

---

[1] Remember, the BSP was introduced in Chapter 3. It is a semistructured teaching protocol. Essentially, it asks teachers to gather students to discuss "What are your/our barriers to this work?" and then "What strategies can we use to be more successful?"

EFs AND THE ACHIEVEMENT GAP

Differences in school achievement related to socioeconomic disparity exist around the world (Mullis, Martin, Foy, & Hooper, 2016). The following discussion will make a connection between these gaps and EF. We will suggest that the support of EFs in school should be considered a moral imperative for those hoping to educate fairly, remove barriers for all children, and empower the most traditionally disadvantaged learners.

First, let's take an imaginary field trip to the achievement gap. We load our students onto a bus, count heads, and drive half an hour north. Along the way, we turn around to chat with a student sitting alone: "Are you looking forward to the trip, Sean?" Hearing the roar of his classmates' voices filling the bus, and feeling a little motion sick, he looks up weakly and gives the tiniest nod. Sean seems so discouraged, even before the day has begun. Upon arrival, we park, visit the washrooms, and then head off through the woods. As we approach the gap, we see that it is wide and will be quite challenging for some to cross. Before we even have time to provide instructions, however, one or two of our students take a running start and leap boldly across. While the others watch, the successful jumpers celebrate—play, climb trees, chase each other around—becoming the best of friends. A few others are encouraged by this example and take the leap, joining immediately in the celebrations on the other side. Still others are urged across with a few words of advice. We spot Sean among a small group on the near side.

In many ways, this is a trip we make every day at school. The day begins, we present some kind of a challenge, and students begin to respond. Both in school and on our imaginary field trip, there are a handful of students who need an extraordinary amount of help to cross the achievement gap, some who will not make it, and some who will not even try. Work that relies heavily on EF, such as learning to read, completing mathematical problems, or engaging in critical thinking or collaboration, will be the most challenging. How do we respond? On our imaginary field trip, would we walk the stragglers down to the shore, find a bridge, and pass over? Would we carry students across one by one? Or would we set up camp on the near shore with this small group and come up with another engaging activity? All of these options avoid or replace the challenge of crossing the gap. Though we endeavor to support these students with encouragement and reassurance, the alternate activities we offer day after day will come to feel like failure for many.

Looking back at photos of this field trip, we might notice several things. First, we might notice that the students who made it across the achievement gap were all romping around in a comfortable pair of shoes, while the discouraged few had none at all. This would represent an *opportunity* gap, an unequal distribution of resources; the unsuccessful students may actually be powerful jumpers who are only disabled by the stones and prickles under their ill-equipped feet. This is a good comparison to the many children who arrive at school lacking (to varying degrees) another fundamental piece of equipment—their EFs. They are in possession, often, of adequate or even exceptional knowledge, wisdom, and creativity but are severely disadvantaged by their inability to manage and execute. Imagine, for example, a math class focused on problem solving.

For example, equipped with an average level of aptitude and high EFs, Kelsey will pay attention to instructions and get started right away. She will find the mathematics challenging but will stay calm enough to persist by asking her teacher for clarification. Meanwhile, Sean, who has an extraordinary aptitude for math but lower EFs, might lose focus during his teacher's instructions and delay getting started. After he starts, he might tackle the work using a self-designed approach that is ingenious but time-consuming. Any frustration he experiences will further suppress his

EFs. Add to this how alienated he might feel if his teacher walks by and suggests he is on the wrong track. Without classroom support to manage this spiral, it is very likely that Sean, despite his superior aptitude for math, will not succeed and enjoy the fruits of his talents. In fact, he will probably end up in trouble. Kelsey, meanwhile, will experience success, receive positive feedback from her teacher, enjoy admiration from her peers, and perhaps wind up in a group with other optimistic high achievers. "Kelsey is a hardworking student," we will all agree, and "Sean is often off track and needs to put forth more effort." How might our responses change if the disability represented by a weakness in EF was as obvious as a missing pair of shoes?

Looking at photographs from our trip to the achievement gap, we might notice something else. Most of the children, girls and boys, who are huddled around the teacher doing alternate activities on the near side of the gap are not White. Weakness in EF is a selective disability. In the United States, ethnic minority students, and particularly male ones, are at the highest risk for inattentive and hyperactive behaviors. Researchers believe, however, that almost all association between ethnicity and weak EFs is explained by a third factor: low socioeconomic status. Poverty, through its association with household chaos, grinding stress, and instability in parental care, interferes with the normal development of the prefrontal cortex and impairs EF (Martel, 2013). Meanwhile, wealth, though not always a guarantee of attentive parenting or low stress, is associated with enriching preschool care, specialist lessons, and tutoring (Chmielewski, 2019). Each day in schools, therefore, the most economically privileged children are often better equipped to leap across achievement gaps; enjoy the satisfaction of expressing their knowledge, wisdom, and creativity; and reap praise. Meanwhile, the least privileged cope with, yes, not only the daily challenges associated with their socioeconomic status but also the discouragement, shame, and fatigue of trying to operate with neurological equipment that, *as a result*, just doesn't function as well.

If our children were *literally* jumping across the achievement gap, and some of them *literally* had no shoes, the discrepancy would be plain and our response would be automatic. We would do everything possible to provide each child with such an essential piece of equipment. As educators, we should elect leaders that support young families, but we can also intervene by making EF development and support a core focus in our classrooms. To level the playing field, we can support the slow, steady development of core EF by providing joyful, structured, and stimulating classroom environments (see Chapter 1). Also, we can help students to build the compensatory strategies necessary to use what EFs they do have more efficiently and effectively. So, while we can't give them all the exact same shoes enjoyed by the most privileged in their class (and may not move the needle much on their core capacity for, say, attention) we can teach them strategies for crossing the gap no matter what shoes they are in (strategies to pace, manage, and optimize what attention they can manage). By helping students to become EF literate, we can alert them to the biggest and sharpest obstacles they will face (see Chapter 2). Each time we work with students to notice the EF challenges in a task, we can make them more adept at quickly spotting and avoiding them in the future. When we gather students together to discuss both these barriers and the strategies they can use to be successful, we can build morale, courage, and skill (see Chapter 3). Then we can reorient our observation, feedback, and assessment systems to notice, cheer on, and reward their progress (Chapters 4, 5, and 6). "This is really challenging," we can tell them. "To cross this gap, you will have to work extra hard to manage your executive functions." Through our EF-literate teaching, our most vulnerable and disadvantaged students can learn the complex adaptive skills to cross the gap no matter what "equipment" they arrived with.

EF-LITERATE TEACHING AND 21ST-CENTURY LEARNING

Around big family dinners, the conversation inevitably turns to the new and surprising deficiencies of "kids these days": they're glued to their phones, they don't do enough chores, and they don't seem to want to grow up. When the conversation shifts to what to *do about them,* you can be sure there will be little agreement. Grandma and Grandpa may advocate strongly for a back-to-basics approach, through which children learn useful skills like sewing, cooking, mechanics, and balancing a checkbook. Uncle Lionel, frustrated by his lot in life, may feel education should focus primarily on money, the law, and business. For their part, kids often envision a future of YouTube stardom or gaming glory. As the educator at the table, your family may look to you for guidance. The following discussion will give you a few points to share regarding the aims of education in the 21st century, as well as a clear breakdown of how our process-oriented approach is aligned. We hope, at the very least, it will help you to navigate your holiday dinners.

The first point you should make is that it *is* unusually difficult at this moment in history to figure out which skills and knowledge to focus on in school. Many believe it is crucial for students to learn to code and handle data, and others emphasize the importance of training in STEM (science, technology, engineering, and mathematics) and AI (artificial intelligence), while others are focused on the importance of social sciences, such as history, psychology, culture, and environmental studies. Each of these disciplines, on its own, is a tall order and may be more complicated than what educators have traditionally been responsible for teaching. As well, each of these disciplines is constantly changing due to rapidly evolving technology and far-reaching environmental change; even if we hit a few of these moving targets in school, and we will surely try, it is doubtful that the specific skill sets and knowledge we impart now will be wholly useful in the future. The Python computer programming language commonly taught to seven- and eight-year-olds at school, for example, will probably not be the one they use as engineers at Google.

For this reason, you can confidently reassure your relatives that even among experts, a specific curriculum of skills and training hasn't been fully agreed upon. Before they throw up their hands, however, reassure them that among experts, a plan has begun to form. We're going to teach children *not* as if we're programming microwaves, each with the same fixed set of functions, but as if we're programming super modern robots who can adapt, learn, and respond to a variety of challenges. If you'd rather, we can just agree to teach them, for the first time, like they're "humans." (Whaaat?) This is the second point you should make: that we're going to teach children to use their full potential as human beings. A group of experts based in the United States ("Framework for 21st Century Learning," 2016) have agreed that, in addition to subjects like math, science, literacy, social sciences, information technology, and media literacy, students should learn the following:

- Interdisciplinary themes such as global awareness, as well as financial, civic, health, and environmental literacy
- Learning and innovation skills, such as creativity, innovation, critical thinking, problem solving, communication, and collaboration.

So, to recap, the vision for 21st-century education includes traditional school skills, unified by several global and environmental interdisciplinary themes, and powered by a set of learning and innovation skills. That power-up is where we come in, because those skills are distinctly not *things to learn* but *ways to learn things.* Any time we talk about the *ways* students do things, we're talking about *execution* or executive function. Table 7.1 presents just a few of the most obvious connections between 21st-century learning and innovation skills and EFs.

The idea of teaching learning and innovation skills should be pleasing to those with a back-to-basics perspective. Back in the good old days, before life became so automated and simple, they were like the "frontier" skills that any ordinary person needed in order to survive. When instilled, they will allow graduates to retrain and quickly figure out new technologies, and also to manage unexpected change. They will enable the next generation to adapt to and even capitalize on the myriad shifts and changes to come. For example, our students will be pioneers in the retrofitting of homes that must endure extreme weather conditions. Or they may work toward needed efficiencies in the distribution of personal protective equipment during a global pandemic. Even in their own homes, our students will need to troubleshoot: new remedies, the switch to renewable power, and the conservation of water, to name a few. After the Cold War, the U.S. military coined the term "VUCA" to describe the quality of these particularly Volatile, Uncertain, Complex, and Ambiguous problems. VUCA problems typically arise when we don't know exactly what situations we will have to confront and are unable to anticipate the results of our actions. To manage a future with these kinds of challenges, our students will need to hit the ground running, equipped with learning and innovation skills that can be adapted to pass a wide variety of novel tests.

The third point you can make is that we will achieve this level of independence and problem solving by teaching it directly. It won't be enough to simply tell children about learning and innovation skills—we're going to have to provide them with direct guidance to develop and apply them. In the landmark book *Four-Dimensional Education,* Fadel, Bialik, and Trilling (2015) provide what many believe to be the best available advice for forward-looking educators. Focus your efforts at school on knowledge, skills, and character, they suggest, but also surround these efforts with an emphasis on "meta-learning." Across most major international education planning organizations, they explain, meta-learners have been characterized as versatile, reflective, self-directed, and self-reliant individuals who know *how* to learn. Fadel and colleagues caution, however, that to instill

TABLE 7.1. Connections Between Learning and Innovation Skills, and EF

Creativity and innovation	• *Flexibility* to imagine/consider a range of new ideas. • *Response inhibition* to resist distraction. • *Goal-directed persistence* to carry a vision through to completion. • *Emotional control* to tolerate ambiguity calmly.
Critical thinking and problem solving	• *Organization* to understand and analyze complex situations. • *Planning and prioritizing* to tackle multistep problems. • *Response inhibition* to resist jumping to conclusions. • *Goal-directed persistence* to stick with challenges and *time management* to meet deadlines. • *Metacognition* to monitor and evaluate the impact of different approaches and solutions.
Communication and collaboration	• *Flexibility* to see other points of view and explore opposing models. • *Working memory* and *sustained attention* to listen to, understand, and respond to others. • *Response inhibition* to take turns and share ideas. • *Emotional control* to manage disagreement and tension.

this capacity teachers must go beyond the simple delivery of prescribed strategy toward the development of deep growth mindsets, self-monitoring, and persistence (p. 96). Practical approaches to mobilize this ambition have been explored and explicated throughout Chapters 2–6 of this book. We're advocating for classrooms in which children regularly stop to collectively monitor problems, plan strategic approaches, and optimize their executive function. We believe that, with daily practice, all children can learn to approach novel problems not with their hands up, waiting for help from an expert, but with the ability to stand on their own two feet and strategize.

Finally, you can wow your family with the idea that because school is going to prepare children for unknown problems in as-yet-unseen global conditions, it's going to be a little bit like astronaut training. Chris Hadfield (2013), a retired Canadian astronaut, has penned a few useful lessons. In his book, *An Astronaut's Guide to Life on Earth*, he describes a type of readiness that sounds an awful lot like 21st-century skills: "Competence," he says, "means keeping your head in a crisis, sticking with a task even when it seems hopeless, and improvising good solutions to tough problems when every second counts. It encompasses ingenuity, determination, and being prepared for anything" (p. 26). He explains that "astronauts have these qualities, not because we're smarter than everyone else . . . [but] because we are taught to view the world—and ourselves—differently." At NASA, it turns out, in addition to learning how to fly and maintain a space shuttle, perform basic medical procedures and science experiments, and speak Russian, astronauts are given training in "survival." Their journals, published online at *www.NASA.gov*, describe learning to use imagination, common sense, and trust among team members to improve collaborative problem solving under the toughest of conditions. This is how we need to train children in school: like bold adventurers who are ready to enter radically new spaces and times, feeling in control of their cognitive resources, and ready to manage whatever challenge they may encounter.

EF-LITERATE TEACHING FOR AN EQUITABLE AND MULTICULTURAL CLASSROOM

For many children, school is an unreceptive place. They arrive with a lifetime of skills, strategies, tricks, experiences, and interests, and realize that their wisdom is foreign. Even working with the best of intentions, the average teacher will not meet the needs of unusual or unfamiliar students. We hope to provide the many teaching teams, school committees, and camp staffs working on this challenge with a powerful new idea that is practical enough to understand, share, and attempt right away. The following discussion will state the case for adding the BSP to your multicultural teaching approaches. To do this, we will summarize the importance of equitable and multicultural education and describe the challenges that many teachers are facing while trying to achieve it. We hope to help broaden your appreciation of equity in a classroom, summarize the time and resources generally recommended for achieving it, and convince you that the BSP offers excellent value for your effort.[2]

First, let's get grounded in what multicultural education really means. Consider a hypothetical student named Aarav: One morning he spat into a vial, capped it, enveloped it, and signed

---

[2] Remember, the BSP was introduced in Chapter 3. It is a semistructured teaching protocol. Essentially, it asks teachers to gather students to discuss "What are your/our barriers to this work?" and then "What strategies can we use to be more successful?"

across the label. Six weeks later, he found out he was part Welsh and had a half brother in Pennsylvania. In addition to these *new* discoveries, Aarav has a sister with a severe illness, is intellectually gifted but a little disorganized and intense, loves learning languages, went to an arts-based grade 6 program in Mexico, and, like his mom, is quite drawn to math and computers. He is a rich and complex individual, and he shifts between his many ways of knowing depending on who he is with and on what he is working. If you ask him for advice, he may respond with sensitivity, suggest a technical work around, or steer you away from confrontation.

We believe identity is about more than just race. It also encompasses, for example, religion, sexual orientation, class, gender, or income level. Each one of us, like Aarav, is blessed with a different combination of background, interests, talents, skills, and challenges. Rich in emotional connections, powerful memories, and formative experiences, this intersectional framework is a lens through which we will process almost every new opportunity we encounter (NASEM, 2018). Each of these unique qualities, however, creates the opportunity to feel marginalized and misunderstood among a group of more typical-seeming peers.

Aarav's parents immigrated from Bangalore in South India when he was a baby, so, like *more than half* of all U.S. children, he is part of a non-White ethnic group (U.S. Census Bureau, 2015). Canada is expected to hit this milestone by 2036 (Statistics Canada, 2017), while the United Kingdom projects 30% by 2061 (Rees, Wohland, Norman, & Lomax, 2017). These changes to the composition of our schools will pose complex social and academic challenges. Socially, we know that while most children go through phases of feeling they don't fit in, girls, immigrants, students of color, and students with low socioeconomic status tend to report these feelings most consistently. On a scale of 1 to 5, they circle high scores when asked if they feel like an outsider, feel left out of things, have a hard time making friends, feel awkward and out of place, suspect that other students don't like them, and feel lonely at school (OECD, 2017). Consider also the profound effects that loneliness and isolation have on learning. Children who don't feel accepted, valued, and included experience a reduced sense of safety, which can close the door to optimal EF, the pursuit of high goals, and the taking of academic risks (Brownlie & King, 2011). Meanwhile, researchers have demonstrated that feeling interesting and important to others, or as though you "matter," is a crucial aspect of overall well-being, and a shortage of it is associated with delinquency, depression, and anxiety (Rosenberg & McCullough, 1981). Schools need to adapt to meet the needs of their changing populations.

At school, students with a sense of cultural isolation may also endure ill-fitting academic experiences. International students, for example, often arrive in classrooms that bear little resemblance to the learning environment they are used to. They may suddenly find themselves among teachers with pedagogical styles and teaching approaches that differ considerably from those to which they previously became accustomed (e.g., constructivism, student orientation, discipline, collaboration, and use of resources; OECD, 2009). Moreover, in order to fit in, students often *discontinue* important cultural- and value-based learning preferences and practices they have mastered from their elders, in their home communities, or from their cultural teachings (Tyler et al., 2008). To whatever extent a sense of *disconnect* persists between a child's roots/home life and the dominant culture at school, a risk exists for reduced emotional well-being, efficacy, self-esteem, and GPA, and increased anger and self-depreciation (Arunkumar, Midgley, & Urdan, 1999). Also, academic topics, examples, or materials that are unfamiliar and do not engage students' preexisting knowledge make it difficult for them to fully grasp and remember new learning (NASEM, 2018). How many of your students experience these challenges?

Before we propose a solution, let's add up the time, resources, and attention equitable teaching may require. Even if you begin with the basics, it's a fairly tall order. The first thing you should do, according to the most well-accepted frameworks (Gay, 2000), is validate each student's identity. That means making their cultural, linguistic, and social uniqueness your business, and also getting to know their particular dispositions, attitudes, and approaches to learning. Considering the complex range of origins and cultures in our classrooms, and the natural limitations of our ability to gather, learn, and remember information, this will be quite a task. "Oh shoot," we may think, "is Aarav the one who grew up in Mexico, or is that Juno?" Your second job is to purposefully incorporate these qualities into the curriculum and skills taught, the materials used, and the manner of instruction applied in the classroom. The goal is to know enough about the cultures among your students to intentionally plan learning that incorporates them. The most respected voices on this topic encourage educators to develop not one or two new techniques, units, or lessons but a multifaceted approach that will transform the school day and allow a broad range of students to succeed (e.g., Hammond, 2015). Toward this goal, teachers will do all of the usual tricks: build a nice collection of mentor texts and teaching manuals, follow certain blogs, and attend workshops to get ideas from other educators. This is such important work, but how will we "afford" such a deep and broad change when our time, resources, and attention are already so stretched?

We don't blame you for feeling overwhelmed. This is a lot of work for one teacher to do in the background while integrating the demands of a language, math, and social studies curriculum. We believe, however, that you can succeed if you stop taking all of the learning about the multiple cultures in your classroom upon yourself and instead share the process of learning and, more importantly, *some of the control* with your students. Our advice is to move your approach further upstream—past topics and different delivery techniques—toward the way you *regulate learning in your classroom.* Using the BSP, you can regularly incorporate meaningful and authentic opportunities for your students to voice their perspectives. This theory may take a moment to wrap your mind around, so look at the practical examples in Table 7.2. Each vignette contains a blow-by-blow account of three different types of learning regulation for the lovely Aarav: a self-regulated learning style through which he manages his own performance, an externally regulated learning style through which his teacher takes over and regulates learning for him, and a socially shared learning regulation style (see review in Panadero & Jarvela, 2015) through which he is encouraged to bring his culture and experiences to bear on the learning regulation taking place among the peers in his class. We had fun piecing together the scenarios and think they nicely capture what can happen in a typical classroom.

With our little tweak toward socially shared learning regulation, we are interested in using daily classroom challenges to actively distribute voice, participation, and authority evenly among all members (Perry, Yee, Mazabel, Lisaingo, & Maatta, 2017). By using the BSP, Aarav's learning problems will no longer be solved by a single teacher who puzzles and scrambles and worries over how to correctly and deeply incorporate his unique cultural background and range of skills. Rather, Aarav himself will be pulled into the process and invited to weigh in alongside his peers and teachers. For example, instead of his teacher alone trying to figure out how to make the solving of math problems culturally relevant, she can gather Aarav and his peers to ask, "What are our barriers to this challenge?" and "What can we do to be successful?" In response, Aarav and his classmates can share a diverse range of strategies and solutions for handling EF challenges. This process becomes even more aligned with the goals of equitable teaching when a teacher or peer stops to ask Aarav, "Where did you learn that?" and provides reassurance that his ideas are valid

TABLE 7.2. The Impact of Self-Regulated, Externally Regulated, and Socially Shared Learning Regulation on "Aarav's" Experience at School

Self-regulated learning: *Students individually monitor problems, create solutions, and reflect on process.*	Externally regulated learning: *Teacher monitors problems, creates solutions, and reflects on process.*	Socially shared learning regulation: *Collaboratively, class monitors problems, creates solutions, and reflects on process.*
First period (math): Aarav is overwhelmed by a crowded math page		
To calm himself, Aarav works with a partner. Like his mother does, Aarav methodically rewrites each question on a separate piece of paper to make it less overwhelming. This takes a long time, but he uses a similar process later, in science class.	The teacher believes the room is too noisy for students to focus. They are asked to work silently. Aarav becomes frustrated and leaves the room for 20 minutes. Reflecting on the success of this approach, the teacher uses it again the next day.	The teacher asks the class to share barriers and strategies, and many do. Aarav shares his mom's approach of rewriting questions and also uses a peer's idea to cover adjacent questions. Later, the class reflects that Aarav's approach takes longer.
Third period (history): Aarav's notes are disorganized and he is a little behind		
Like his grandfather, Aarav takes a deep breath and talks himself though the organization of his notes: "Okay, this goes first, and I'll put this in a folder, and this is garbage." Fifteen minutes later, he's ready to start.	The teacher calls Aarav as well five other students to her desk at the beginning of class. She gives them a special folder and tells them she will keep their notes behind her desk after class each day.	The teacher asks the class to share barriers and strategies, and many do. From a friend, Aarav learns to number his pages; he won't have such a mess to deal with next class. Three girls start using his self-talk strategy.
Fourth and fifth period (science): Aarav builds a bridge with a team of peers		
Aarav uses a computer program to plan the structure of his bridge. This takes a long time, and his group builds a different structure without him.	The teacher gives 20 minutes of detailed instructions on exactly how to manage materials, plan the structure, and collaborate with others.	The teacher asks the class to share barriers and strategies, and many do. Aarav demos the planning program he likes. His group combines it with another idea for organizing materials.
After-school diary entry:		
Today I felt lonely. Nobody listened to my ideas for building the bridge. It was nice to use Grandfather's trick for getting organized, but nobody really noticed.	My teacher doesn't understand me, and she doesn't like me. Nobody wants to be my partner. The girls said I'm a mess.	Chen-Ling's numbering strategy is my new favorite, and Marci, Ami, and Tonika loved Papa's self-talk strategy. I taught my whole class how to use Sketcho. I felt so proud.

and useful. "That is so cool, Aarav," one might comment. "I wish *I* grew up in your house." While this may sound overly sunny and ideal, we often overhear comments like these among children who have been given the chance to deeply appreciate the value in each other's differences: "I wish *I* celebrated Diwali" or "I wish *I* could go with the reading teacher," or observing a particularly creative use for a leg brace, even saying, "I wish *I* had a broken leg!"

This approach places problem solving into the social arena of the classroom. When children's perspectives and strategies are validated on this stage, it cements their feelings of autonomy and competence in the third essential factor for motivation: relatedness and a sense of belonging (Deci & Ryan, 2000). In contrast to feeling alone, unknown, and unimportant, a child can share an old family organization trick, a calming strategy they learned from their grandparent, or a mindset they learned in their place of worship and feel appreciated for their most personal qualities. Furthermore, by providing communal space for classmates to participate in the regulation of their learning, we make it possible for children with many different backgrounds to help one another on a strategic level. By this approach, when a learning problem arises, the processes of understanding it and figuring out what to do next are no longer tethered to the experience, habits, and biases of one particular teacher. Rather, within open large-group conversations, students are free to share ideas that may be worlds apart from those of their teacher. This process allows students to belong *in their fullness* in the classroom.

How often do you think self-regulated learning actually happens when students are faced with challenging problems in your classroom? Failing that, how often do you think you wind up taking over and switching into externally regulated learning? If you think you might support students with external regulation as a go-to, it is interesting to consider whether they are discouraged by it and if they may quickly be reinvigorated by a more communal, socially shared approach. By interrupting your habitual teaching practices several times a day to actively recruit your students' expertise, knowledge, creative thinking, and voice, you place your own power, biases, and perspective in check. You also create authentic and meaningful opportunities for cultural learning among your students and for yourself.

You might know an extraordinary teacher who has transformed his or her classroom, materials, and teaching practice and is making huge strides toward multicultural education. You may have seen their posts on social media or listened to them speak at a conference, and you may feel inspired by their work and called to action. We think it is important to remember that multicultural teaching is not only for those who eat, breathe, and sleep the issue. Our schools will be truly equitable when multiple cultures can flourish and thrive in *every* classroom. While the BSP is a powerful practice for *leaders* in multicultural teaching, it is also a great, self-contained starting point for teachers with more general interests. It can be adapted to an almost infinite variety of classroom situations and is compact and manageable enough to be used by regular ed. teachers. Using the BSP, teachers can begin to offer students' experiences, cultures, backgrounds, and unique wisdom the voice and power they deserve in the classroom.

EF-LITERATE TEACHING
AND INDIVIDUALIZED EDUCATION PROGRAMS

In the following discussion, we will speak rather generally about "IEPs" (individualized education programs or plans); by this, we mean to evoke a variety of structured, legally binding documents created and monitored by parents, teachers, administrators, and district representatives to support a student who is experiencing difficulty. This document consolidates assessment results, interventions chosen, and a timeline for the accomplishment of specific goals, and is revisited several times per year to ensure progress and make adjustments. Sometimes the target students are involved in this process, but often they are not. In your part of the world, these may be called IEPs or 504s or something else—we are writing for an international audience, and while the procedures are quite similar in essence, the details and logistics vary.

In a perfect world, a student with special needs could enter any mainstream classroom armed with one of these IEPs and receive the support required for success. For a handful of reasons, however, this doesn't always happen. In the following discussion, we'll describe three complex challenges regarding the delivery of special education. We'll do this in order to set a stage on which the contributions of an EF-literate teaching approach can be fully understood and appreciated. As lifelong teachers and advocates for children, we don't challenge the established special education approach lightly; throughout the history of public education, students with special learning needs have been terribly underprivileged at school, and the essential rights and protections offered by IEPs are vital and hard won. Our goal is to propose ways that this system may be complemented and strengthened by our approach.

Challenge 1: IEPs That Aren't Specific Enough

IEPs are based on top-notch diagnostic approaches and are meant to contain specific, measurable, achievable, realistic, and time-bound goals. To determine these goals for each student, a team will weigh current academic achievement as well as unique learning challenges. While the diagnosis and targets are specific, the recommendations for accommodation and intervention are often less so. They tell us clearly where the student is and where he is going but include less detail about *how to get there*. Odds are, if you have four students in your class with an IEP, they share a handful of similar accommodations: preferential seating, time and a half for tests, and the provision of quiet space and release time for an additional service like occupational therapy. These are just a few of the most common ones. With 10 out of 25 students jammed into a preferential front row that winds up being loud and chaotic, however, you might wonder if there is anything missing in the IEPs.

In fact, students' needs shift and change in ways that are often not included in an IEP. Imagine Jana, a student with a language-based learning disability and anxiety. Her IEP prescribes accommodations for extra time and a computer and suggests that she practices mindful breathing when she feels overwhelmed. We know, however, that students with special needs often have a cluster of challenges that interact in complex ways (Aitken et al., 2017). On Day 1 of a group project assignment, Jana may actually require support to manage the interpersonal aspects of the work. On Day 2 she (and others) may be bogged down by the organization of the project and benefit from a filing or labeling strategy. As the project evolves, it may tax Jana's abilities in a slightly different way each day. While her accommodations for time, technology, and breathing will be essential to her ability to succeed, they may not ensure her success as she navigates specific tasks.

To optimize student success despite these multidimensional and dynamic challenges, experts believe that diagnosis and intervention should be conducted in the context of daily performance (Fletcher & Grigorenko, 2017). That means "Hey teachers! It would be really great if you could conduct a separate assessment for each new challenge and then provide the specific and tailored accommodations that each of your students really needs." When publishing this finding, Fletcher and Grigorenko may have paused to wonder how it would be useful to mainstream teachers responsible for large numbers of needy students. "Let's put this in the highly theoretical, for-use-in-a-perfect-world pile," they may have thought. We agree. This recommendation sounds almost impossibly precise and time-consuming, but we think our EF-literate approach comes pretty close to pulling it off.

Consider how the BSP accomplishes frequent diagnosis and intervention in the mainstream.[3] When we assign groupwork, for example, and ask our whole classes to explore the types of barriers they will face, Jana will have a chance to describe her worries about sharing responsibility, and she may hear a peer's concerns about handling disagreement. Her teacher, otherwise focused on fulfilling the specific recommendations mentioned in her IEP, may be surprised. Students in the class may agree to assign roles within the groups, use timers, or create to-do lists. One class we worked with suggested using "safe words." Regardless of what is discussed, when the class works together to identify strategies that may intervene on these specific challenges, Jana will receive the type of personal, just-in-time special education support that is recommended by Fletcher and Grigorenko (2017). The following day, the protocol may reveal a fresh range of challenges and suitable interventions. In this way, the use of our EF-literate approach may provide more precise, specific, and timely support for students with special education needs. It may also be a big help to students who have not been formally assessed but who have special learning needs and could do with the support.

Challenge 2: IEPs That Seem Contradictory or Are Confusing

There is a big difference between a teacher and a psychologist; cognitive processes are complex, and it takes years of training to really understand how each little component works. Unfortunately, this complexity can be hard to decode on a psychologist's report, and the confusion often trickles onto the IEP. For example, imagine Logan. He has a "strong visual working memory" in math (He can hold numbers in his mind during arithmetic?) and also "struggles with reading comprehension" (He can't hold words in his mind when he reads?). You may wonder why Logan can hold numbers in short-term memory but not words. If we could get it all straight, we might start using a certain approach with him across many subjects. Given the contradiction, however, we may feel overwhelmed and end up not doing much of anything at all.

This is another time that the BSP may prove useful. Using a regular whole-class check-in regarding the barriers presented by different tasks, and which strategies might be helpful, teachers can build on their understanding of how each student learns. In fact, we'll argue after using the BSP for a few months, teachers can substantially enrich and extend the insight of psychologists and IEPs. This is easy to appreciate when you consider the high degree of context-, subject-, emotion-, and peer-group specificity available to a teacher as a result of these conversations. For example, by December, Logan's teacher might understand that his working memory struggles most when he's reading, except if it's a poem or song, especially if he works with a partner, more so in the morning, and less so after a good breakfast. Similarly, she may realize that Logan automatically translates

---

[3] Remember, the BSP was introduced in Chapter 3. It is a semistructured teaching protocol. Essentially, it asks teachers to gather students to discuss "What are your/our barriers to this work?" and then "What strategies can we use to be more successful?"

mathematical information into mental pictures, and that this is why his working memory seems better with numbers. Even better, Logan may understand this too! The BSP offers teachers (and students) an almost infinite opportunity to clarify and build upon IEPs that may be confusing or seem contradictory.

Challenge 3: IEPs with Recommendations That Aren't Feasible

Have you ever received an IEP with recommendations that rely on technology that hasn't arrived, materials that are scarce, or space you don't have? For example, it can be tricky to provide a calm, quiet, or private workspace in a room that barely has enough space for desks. While we do everything possible to adapt and make do, it can be challenging to meet the demands of an IEP created outside of your classroom context. For this reason, the work done by your students during daily barriers and strategies conversations may be extremely helpful for fine-tuning student accommodations.

For example, in a really squishy classroom, a recommendation for calm, quiet space to help manage attention may seem as if it can only be accomplished with the use of headphones. During a BSP, however, students may discover alternative strategies that also work. As a team, they may realize that a calming effect also results when students work in partners and talk each other through math problems, run the stairs between every three problems, or focus on smaller chunks of work. While some students may be happy to calm down while using headphones, others can explore strategies that feel perfect for them. For example, our friend Stacey Falconer has a student who invented a strategy to address an almost impossible combination of needs.[4] He required both "proximity to teacher" and a "quiet workspace." Eager to make use of a study nook in the back of the room, this student rigged up a camera that projected his image, larger than life, onto the classroom whiteboard. In this way, he was able to enjoy the calm workspace while still benefiting from the feeling of close supervision. A student like this would never otherwise have had access to the study nook. Even the very best IEP committee cannot match the innovation possible when a whole class of students looks around their environment, thinks about the resources available, and flexes their playful and creative problem-solving skills.

We've discussed the ways an EF-literate approach can fortify three critical weaknesses of the IEP process. In general, we believe you can use the BSP like a mini, *auxiliary IEP*: It revs up and kicks in when more powerful and precise navigation is required. Over the course of an academic term, the learning will accumulate for both teacher and student. A hyperactive student with a September IEP specifying motor breaks, computer access, and a quiet workspace may head out for winter holidays regularly using a handful of alternative, student-styled, precise little strategies. These may include the following:

- Tape box around desk. If I'm in it, I'm on the right track and counted as "in my seat."
- Use of a 10-minute timer to plan out breaks.
- Read instructions on math tests to myself in funny (and friendly) voice.
- Watching a very calm student to figure out how to behave.
- Reading while walking around or reading with my feet up the back wall.

---

[4] Stacey Falconer teaches at Lakeshore Public School in Burlington, Ontario, Canada. Used with permission.

Under ideal conditions, students themselves would have a starring role in the creation of their IEPs. When this isn't possible, the work done by teachers and students within BSP conversations can provide similar benefit. And after doing so much work to understand students' learning, classroom teachers and students themselves will be much more prepared to take an active role in interpreting and offering suggestions for updates to an IEP. In this way, the BSP becomes like a daily IEP workshop in which students see themselves as frontline field testers and innovators, bringing meaningful insight about what works and what doesn't.

EF-LITERATE TEACHING AND UNIVERSAL DESIGN

Throughout this chapter, we have emphasized the way the BSP, our method of socially shared learning regulation (see review in Panadero & Jarvela, 2015), promotes equity, student voice, and empowerment. The following discussion will present similar arguments but will align them specifically with the objectives of UDL. We know there are quite a number of schools focused on UDL, and we hope to serve up the exact information you need to present our EF-literate approach to your team as an option. In a nutshell, we think our approach moves a step beyond conventional UDL practices. Using the BSP, our approach supports a more adaptive, unbiased, and data-based version of universal design.

First, let's agree that UDL is a method for making your educational environment usable and supportive to the widest range of students. It encompasses everything we can control in the classroom, including the means of representation (how students acquire info), expression (how students demonstrate learning), and engagement (the way we motivate and interest students). UDL asks us if there are things we can install in our core approaches, environments, and materials that will make learning more universally accessible.

If you read the previous section about IEPs and accommodations, you may agree that a discussion of UDL is a perfect next step. As we come to terms with the requirement for individualized support and intervention, we may feel as though we've opened a Pandora's box; while some students are extraordinarily needy, almost every single one could do with *some* individualization. Accordingly, teachers strive to provide fully differentiated instruction, through which many different versions of their materials, tasks, objectives, and instructions are available (Tomlinson, 2001). In stark contrast, UDL is satisfying because it promises efficiency; we can throw away our elaborate lists of exactly who needs what and simply install a few good universal solutions. For example, we can stop providing four specific students with lesson goals and simply post them for everyone. The more we can universally design our spaces, the less time we'll spend organizing and managing one-off accommodations and differentiation.

How can we achieve more through Universal Design? We believe that a move toward socially shared learning regulation holds great promise. Previously in this chapter, we talked about the difference between socially shared learning regulation, self-regulated learning, and externally regulated learning (see Table 7.2). This is not as complicated as it sounds. While students are learning to *self-regulate,* to go about their day managing their own attention, inhibition, and organization (for example) independently, we typically boost their performance by supplying *external regulation.* We intervene on learning regulation that is immature and often a little chaotic to give specific instructions for how to regulate. For example, after having assigned a one-page book summary, a teacher (let's call him Mr. Martin) might notice that many students in his class have failed to settle down and pay attention to the task. Supplying some external regulation, Mr. Martin may ask his whole class to work quietly to support their ability to focus and get the work done. Or he might suggest they all organize their summary using a Venn diagram, which is a strategy that always works for him. While these methods will be very useful for some students, they will not provide a differentiated environment that is suitable for all learners. For example, what if one of the students he's asked to work silently is low on energy and desperately needs the stimulation of a partner? Or imagine that there is a student with visual or spatial impairment who might organize an essay more effectively by talking through its structure. Externally regulated learning is our default, but it isn't very differentiated or universally supportive.

It is interesting to consider what drives our decision making when providing learning regulation instructions for students. When we rely on external regulation of learning, we may design our classroom in a way that is suitable for our *own* instructional and learning preferences. Mr. Martin, for example, may have chosen silence and a Venn diagram because those two strategies work for him. We all do this from time to time, and for good reason. We're operating based on a genuine desire to help and support, but according to a "false consensus bias," we truly think our own preferences, habits, and thoughts are typical and shared by others. As Mr. Martin watches his students working silently on Venn diagrams, he assumes they are as satisfied and well served as he would be. Now that you know about this bias, you may be thinking you can (or often do) consciously override it. Even *that* assumption is biased. That feeling arises from another form of bias called "illusory superiority," through which we believe we have a superior level of insight and self-control to those around us. In actual fact, unless you're doing something really radical to interrupt your habits, these biases are almost impossible to ignore (Katz & Dack, 2013). Don't worry though. Both of them are perfectly normal, and we will shortly recommend a detour. We only raise them to suggest that our default to external regulation of learning leaves our classroom environment rather narrowly designed—perfect for the handful of students who think just like us. Fascinated by this? We discuss teacher bias at greater length in Chapter 3.

We think teachers can use our approach to socially shared learning regulation, via the BSP, to create universal designs that are *truly* universal. If Mr. Martin can interrupt his own biased assumptions for just 5 minutes, he can conduct a BSP and do some real learning about his students' needs. When he asks, "What are our barriers to this specific task?" he has the chance to gather data from not one or two but every single student in his classroom. He may be quite surprised by the information he gathers and gain some unbiased insight about the needs of his students. "I had no idea that silence could be so unproductive! Some students need movement and conversation to stay focused and feel confident," he may think. Similarly, when he asks, "And what strategies might we use to be successful?" his entire class will have a chance to voice their suggestions and approaches. Based on this, Mr. Martin may discover the most unexpected and kid-friendly approaches for the regulation of learning. In addition to showing the students his Venn approach, he may learn that Mark organizes written tasks using a list, Leisl would love to make a giant mind map on the board, and Malia once spoke her history assignment into a recording app and it seemed to really help. These student-created strategies may be much simpler and more efficient than Mr. Martin's suggestions, and easier to add to his universal design. In fact, he may post a list of these strategies and announce, "Anytime we do a writing task, you can use these strategies."

It is so easy to misregulate learning on behalf of our students. Indeed, while perfect silence and Venn diagrams may work as a treat for most of the class, these options may be uncomfortable and unproductive for others. It is only through the continual and routine collection of data that we can interrupt and correct our misconceptions about what students need. And we need to do this not once at the beginning of the term, not from only the loudest and most vocal students, and not from only those whose parents call us with requests but from everyone, every day, for many different tasks. You can accomplish this using the BSP.

We are reminded of our experience with a grade 2 student, who huffed and rolled her eyes at our suggestion that she ought to repeat a positive affirmation before heading out to recess. The boys had been excluding her from their game of BUMP, and she seemed to get bonked on the head with a basketball every single time she stepped onto the court. Unlike so many students, she managed to correct our mistaken assumption. Head tilted to one side, lips tight, and eyes squinty, she seemed to be thinking, "Oh goodness. Here we go with the meditation and mantras." What she actually said was: "I JUST NEED TO LEARN THE RULES TO BUMP!" Promoting this type of voice among all of our students would be the ultimate universal design.

EF-LITERATE TEACHING AND BURNOUT

In the last several pages, we've discussed the ways our approach may affect the achievement gap, global competencies, equity, IEPs, and UDL. With space for one last discussion, we checked in with our community on Twitter: "Here's what we've already covered," we said. "Is there anything else that you wouldn't want us to miss?" Below, you'll see a list of their replies. We didn't steer these responses in any particular direction, but almost all of them followed the same theme. No joke—it happened to be the exact one that we had in mind.

- What about the benefits of an EF approach on the wellness of all stakeholders in a school?
- How about teacher burnout? How does this approach support teachers by decreasing their mental and emotional load?
- Please talk about how we can better support students when we feel good ourselves.
- I'm excited about the way your approach develops efficacy in both students and teachers.
- We really think that EF-literate teaching makes the support team around a child more well informed, capable, and strong. Can you talk more about that?
- Can you talk about how EF teaching can renew teacher energy and reduce burnout?

These responses came from people who were already doing EF-literate classroom teaching. Like so many educators we work with, they were saying, "I know what this seems to do for me, but I want to understand exactly why." We set about explaining the connections between EF-literate teaching and a reduction in feelings of burnout. Much of what we found reflected the very same issues of emotions, efficacy, and "mental load" that had been raised by our community, so that is what we'll tackle in the discussion below. We won't deal much with the straightforward remedy of overall wellness, but please know it is heavily represented in the literature. You should definitely keep hustling to make those smoothies, pack a lunch, go to bed early, and exercise regularly. You know, in all of your free time.

Burnout

To begin, let's define this term. Traditionally, "burnout" is seen as a combination of emotional exhaustion, a reduced sense of personal accomplishment, and feelings of depersonalization (Maslach, Schaufeli, & Leiter, 2001). That means, yes, feeling wiped out and frustrated, but also distant, unsympathetic, and out of touch with the value and uniqueness of the individual children in your class. Recently, arguments have been made that because burnout shares many of the symptoms of depression—including moodiness, weight gain, excessive sleepiness, and something called "leaden paralysis," good grief—it should be treated as such (Bianchi, Schonfeld, & Laurent, 2015). Burnout is caused by excessive workload, lack of control, unclear expectations, troublesome politics, lack of support, and chaos, as well as "moral distress." While moral distress is often ascribed to nurses or medical professionals, it is just as applicable to teachers. It happens when you believe you know the right course of action, but some kind of institutional barrier, such as a lack of resources, stands in your way (Raines, 2000). You may not be fully distressed and burnt out, but odds are you've had a few questionable days, months, or even whole years. We all cope in different ways. While the first thing we may try to focus on is the management of our *physical hygiene* (sleep, diet, and exercise), research suggests we should be just as concerned about interpersonal factors that may be more related to *emotional hygiene*. We'll focus on the ways our EF-literate teaching approach may support your emotional health and ability to thrive in the classroom.

Emotional Intelligence

We are all sensitive and emotionally intelligent, but this is a skill that comes more naturally to some people than others. It turns out, despite the conventional wisdom that it takes a "thick skin" to survive as a teacher, it is the most sensitive and tuned in among us who tend to suffer the least burnout. In a study examining the role of high emotional intelligence, teachers who most effectively paid attention to and subsequently met students' needs ended up becoming the least burned out. Increased sensitivity reduces burnout because it allows teachers to deal with problems before they escalate and become more complicated. This finding, however, is not a silver bullet. After reading this, you probably shouldn't expect to switch up your approach and immediately see a big improvement. While a more sensitive teacher will not prevail in each and every individual situation, research shows that those who are generally oriented toward more sensitive responses tend to respond to students just a little bit more effectively and report less burnout over time (Nizielski, Hallum, Schütz, & Lopes, 2013).

Consider how our approach may improve teachers' sensitivity and responsiveness in the classroom. First, by becoming EF literate, teachers gain a new lens through which to see and understand student performance. When appraising a student doodling on his math assignment, for example, teachers may begin to query potential EF obstacles rather than assuming defiance or lack of interest. They may wonder, "What is really happening? Did they lose attention during the instructions for the task? Are they unable to plan the next step?" Even EF-literate teachers, however, are often surprised when they take the time to probe deeper with a barriers and strategies conversation (Chapter 3).[5] A doodling student may be using a focusing strategy learned

---

[5] Remember, the BSP was introduced in Chapter 3. It is a semistructured teaching protocol. Essentially, it asks teachers to gather students to discuss "What are your/our barriers to this work?" and then "What strategies can we use to be more successful?"

from a therapist, applying an unfamiliar counting strategy, or attempting to sketch the problem. We may be experienced and sensitive, but we are not mind readers! In fact, we know a teacher who directly admits to students that she sometimes misses important things and makes incorrect assumptions, and that she uses the BSP to get at the truth. Remember, researchers tell us that the more you know about your students, and the more responsive you can be, the less burnt out you will feel.

Relationships

Ever had a year of just *not getting along* with one or a handful of students? Relational conflict is especially wearying; it is the type of teaching stress most associated with emotional exhaustion, depression, and quitting (Skaalvik & Skaalvik, 2011). Knowing this, it seems understandable that teachers sometimes put a little distance between themselves and their most challenging students. You may recall saying something like this: "I know she's cutting her eraser into tiny pieces and dropping them all over the floor. I've decided to ignore it because I'm going to go crazy if I have another confrontation with her today." "Avoid the conflict, reduce emotional exhaustion, and have more bandwidth for the other 27 students who need me," we think. Researchers, however, have suggested there is something that may be even more productive than avoiding and reducing conflict: building close relationships (Corbin, Alamos, Lowenstein, Downer, & Brown, 2019). Close relationships with students are well reported to be the main source of enjoyment, satisfaction, and motivation for teachers (Quan-McGimpsey, Kuczynski, & Brophy, 2013), and having achieved them makes teachers feel a sense of professional accomplishment (Chang, 2013). It seems counter-intuitive, but we should run toward our challenging students, not away from them.

You *could* form closer relationships with your students by hosting special, add-on experiences. For example, you might host a fun little pizza party, do an "All About Me" project, or go on an exciting class excursion. During these atypical events, however, your most challenging students will still be challenging (and maybe even more so). Furthermore, after having gone out of your way to reach out to them, you may find yourself engaged in conflict that is even more disappointing than usual (Rodríguez-Mantilla & Fernández-Díaz, 2017). Haven't we all had those days? You drag yourself into the teachers' lounge at the end of it all, perhaps covered in paint, or cupcake sprinkles, or soaked from a rainy excursion, flop into the hermetically sealed vinyl couch, and say, "I give up!" These big efforts are sometimes successful, and they can be truly wonderful, but we think there are more steady and routine ways to build relationships with your students.

In terms of a regular, low-stakes, and feasible way to get closer to your class, you could do a lot worse than the BSP (Chapter 3). You only need 5 minutes and an interesting shared challenge to unify your students in an authentic little "getting to know you" experience. By asking students to tell you about their barriers, you are expressing interest and compassion, and by asking them about their strategies, you are expressing respect and appreciation for their wisdom. Not only will you gather information and build relationships during the 5-minute exchange, the frequency with which you can use the BSP may allow you to normalize a tone of sharing and care. And who knows, this type of rapport may seep into other, less structured, interactions. You may find your students approaching you informally to tell you about other difficulties or bright ideas. While this won't necessarily eliminate conflict in your classroom, it may allow you to walk a more positive, emotionally fulfilling path with even the most challenging of students.

Efficacy

If we apply the *job demands–resources* model (Demerouti, Bakker, Nachreiner, & Schaufeli, 2001), the well-being of teachers relies on the balance between the effortful work we do and the physical, social, or organizational assets we have to achieve goals, ease strain, and thrive. The more of these advantages we have, the more energized and dedicated we will feel, and the more we will be able to deal with the exhausting effects of a classroom (Bakker, Demerouti, & Euwema, 2005). Yes, of course teachers benefit from supportive supervisors and adequate physical materials and space, but the personal resources of a teacher also count. Again and again, researchers confirm that the most important personal resource for reducing teacher burnout is self-efficacy (e.g., Bermejo-Toro, Prieto-Ursúa, & Hernández, 2016). This refers to our sense that we can successfully instruct, manage, and engage our students, and also that we can develop and sustain positive relationships with them. If self-efficacy can tip the balance of our burnout level, it is worth pursuing.

You will not be surprised to hear that we think the BSP (Chapter 3) can help you build self-efficacy. We'll present two approaches—the first more obvious and the second a little more novel. First, we would like to suggest that the BSP provides data that even the most well-trained teachers need to rack up teaching "wins," avoid frustrating "losses," and cultivate self-efficacy. Consider the way teaching challenges are ordinarily diagnosed and tackled. To manage a group of students who can't perform 2-digit subtraction with borrowing, for example, a teacher might gather her class to reteach the lesson using base-10 manipulatives and a story about how we borrow from neighbors. This "best practice" intervention could take 10 minutes to plan and prepare, as well as 20 minutes to execute. Any teacher of mathematics, however, knows that even the very best practices sometimes mysteriously flop. We return to school fresh from a math training course with innovative approaches that yield the same blank stares and wrong answers. This is a big drag on our self-efficacy.

Alternatively, the same teacher can use the BSP to ask her students for precise information about the barriers they face. She may discover that most of the class understands the concept of borrowing and base 10 but are actually struggling to keep the digits in each problem straight and tidy. After supplying a different-sized graph paper and assigning double-check partners, as the students themselves have suggested within the BSP, she can deliver tailored "best practice" support to the small group who really need it. Knowing more about these students, it is no surprise that the standard "best practice" approach was unnecessary for most of them. Using the BSP to gather data about her students' precise needs, this teacher has not only a greater chance of success but also a lower chance of mysterious failure; she increases *and* protects her sense of self-efficacy.

Another route to a reduction in feelings of burnout may be through *class collective efficacy*. This term refers to how capable we feel, as a team, of working together with students to achieve learning goals (Bandura, 1997; Chen & Chin, 2006). Around a school, teachers often talk informally about their class collective efficacy. You might hear, "I have to keep a close eye on this class. We just can't seem to get it together" or "This is an amazing class. I feel like they can handle anything." In much the same way that self-efficacy grows, perceived collective efficacy is also thought to grow when we work together to master new challenges, watch others master new challenges, and work together in a social climate of goal striving and success (Bandura, 1997). Your personal success and self-efficacy can protect against burnout, and so can the success and efficacy you feel as part of a team with your students.

We think the BSP can guide you toward greater class collective efficacy by providing more structured, scaffolded opportunities for communal problem solving. Whereas a teacher might ordinarily struggle with intervention ideas, accommodation plans, or instructional challenges independently, the BSP moves more of this work into the collective space. Within daily conversations, whole classes can wrestle with shared problems and enjoy small victories together. "We can do hard things," our teachers often reassure their classes. "It doesn't matter how hard the task; if we work together and share strategies, we can do anything."

Teacher burnout is a significant concern for the profession. Too many seasoned educators, who should be in the prime of their careers, providing guidance, leadership, and mentorship to others, are instead either lingering resentfully in classrooms or limping off on medical leave. Our wonderful teacher friend Paula Barrow swears that discovering an EF-literate teaching approach after 22 years in the classroom pumped her up for another 15.[6] Are you at the end of your rope? Before you start packing boxes and filling in job applications, why not try just one more little thing?

---

[6] Paula Barrow teaches at Fenelon Township Public School in Cameron, Ontario, Canada. Used with permission.

CHAPTER 8

History and Reflections
Our Work with Teachers

CREATING AND NAMING THE PROJECT

Sometimes, after a talk or a workshop, an educator hangs back to ask us, "How did you get from your teaching jobs to where you are now?" Practically speaking, the approach we describe has been in development since 2010. The BSP first took shape in Laurie's classroom after a vice principal introduced the idea of EFs to the whole staff. Then, feeling very enthusiastic about the potential of the approach, she began sharing the idea in blogs, a website, and at teaching conferences. Adding up to almost 40 separate engagements over 3 years, the presentations were rough and experimental, and almost every one of them had a moment of reckoning: Teachers coping with really challenging classes are tough customers. "You don't know my students," they would say, or "You don't know my school day." A big, strong gym teacher told us, tearfully, "You don't know my *stress level.*" We learned how badly teachers needed solutions for managing students' self-regulated learning and stress, and also how dynamic and shatterproof the solutions needed to be. We were so grateful for this early learning.

While teaching, Laurie met Peg Dawson and Richard Guare, who took an interest in her work, provided guidance and moral support, and later devoted a chapter of *Executive Skills in Children and Adolescents* to Laurie's description of the emerging approach (Faith, 2018). They invited Laurie to participate in more high-profile speaking engagements, mentioned her work on their own speaking rounds, and facilitated many interesting introductions. In 2014, Laurie discovered the work of Gabrielle Oettingen and Peter Gollwitzer. After 17 years in the classroom, she left her teaching role and set off on an academic path. Oettingen and Gollwitzer's research on "mental contrasting with implementation intentions" seemed to substantiate the barriers and strategies conversations. This work, alongside the well-established scholarship on self-regulated learning, plus several important studies on EFs and growth mindset, fit together into a research basis for the approach. So much powerful insight was there for the taking; all it needed was an educator's eye to assemble it and mobilize it into a classroom.

With a chapter published by Dawson and Guare, and a PhD in the works, Laurie had the opportunity to present, collaborate, and network on a larger scale. Another big breakthrough came in the form of a five-person team of teachers from Trillium Lakelands District School Board in Ontario, who approached Laurie at a teaching conference. These experienced teachers wanted to learn more about EFs in the classroom, so had applied for and received an Ontario Teacher Learning and Leadership Project (TLLP) Grant. They used their funding package to pay for release time for themselves and their colleagues, and were then able to engage in several workshops and other collaborations with each other and with Laurie. Two other teams from the same school board later applied for and received TLLP grant money to build upon this work in design-based teaching and in the arts.

Collaborating over the next few years with teachers from the Trillium Lakelands District School Board—getting to know them and their students—allowed for deep learning. It was fascinating to support teachers as they adapted to various challenges, steadily honing a whole range of EF-literate approaches that were both practical and powerful. Many of those teachers are the stars of this book. From this work, a team of 11 especially keen teachers emerged and helped to fine-tune a slide deck and workbook of materials used for training other schools in the board. This team also helped to coin a name for the movement: "Activated Learning." Following this, several other school boards requested training, talks, and partnership.

During this time, Laurie was building a relationship with a group of U.K. psychologists and educators called Connections in Mind. Over 2 years, Laurie visited London several times to collaborate on an EF-literate approach for local teachers, coaches, and parents. Finally, through this organization, an introduction between Laurie Faith and a very experienced educator with both U.S. and U.K. experience was made (Carol-Anne Bush). Carol had just left a 10-year post as an administrator, was seeking a big creative project, and was reenergized by the potential of EFs in the classroom. Laurie and Carol quickly formed a partnership, with Carol's skills complementing Laurie's perfectly. Around the same time, Peg Dawson and Laurie had been talking about the success of Laurie's website, and before you know it, Carol, Peg, and Laurie were crafting a pitch to document the whole project in a book with Guilford Press.

The task of naming this project has haunted us. In the 2018 Dawson and Guare chapter, it was called "EFs 2 the Rescue Pedagogy." Later, teachers called it "Activated Learning" and "#EF4ALL." For now, we're holding on to the name "Activated Learning" so it can be located on the Internet and referred to, with the understanding that new teams of teachers may continue to rename it as they like. The whole challenge around naming arose because, technically, we didn't really know what the project was or should be. A program? A practice? A movement? Anytime you make something cool, even if it's just cobbled together from scraps of research and ordinary classroom practices, people start to worry about these things. Any creation that seems like a commodity triggers pressure to name it, hoard its ownership, and hurry up and monetize it before someone else does. Even our most relaxed friends tracked us down, looked us in the eye, and tried to talk some business sense into us. "Well . . ." we were warned, "you don't want to have any *regrets*." Our neighbors told us to apply for a trademark. Our grandmas told us to get a lawyer. At one point, someone suggested we should *patent* the idea. "A patent," an expert cheerfully informed us, "kills trade secrets and independent creation." We had a good laugh at the absurdity of this: The contents of this book, and its overall ambition, are based on the *thriving* of teachers' independent creation and trade secrets. Even so, in this context, the threat of being taken advantage of, *somehow*, prompted many discussions and kept us up at night. Around this time, Laurie had a call with Carol Dweck to discuss these concerns. "This is what scholarship is all about," she advised. "Share it and move on to your next idea." So, after much contemplation, we realized that to hoard this idea would stop it, and us, in our tracks. It was a growth mindset moment. We decided: Let's be thinkers, learners, and collaborators rather than owners. Indeed, for any decent educational invention, and particularly those operating on teachers' daily, ingrained, pedagogical habits, the biggest goal should be *user* ownership. Therefore, we're placing this idea into the public sphere and truly hope that any educator who wants it will grab it up and run with it.

MEETING TECHNICAL *AND* ADAPTIVE NEEDS WITH PROFESSIONAL DEVELOPMENT

Starting around 2015, references to EFs started coming from all sides: in the news, on psychoeducational reports, in staff rooms, and at conferences. When teachers learned the technical name for the off-track, disorganized, and inattentive behaviors they were so familiar with, they wanted to know a lot more. "How do we address this in the classroom," they wondered? Requests for after-school training, 1-day workshops, and other forms of professional development (PD) started pouring in.

We took meetings with superintendents, directors, principals, and teachers to understand what our training should look like, but the opinions were often contradictory. First, we listened to teachers, who told us, "Give us as much as you can. Supply us with posters, lessons, and anything else you have to make our job easier." We also listened to several administrators, who told us, "The last thing we want is another binder or spiral-bound curriculum. Hundreds of those land on our desks every year, and they are rarely useful. We want something that teachers can muddle into and adapt to their own classrooms." Both muddly *and* easy? This stumped us for a while. Should we provide premade materials or not?

One thing we knew for sure was that teachers don't show up to work hoping to solve as many elaborate problems as possible. If a simple, one-size-fits-all solution exists and will make the day run more smoothly, teachers tend to use it. Who can blame them? For example, teachers often share tried and tested worksheets, easy lesson ideas, or activities. They share ideas for how to best organize a classroom library and borrow each other's lineup tricks. Solutions like these are essential, but they only go so far. How do we respond to children who are off track or whose behavior surprises us? There is no worksheet that will help us, for example, when we walk in the room and Daniel is *lying* on that perfectly sorted bookshelf. No quick and easy activity will support Frida, who has been in remedial reading support for 6 weeks and hasn't made any progress. These are pedagogical aspects of teaching and cannot be handled with a quick photocopy or a premade lesson. Experts call these *adaptive* rather than simple *technical* challenges, and they require problem solving (Heifetz & Linsky, 2002). While some parts of our approach are technical (teaching children new EF terminology, for example, is pretty straightforward and can be done with simple, premade lessons), some of it is adaptive. The BSP must be administered creatively, flexibly, and using teachers' judgment. We realized that the most effective day of learning would include some sharing of quick and easy technical solutions, and a lot of guidance to support the necessary adaptive (muddly) problem solving.

On this basis, the training evolved toward providing a half day of technical solutions for teaching EFs plus a half day of exploring ways to adapt the BSP. In the morning, we'd playfully dig into the materials you'll find in Chapter 3, using the surveys and posters for practice. We'd show pictures and tell stories of the many ways other teachers had taught EFs. We'd lead participants through the "11 Lessons to Teach EFs," modeling a few of the activities. This allowed our participants to gain a deeper understanding of EFs, and also to get ready to use these materials in their classrooms. Then, in the afternoon, we led participants through three or four different BSPs. Again and again, we noticed smiles, laughter, and a sense of connection among the teachers as they opened up and shared their personal barriers and strategies. It seemed like a good balance.

A problem arose, however, when these teachers headed back to their classrooms. Through extensive follow-up consultation, we noticed they were getting stuck, often focusing for a long time on teaching EF knowledge. Teachers would spend weeks slowly administering the 11 lessons, developing special folders to collect EF activities, or creating elaborate bulletin boards to display facts about EFs. They would linger, trying for perfection. While these initiatives demanded a lot of technical work—photocopying, scheduling, planning, and organizing, not to mention time—we realized they did not require much change to the most ingrained and fundamental pedagogical habits. This pattern fit perfectly into Piaget's theory of learning, which tells us that as humans, we are much more comfortable assimilating new ideas into preexisting schemas than making fundamental schematic change (Piaget, 1952). When they were teaching EF knowledge, teachers were using a well-established schema: Learn some information, prepare a lesson, and deliver the lesson. In order to administer the BSP, however, they would have to undergo an uncomfortable *cognitive dissonance* resulting from the fundamental change to their schema for pedagogy. Instead of responding to off-track students by supporting, redirecting, or reducing their expectations, they would have to *accommodate* a brand new approach. Muddling isn't easy; learning a new way to respond to students isn't easy.

After making these observations, we made a few changes. First, we took the time to acquaint teachers with the importance of a little discomfort and cognitive dissonance. "This will feel uncomfortable because it is real, deep learning. Don't let the discomfort scare you off—it's a sign you are learning and doing something new." We also moved all of the tempting *knowledge-based* content to an afternoon slot. While we continued to provide a basic education on the science of EFs, we were careful not to overemphasize knowledge teaching. We stopped showing our favorite 15 or so slides of teachers with perfect bulletin boards, and instead showed one slide of a really straightforward display. We decided to frontload the BSP. This allowed us to kick off our PD with the smiles, laughter, and sense of connectedness it brought. It also provided authentic opportunities to explore EFs. We often, for example, asked teachers to consider a familiar and personal issue, such as how to get report cards done on time, or how to stick to a new exercise routine. Through these conversations, key EF vocabulary often came up naturally. "I am a terrible procrastinator, and I leave my reports to the last minute," they might say. When we responded by asking, "Does it feel more like stress, or timing, or attention?" a conversation about EFs would arise. We also spent more time helping teachers mentally prepare for the big pedagogical shift. We asked them, "When do you think you might first use the BSP?" We made long lists of all the triggers, moments, and opportunities: when there are a lot of mistakes in math calculation, when editing isn't being done, when groups can't work well together, when a supply teacher is coming, or when a big project is about to start. We even conducted BSPs on doing the BSP. We asked, "What will stand in your way of starting this? What will stand in your way of doing it a second time? And how will you be strategic to meet your goal?" They told us, for example, that they planned to work in teams, consult one another, try "small starts," and start at less stressful times. We also helped teachers practice several universal and simple applications. For example, we made sure every teacher left our training with experience doing a BSP on "getting homework done on time," "having a good recess," and "reading to understand." We challenged each trainee to try a BSP on their first day back in the classroom. Our goal was to reduce the inertia that would slow down their first try, and then load them up with coping strategies to ensure they followed up a second, third, and fourth time.

We also reoriented our delivery of technical, premade materials. We added a range of teacher-created materials to the website that could be freely accessed on an as-needed basis (*http://activatedlearning.org*). If a teacher wanted a certain poster, lesson, or survey, they could simply pop online and print it out. We also established a Twitter community under the hashtag #ActivatedLearning that focused on sharing a wide variety of classroom approaches and tools. No longer simply teaching 11 lessons over a few months, teachers began to follow and adapt to the needs of their own classrooms. In this way, we avoided superimposing a rigid approach on top of the local diversity. Rather, our training followed established best practice by being simple and flexible, allowing users to organize their own approaches, and encouraging sensible and personal choices (Lanham et al., 2013). The teachers we worked with seemed more energized, curious, and satisfied by their efforts.

GROUNDING PD IN GENUINE PROBLEMS OF PRACTICE

Every time we gave a workshop, we would stimulate a cautious change among a majority of typical teachers and completely *light up* a handful of the more unusual ones. Alongside the steady pace of the masses, those early adopters would leave our sessions at a run. Back at school, they'd fabricate time and energy as if by magic, play fearlessly with the BSP, explore new ways to build EF literacy, and mobilize motivation psychology in ways we hadn't anticipated. Then, they'd stop us in school hallways to give us breathless feedback or email us with loud and enthusiastic testimonials. "This is amazing!" they'd say. "This process is so easy!" or "I feel like this is the most natural thing in the world!" When this happened—let's be honest—we'd feel quite excited and satisfied. We'd make time to visit their classrooms, arrange phone interviews, and beg them to Tweet out pictures to share their learning. We were delighted to have new creative partners, and we knew these daring few could help other teachers understand the approach and feel motivated to try it (Hall & Hord, 2001).

As much as it was thrilling to discover an Activated Learning superstar, however, we knew they had very little to offer us as representatives of typical teachers. *Outlier, outlier, outlier,* we'd remind ourselves. While these teachers were thrilling to learn with, we knew that if we wanted to reach the majority of students, we had to gear our training 100% toward the needs of more typical educators. Knowing most teachers leave PD sessions feeling as though the demands placed on them have been unrealistic (Fitzgerald, Danaia, & McKinnon, 2019), we set about equipping every single attendee with a *feasible* approach.

The principals and superintendents who booked us always reinforced this concern. Having witnessed many cycles of unproductive PD, they took very seriously the basic learning needs of their teachers. Seemingly on cue and in perfect harmony, they were all quoting the same kinds of concerns. Teachers wondered, first, "Who is this expert, and so soon after the last one?" They complained of being tight on time, overwhelmed, and for that matter, *still trying to implement that last great new thing*. They felt as though new approaches presented in PD were often random, seemingly disconnected from what they were genuinely concerned about. Furthermore, they confided that PD often carried the suggestion that they were doing it all wrong and ought to start from scratch. If you don't address these challenges, we were warned, you're going to have a room full of frustrated and checked-out participants.

Inspired by these conversations, we dug deeply into the issue of feasibility and connectedness. We studied the literature on classroom implementation and discovered we needed to connect what we were sharing to a professional problem teachers were genuinely frustrated by, stuck on, or fed up with (Marzano, Pickering, & Pollock, 2001). We also needed to ensure our approach was sensible, achievable, and not too intrusive (Kazdin, 1980; Lakin & Shannon, 2015; Reimers et al., 1987). Teachers needed a lot of good reasons to believe us when we said, "This will help, and it is something you are more than capable of doing." These considerations guided the training, and if you have been reading this book from cover to cover, they will be familiar because they have guided our written approach as well.

As it turned out, helping teachers to recognize and get behind the problem we were trying to solve was easy. We quickly discovered how enthusiastic—riotous, even—teachers could be when asked to describe classroom challenges related to EFs. Accustomed as we were to trying anything to connect with our audience, no matter how quirky, we once brought a whole bunch of bells, whistles, and other noisemakers and asked teachers to sound off when they heard something familiar. "Reexplaining instructions to students who weren't paying attention!" we'd call out, to a cacophony of Ding! Ding! Dings! "Helping students to solve disagreements! Putting students' notes in order! Getting students going again when stalled!" Watching an exhausted fourth-grade teacher smile with satisfaction while repeatedly ringing a chrome-plated customer service bell is a sight we will not soon forget. Eventually, the bells broke, and we retired the activity. To replace it, we asked teachers to sticky-note all of the little snags, challenges, and obstacles they faced while moving students from instructions to goal completion each day. From a roomful of educators, hundreds of these little papers would be amassed and then slapped onto big chart papers representing different EF categories. "I can't believe how many of these problems relate to EFs!" the teachers would recognize. It was never hard to convince teachers that lagging EFs and self-regulation were absorbing most of their attention and energy in classrooms.

We also helped teachers appreciate that they were *already doing* a lot of EF and self-regulated learning support. First, we described the way incremental, rigorous challenges in a calm, structured, stimulating, social, and joyful environment supports EF development (Diamond, 2014). We asked teachers to consider all of the ways in which they were already meeting these needs; they made long lists of every carefully planned lesson, organized learning space, special club, and extracurricular activity they took the time to put in place. To emphasize how much self-regulated learning support was already happening, we simulated the way teachers often rush from student to student, quickly moving through a cycle of plan, act, and reflect with each one: "Hi Sam. What's your problem? Whataya gonna to do about it? No ideas? Hmm. Try making a list! Great. Go!" In training, we moved around the room kneeling and bending over our attendees one by one as we tried to imitate the daily madness of trying to *regulate* for not only oneself but also 20 to 30 students. "It's like playing Whack-a-Mole," we said. "You get Sam going, move through six other students, get halfway across the room, and look back to see that Sam has fallen apart again!" Or we compared it to spinning plates, joking about how impossible it was to constantly keep them all balanced and moving. While these ideas felt a little exaggerated to some, they were bang on to others. We seemed to be hitting a nerve. Teachers were gratified by how vividly we could describe their classroom experiences. They could see the connection between what we were presenting and what they were already spending most of their days working on.

Freshly reminded of their daily work to support student EFs and self-regulated learning, teachers could interpret our suggestions as *efficiencies.* They explored our approach not as a "start from scratch" but as a way to consolidate and front-load a process they were already doing. By doing a BSP with the whole class, we suggested, teachers could get students started on tasks with potential obstacles and strategy ideas already in mind. "Then, instead of playing Whack-a-Mole, you can stand back and become an observer," we encouraged. We modeled the way teachers could migrate from kneeling beside desks to standing up straight. "You will have more time to observe, pay attention to your students' process, and provide 'notice and name' feedback." We didn't suggest it would be a perfect process right away. We acknowledged it might take a while for certain classes to relax enough to engage fully in conversations about their barriers. And while we admitted that they, themselves, might sometimes feel nervous to engage with students on such a personal and vulnerable level, we also reassured them that starting right away and practicing a little bit every day would pay off.

Experts agree there is a right and a wrong way to deliver PD: Be content focused, they say. Allow for active learning, provide feedback, involve collaborative examination of student work, and provide long-term follow-up (Ingvarson, Meiers, & Beavis, 2005). Accordingly, at each training, we asked teachers to spell out their most troublesome content areas so we could delve into their unique EF barriers and practice creating useful compensatory strategies. We created opportunities to journal, talk, move, and create. When it was all over, we set up videoconferences and return visits to provide follow-up. Despite these provisions, however, we all agreed that even the most skillful and captivating presentation is a complete and utter waste of time and money if it is unnecessary, unwanted, or impractical. Providing feasible training that was grounded in urgent problems of practice was our number one priority.

FINE-TUNING THE FORMAT AND DELIVERY OF PD

Having fine-tuned our training, we began to question the format of our delivery. We knew we had a role to play with educators, but it took a while to understand exactly how to play it. On one hand, we were getting great reviews on our workshops. We had developed an engaging 4-hour program that left teachers feeling enlightened and excited. We were aware, however, of the very bad press surrounding "one-shot" PD. We could not deny the well-known fact that one day of learning rarely leads to lasting change (Garet, Porter, Desimone, Birman, & Yoon, 2001). Over time, we realized that in addition to offering the training, there were three supporting pre-, during-, and post-workshop factors that were within our control and that needed to be in place.

First, we realized that our workshop groups were engaged in very different preparation prior to our arrival; sorting through requests from teacher teams, principals, and school boards, we became adept at detecting training engagements that were headed for disaster. If an organizer wasn't calling on behalf of the majority of our "trainees," we suspected the crowd would be divided into two polarized groups who were frustrated at one other. If a principal called us because he had heard about the workshop from another principal, we knew we might arrive to a bewildered staff caught completely unawares. And when a small group of teachers called, hoping we could come in to transform the rest of the staff? Just . . . yikes! All of these situations involved us dragging tens of teachers backward through hours of learning they didn't ask for, didn't necessarily want, and might resent as a distraction from their actual priorities.

The kinds of organizers we looked for tended to tell different stories. Some explained that EFs had emerged as a major area of concern in a staff meeting, while others revealed they had been reading about growth mindset as a whole school team and felt ready for the next step. The very best news, for us, was when a school told us they had come together as a group, found EFs to be a major area of concern, and begun to gather data to understand the scope of the problem. Bingo! We knew this was a promising and legitimate training situation, because it mirrored the structure of "collaborative inquiry." Collaborative inquiry, through which educators base their learning *on their own shared experiences and goals,* is a reliable driver of improvement for both students and schools (Vescio, Ross, & Adams, 2008). What did we do with the more worrisome invitations? We suggested they start with a 15-minute whole-staff introduction. In these meetings, both conducted in person and via videoconference, we could quickly explain the challenges we wanted to tackle, the kinds of science we would like to discuss, and the types of approaches to be explored. "Please take a few weeks to think about this and talk it over. We do not want you to waste your precious PD dollars on a workshop that doesn't relate to your most pressing challenges." Almost every single group who received this pitch eventually asked for a workshop, but it was based on the agreement and genuine interest of the majority of the staff.

The second supporting factor we learned to control was the involvement of principals. We began to notice that the groups who went on to engage and change their practice the most were those led by a dazzling variety of hyper-involved principals. This type would come armed with their own books on the subject, or rush off at every break to plan unique applications with groups of teachers, or end the day with five or six questions and a to-do list. In contrast, teams who struggled seemed to have principals who were distracted, were seated at the back of the room, floated in and out during the morning session, or were pulled out unexpectedly during the afternoon. Our hunch was affirmed by a whole lot of science that suggests that engaged, *learning-with* principals bring a crucial sense of relevance and importance to new learning (Ajzen, 1985, 1991; Ajzen & Fishbein, 2000) and can almost double the impact of any other dimension of PD on student achievement (Robinson, Hohepa, & Lloyd, 2009). Before booking a workshop, therefore, we made sure to explain and emphasize these realities with principals. "Ugh. I know. I'm so sorry. I have so much on my plate . . ." they would tell us, with genuine regret. Indeed, distracted principals are almost never shopping for vacations and new sneakers online—in our experience, most are simply overloaded and putting out one urgent fire after another. We wondered if it might make sense to have principals fill in a barriers and strategies reflection prior to training. We prompted them by saying, "My goal is to be fully present and engaged during today's training. What barriers might I face? What strategies can I use to be successful?" In response, principals sometimes made different arrangements to handle unexpected interruptions, such as sharing the responsibility with a senior teacher. When principals were reminded that their participation would have a ripple effect throughout the staff and determine the overall success of their initiative, they often found creative ways to remain engaged.

The third factor we concerned ourselves with was follow-up support. We wanted to make sure that, after participating in a workshop and attempting to implement new approaches, a teacher had someone with whom to problem-solve. We also wanted to encourage a culture of ongoing adaptation, personalization, and ownership. This has been called "generative professional development," and it treats teachers as free-thinking individuals who can take an active role in their own learning (Flint, Zisook, & Fisher, 2011). While our engaged principals carried much of the load, and teachers often sought each other out for help, we also tried to provide a system of as-needed, 20-minute videoconference check-ins before and after school. Teachers from larger workshop groups were offered semi-private meetings in groups of three to four, while smaller training teams were spoiled with private meetings. We learned a lot. Contrary to our assumption, the teachers who met in *groups* thrived and persisted the most. Spending more than half of their "consult" time either listening to other teachers or being overheard didn't bother them. In fact, they seemed to enjoy it. We did some reading and realized that, yes, while most real change to teaching practice happens when teachers are encouraged to experiment with new understandings (Guskey, 2002), they benefit equally from interactions with colleagues (Penuel, Sun, Frank, & Gallagher, 2012). By offering private consultations, we were encouraging their experimentation but isolating teachers from each other's expertise and experience. Going forward, we made sure to create online opportunities that would cluster at least three teachers into one conversation.

As we move forward, we are looking for ways to more fully empower teachers as learners. One of our new directions is to remove the full-day workshop entirely and replace it with a number of shorter engagements. By doing this, we hope to enable more use of videoconference, which will increase our reach, reduce travel, and almost eliminate costs due to teacher release time. Even better than the logistical advantages, however, is the fact that with more frequent, short meetings, we can support an entire cycle of collaborative inquiry. Over several months, we can help teachers gather data across four stages: first by identifying a challenge of practice, then researching and establishing a suitable solution, then implementing the solution, and finally determining the success of the solution and making plans for next steps. In this way, we hope to retreat almost fully from being a one-shot, sage-on-stage performance and focus more on facilitating the hypothesizing, creativity, and adaptation that will be most meaningful and useful to teachers.

OVERALL TAKEAWAYS FROM OUR WORK WITH TEACHERS

Below, we summarize a list of the most important lessons we have learned about supporting teachers' professional learning. Within each lesson, we realize, is a factor that is well established in the scientific literature of effective PD; taken individually, these lessons do not break new ground. In this condensed format, however, we hope our list provides guidance as to which specific, research-based factors you should focus on to best foster our particular brand of EF-literate teaching.

- *Heck, yeah!* Conduct workshops, training, and so forth, *only* if the learners believe it will address an urgent problem of practice. A quick introduction of the proposed learning should yield a "Heck, yeah!" response. Otherwise, you should circle back to figure out what your problems of practice actually are and address those things.

- *All aboard:* Conduct whole-school professional learning only when a principal is on board. He or she must be fully available to attend the training and willing to participate in implementation in tangible ways. Otherwise, spend your money on the lunch program or new basketballs, or something that will actually make a difference.

• *Are you with me?* Upon starting a workshop or training, restate and characterize the problem of practice as thoroughly and vividly as possible to reenergize learners. Is this the problem you urgently want to solve? Are you with me? The answer should be an emphatic "Yes!"

• *This is that:* Upon starting a workshop or training, clearly establish the time, energy, and emotional resources that are tied up in current practices and balance the proposed solution as efficiencies against these. Faculty and staff should think, oh, this is for *that* problem.

• *Get real:* Professional learning (training) experiences should be tied to realistic, content-based activities that teachers can relate to. For example, during a training day, teachers should practice conducting the BSP for a specific math, reading or writing, groupwork, and social skill so they can see how it really works.

• *No home base:* Teachers should be gently steered away from dwelling for too long on familiar teaching activities, such as delivering lessons on EF definitions. While this is useful, it should not go on for too long. Instead, they should begin the more uncomfortable work of changing their pedagogy . . . stopping students regularly to investigate the barriers to their goals and the strategies to be successful.

• *We can do hard things:* Teachers should be directly informed and reassured about the uncomfortable feelings of cognitive dissonance that will accompany their real, deep learning and change. Tell them, "This discomfort is a good sign. You're on the right track."

• *Plan for a rainy day:* Before heading out to try something bold and new, teachers should work in teams to plan strategies for managing feelings of discomfort, discouragement, or even fear.

• *All the help:* Teachers need straightforward technical information and tools, as well as the inspiration, reassurance, and guidance to attempt and master more adaptive approaches. So balance the provision of photocopies and premade resources with time for teaching, discussion, and practice.

• *Attentive support:* When teachers are back in their classrooms starting new, stressful, or uncomfortable approaches, principals and colleagues should regularly and generously support them. This may feel like "helicopter parenting" until teachers get up and running.

• *Make it your own:* Teachers should be encouraged to continuously modify, change, and adapt new approaches to the special dynamics of their own classrooms.

• *Teamwork:* Ongoing support should ideally happen in community with other teachers and principals. Support from professional experts can be helpful, but if it happens without the involvement of other staff and principals, it may feel irrelevant to implementers.

Strategy Teaching Interventions for Executive Functions

Intervention	Description	Strengths	Limitations
Alert program (Nash et al., 2015)	Aims to develop students with fetal alcohol spectrum disorder's self-regulation of their sensory needs. Twelve 1-hour sessions over 14 weeks. Delivered one-to-one with an occupational therapist.	Students learn about their sensory needs, factors that affect them, and strategies for self-regulating.	No focus on strategies for learning. Not relevant for typically developing students. High duration and frequency. Not delivered by school staff or in school/home setting.
Chicago School Readiness Program (Watts, Gandhi, Ibrahim, Masucci, & Raver, 2018)	Add-on for preschool curriculum. Aims to develop preschool children's strategies for emotional regulation. Teachers receive workshops to manage stress and children with behavior difficulties receive counseling.	Focus on early intervention. Training for teachers and parents.	No focus on strategies for learning. Only for preschool. High time and resource demands.

(continued)

Intervention	Description	Strengths	Limitations
German Marburg Concentration Training (Wimmer, Bellingrath, & von Stockhausen, 2016)	Aims to support difficulties associated with hyperactivity and attention. Activities involve principles of cognitive behaviour therapy, learning strategies, and relaxation techniques. Twenty-five sessions over 18 weeks; two sessions per week (one for 60 minutes, one for 90 minutes). Delivered by two tutors.	Includes physical activity and learning strategies. Delivered in the school setting.	Strategies for learning are not the priority area targeted by the intervention. High dosage, frequency, and duration. Not delivered by school staff.
Intervention for executive processes involved in reading comprehension (García-Madruga et al., 2013)	Strategy learning for reading comprehension for 8- to 9-year-olds. 50 minutes per day for 12 days over 4 weeks. Delivered by two researchers to a whole class.	Focused on strategies for learning. Delivered to the whole class. Intervention involves practicing the strategies during the learning activity.	Focuses on only one area of learning (reading comprehension). Feasibility issues as two trained professionals needed to deliver.
OutSMARTERs program (Hannesdottir, Ingvarsdottir, & Bjornsson, 2017)	Aims to develop social skills, self-regulation, and EFs for students with ADHD (ages 8–10 years). Two-hour sessions, twice a week, for 5 weeks. Delivered by clinical psychologists and occupational therapists (three adults per group).	Training provided for professionals delivering it. Manualized.	Not relevant for typically developing students. Feasibility issues in terms of time, availability of professionals, and financial resources. Delivered outside of typical lessons.
PASS (Planning, Attention, Simultaneous, and Successive; Haddad et al., 2003; Iseman & Naglieri, 2011)	Aim to develop students' use of strategies in learning (research available on reading comprehension and math). Delivered by teacher in small group or whole class. Ten minutes of planning facilitation for between 2 days and 3 weeks.	Focus on strategies for learning. Low dosage, frequency, and duration and delivered by class teacher in classroom context. Supports learning from peers as students make suggestions of strategies.	Focuses only on planning skills. No explicit teaching of EFs or EF strategies for learning (i.e., from teacher).

(continued)

Intervention	Description	Strengths	Limitations
PASS (*continued*)	This entailed asking questions that elicited strategies that students could use.	Suitable for students with and without additional learning needs.	
PATHS (Promoting Alternative Thinking Strategies; Kusché & Greenberg, 1994)	Add-on to school curriculum. Aims to develop students' social and emotional skills. Three days per week for 20–30 minutes.	Provides strategies for self-regulation of emotions. Delivered in the school setting.	No focus on strategies for learning. High frequency and duration.
SMARTs Executive Function and Mentoring intervention (Meltzer, Basho, Reddy, & Kurkul, 2015)	Aims to develop metacognitive awareness and use of EF strategies through explicit teaching and peer mentoring. Eighty minutes per week for 8 months. Two SMARTs teachers and two assistant teachers per class. (Four weeks of mentor training; then 7 months of SMARTs sessions, i.e., teaching EF strategies.) Secondary school students with learning difficulties, ADHD, and those "struggling academically."	Explicit teaching of EF strategies and peer-supported opportunities to practice the strategies on learning activities. Incorporates goal-setting techniques.	Does not explicitly develop students' understanding of EFs. High ratio of teaching staff needed. High dosage and duration.
Unstuck and On Target program (Kenworthy et al., 2014)	Focus on supporting students with ASD with difficulties associated with ASD such as flexibility in thinking and behavior, and social skills. Twenty-eight 30- to 40-minute lessons by school staff.	Delivered by trained school staff. Other teachers and parents trained to promote generalization. Develops understanding of areas of difficulty and practices strategies of support.	No focus on strategies for learning. Not relevant for typically developing students. High dosage, duration, and frequency.

Note. Table created by Dr. Lisa Carmody for her doctoral research. Used with permission.

EF Basics

A Series of 11 Mini-Lessons to Build Whole-Class EF Literacy (Grade 2 and Up)

Depending on your approach to teaching EFs, you might enjoy the EF Basics Lesson Series. This was created by popular demand, inspired by the outstanding classroom work of our colleague Stephanie Walker at Scott Young Public School in Lindsay, Ontario, Canada. Teachers wanted quick little lessons to directly teach each EF to their students. Each lesson provides two or three simple experiences or mini activities that you can do with everyday materials. They will allow your class to discuss, explore, and understand how each EF feels and affects their performance. We know teachers who use these lessons every day for the first few days, weeks, or months of school. Or some choose to use only a small handful of the lessons because they determined that EFs such as attention and organization, for example, were already so well understood by their students. We also know whole schools that agreed all teachers would cover one lesson per week over a specified period of time. We don't yet know of any schools that have committed to a schoolwide EF Spirit Day, created EF lesson stations, and rotated their whole student body though all of the lessons in one day, but we're hoping to soon! As with everything else, modify and adapt these lessons to your heart's content.

Teaching Guide for All Lessons: EF Basics Mini-Lessons Series

BACKGROUND

Purpose: This series of repeating lessons will build basic EF knowledge and skill for both teacher and students. They can be used alone or in combination with other lessons on EF.

Timing: Any time, but particularly useful at the beginning of the year. May be done daily, weekly, or monthly. Each lesson should take 30–40 minutes.

Materials: Each lesson on the specified EF is accompanied by rich supplementary notes. These notes contain a clear definition of the EF, activity ideas, examples from daily life, strategy examples, and student worksheets.

A set of classroom EF posters will also be useful to have up as you present these lessons, and then to keep up for reference once your class has developed EF knowledge and skill (more poster options at *http://activatedlearning.org*).

LESSON PLAN

Connection: Choose an EF to focus on for the lesson. Gather whole class. Engage students in a short activity to demonstrate how the EF feels (suggestions listed in chart below).

Teach: Keep this clear, succinct, and direct. First, quickly review the "4 Facts" and "What Are . . ." posters. Then display a copy of the Foursquare activity sheet for the EF you are covering. Model how students are to complete this. Write in the definition for the EF you are covering (see chart below). Provide 2–3 examples of how the chosen EF affects performance (see chart below for ideas or share your own). Show students how to draw a moment in which the EF is called upon.

Active Engagement: Ask students to turn and talk with a partner. If you're working on attention, for example, ask, "Is attention challenging for you? Share one time that attention is hard for you."

Link: Provide students with a clean copy of the Foursquare worksheet and invite them to fill it in on their own or with a partner. "You can use some of the examples that we discussed together, or you can create a Foursquare that is personal to you. Your job is to reflect on your own experiences, search your memory for interesting ideas, and make your ideas very clear on your Foursquare."

Feedback to Students: "I see students thinking carefully. I see students coming up with original ideas and making clear notes and drawings. I see students reflecting thoughtfully on their executive functions."

Response Inhibition: EF Basics Mini-Lesson Series
Supplementary Notes for Lessons

EF and definition	Connection activity ideas	Examples from daily life	Strategy examples
Response inhibition Thinking before you act—to resist the urge to say or do things.	*What do you have time for? Mix and match, modify, or simplify. These ideas will get you thinking.* The Marshmallow Test! Will students agree to give up having one marshmallow now (or similar candy) if they are promised two later? This tests whether they can temporarily inhibit their desire for a treat. Look up "Stanford Marshmallow Experiment" to see cute videos. On six blank cards, write the names of six colors (e.g., red, green, blue . . .) each in the wrong colored marker. So you write the word "green" using a red marker, "yellow" using a green marker, etc. Flip through the cards and ask your class to read the names. Flip through again and challenge your students to say the color that each word is written in. Can they inhibit the impulse to simply read the word?	*Try to share examples from your own life, but don't feel you have to exaggerate. Be honest and model self-compassion, self-understanding, and self-acceptance.* Blurting out something that you wish you hadn't said. Asking for help before you really try something on your own. Giving help or advice when someone doesn't really want it. Rushing to the next question before double checking what you've already done. Taking one more shot after the whistle blows in basketball.	*Keep an open mind and be creative. Students will come up with surprising and unusual strategies that might just work!* Apologize right away if you regret doing something impulsively. Take one deep breath before you speak when you're upset. Keep your hands in your pockets. Write "DC" next to each question to show that you've double checked. Try to stay calm: Talk about your concerns before they make you so stressed you can't control your responses. A great mantra to remember: Respond, don't react.

Working Memory: EF Basics Mini-Lesson Series
Supplementary Notes for Lessons

EF and definition	Connection activity ideas	Examples from daily life	Strategy examples
Working Memory Holding information in memory while performing complex tasks.	*What do you have time for? Mix and match, modify, or simplify. These ideas will get you thinking.* Play a paired or group "memory" card game in which pairs of cards are arranged face down and must be found as pairs. Can you hold several different card locations in mind? See if students can remember the last word of three or four sentences you say: "Everyone loves chocolate cake. It is served at birthdays. I always hope to get a corner piece. Corner pieces have the most icing." Can they tell you, "Cake, birthdays, piece, icing"? This tests their ability to hold the last word of each sentence in mind while continuing to listen.	*Try to share examples from your own life, but don't feel you have to exaggerate. Be honest and model self-compassion, self-understanding, and self-acceptance.* Playing chess and holding a series of moves in mind. Remembering all items on a list or in a phone number. Remembering to add your "carries" when performing traditional addition. Copying information from one screen to another on a computer.	*Keep an open mind and be creative. Students will come up with surprising and unusual strategies that might just work!* Jot information down. Make a song out of a list of information. Reduce background noise, slow down, say it out loud. Use a mnemonic: Attach meaning to the information. Visualize what you are hearing. Stay calm.

Emotional Control: EF Basics Mini-Lesson Series			
Supplementary Notes for Lessons			
EF and definition	Connection activity ideas	Examples from daily life	Strategy examples
Emotional Control Managing feelings so you can be productive and successful.	*What do you have time for? Mix and match, modify, or simplify. These ideas will get you thinking.* . . . . Remind students of your work on Zones of Regulation, if your school uses the program. Remind students that they can be more effective when they are calm and under emotional control. Teach "box breathing." Draw a big box on the board, and as students trace the sides with their eyes they breathe for a count of four, hold for a count of four, and out for a count of four. This is a strategy to promote a feeling of emotional control. Do some yoga, exercise, or mindful movement if your class would enjoy it. These experiences may promote feelings of emotional control.	*Try to share examples from your own life, but don't feel you have to exaggerate. Be honest and model self-compassion, self-understanding, and self-acceptance.* . . . . Feeling so worried about doing things perfectly that you can't start your assignments. Getting your stage fright under control. Being so excited and happy that you're way too loud. Feeling as if you can't let go of frustration from something that happened at recess. Staying calm and cool.	*Keep an open mind and be creative. Students will come up with surprising and unusual strategies that might just work!* . . . . Say exactly how you're feeling out loud. "I'm feeling . . ." Make a "good enough" start, even if it is just to get you to your next idea. Try exercise, yoga, deep breathing, and mindful activities. Use self-talk, "I'm feeling a little X because Y, but I can handle it and I'm going to be okay."

Flexibility: EF Basics Mini-Lesson Series
Supplementary Notes for Lessons

EF and definition	Connection activity ideas	Examples from daily life	Strategy examples
Flexibility Seeing many sides of an idea or situation. Being able to change and adapt.	*What do you have time for? Mix and match, modify, or simplify. These ideas will get you thinking.* Ask children, "Do you know what flexibility is? Is anyone very physically flexible? Can you show me?" Make the connection between changing positions and stretching physically and changing positions and stretching your ideas and thinking. Can you change your mind as easily as you can change your body? Draw six simple pictures on the board: a house, a dog, a heart, a cookie, an explosion, and a dollar sign. Ask groups of students to create a story by organizing these details in a certain sequence. Notice how they can be organized differently. Hold up an everyday item, such as a stapler, power cord, or binder, and ask students to suggest all of the different, creative ways it could be used. Can they think flexibly?	*Try to share examples from your own life, but don't feel you have to exaggerate. Be honest and model self-compassion, self-understanding, and self-acceptance.* Appreciating a different point of view in a debate or disagreement. Trying a different method to solve a problem. Being open to someone else's choice of restaurant, project topic, solution, game, activity, etc. Learning a method in math class that is different from the first method that you learned.	*Keep an open mind and be creative. Students will come up with surprising and unusual strategies that might just work!* Come up with three good ideas and choose the best one. Say, "I'm going to put myself in your shoes." Make an effort to try new things at least once.

Attention: EF Basics Mini-Lesson Series
Supplementary Notes for Lessons

EF and definition	Connection activity ideas	Examples from daily life	Strategy examples
Sustained Attention Paying attention even if you're tired, bored, or not interested.	*What do you have time for? Mix and match, modify, or simplify. These ideas will get you thinking.* Show students a shuffled deck of cards, one by one, about one per second. Ask students to clap their hands *unless* they see a king or queen. As their attention wanders, they will be more likely to clap at the wrong time. Go online and search for "change blindness" videos. Find one that is suitable for your group, and see if they can pay enough attention to count all the changes.	*Try to share examples from your own life, but don't feel you have to exaggerate. Be honest and model self-compassion, self-understanding, and self-acceptance.* Listening to teachers' instructions when they are running long. Noticing small errors in written work. Driving past your destination because you stopped paying attention.	*Keep an open mind and be creative. Students will come up with surprising and unusual strategies that might just work!* Chew gum. Stay rested, fed, and watered. Run the stairs or find a way to move. Break tasks into smaller chunks. Remove clutter or distraction. Sit close to a teacher. Talk over your work with a friend or engage with your teacher.

Task Initiation: EF Basics Mini-Lesson Series
Supplementary Notes for Lessons

EF and definition	Connection activity ideas	Examples from daily life	Strategy examples
Task Initiation The ability to begin projects in a timely fashion.	*What do you have time for? Mix and match, modify, or simplify. These ideas will get you thinking.* . . . . Arrange students in a circle, and ask one student to cover her eyes so she can be the detective. Pick a student to be the "starter" and instruct the others to silently follow all actions of the starter. See if the detective can figure out who is the starter. Switch roles. Ask students how it feels to be responsible for starting an action. Give students a fun three-question quiz. "You don't have to share your answers—you can keep score in your head!" Use questions that your students can relate to, such as "Who here brushes their teeth without being reminded?"; "Who here is an early riser, or who needs to be hassled to get up?"; "Who here charges devices *before* they run out of batteries?"; or "Who here starts homework as soon as they get home, and who here leaves it until just before bedtime." Enjoy getting to know your students and sharing your own strengths and weakness with task initiation.	*Try to share examples from your own life, but don't feel you have to exaggerate. Be honest and model self-compassion, self-understanding, and self-acceptance.* . . . . Getting going with work after you're given an assignment. Deciding on the right way to start and feeling confident enough to get going. Starting big projects early.	*Keep an open mind and be creative. Students will come up with surprising and unusual strategies that might just work!* . . . . Try to write the first sentence, or answer, in the first minute. Use self-talk: "Okay. What do I have to do first to get going?" Watch a friend who has already started to see how she began. Decide you will make a "good enough" start, even if it can't be perfect. Get started on work with a partner.

Planning and Prioritization: EF Basics Mini-Lesson Series			
Supplementary Notes for Lessons			
EF and definition	Connection activity ideas	Examples from daily life	Strategy examples
Planning and Prioritizing Creating a roadmap to reach a goal or to complete a task. Deciding what is important to focus on and what's not.	*What do you have time for? Mix and match, modify, or simplify. These ideas will get you thinking.* ······················ What is the most important thing to learn at school? With the class, write 10 ideas on 10 blank pieces of paper or cards. Give students 10 pennies each, and ask them to vote for what they think is the highest-priority learning goal by placing a penny on it. They can put all pennies on one, or distribute them as they like. After they are finished, count the pennies to discover the highest learning priority. Discuss with the class: "How do you make a peanut butter and jelly sandwich?" Make a list of steps, and discuss the decisions you make about the order of those steps.	*Try to share examples from your own life, but don't feel you have to exaggerate. Be honest and model self-compassion, self-understanding, and self-acceptance.* ······················ Focusing on the most important tasks rather than the easiest or most fun ones. Being able to participate because you brought all of the right equipment or materials. Getting ahead on homework on Monday night because you're busy all of the other nights.	*Keep an open mind and be creative. Students will come up with surprising and unusual strategies that might just work!* ······················ Say, "What's the most important part of this project? Where should I start?" Make a to-do list and then start the three most important jobs. When you get an assignment or worksheet, circle the part that will be most tricky and start there.

	Organization: EF Basics Mini-Lesson Series		
	Supplementary Notes for Lessons		
EF and definition	Connection activity ideas	Examples from daily life	Strategy examples
Organization Creating and maintaining a system to keep track of information or materials.	*What do you have time for? Mix and match, modify, or simplify. These ideas will get you thinking.* . . . . Teach students to play the card game Solitaire. Or play Patience online. These games are almost entirely organizational tasks. Ask students to describe how they organize their rooms, their school bags, their desks, or any other areas they have responsibility for.	*Try to share examples from your own life, but don't feel you have to exaggerate. Be honest and model self-compassion, self-understanding, and self-acceptance.* . . . . Keeping a desk, locker, or closet tidy so you can find things when you need them. Making numbers and calculations orderly and easy to follow in written math work. Being able to write so that your ideas on one topic are all in one section or paragraph.	*Keep an open mind and be creative. Students will come up with surprising and unusual strategies that might just work!* . . . . Always find five things to put away, sort, or tidy up. Use baskets, binders, tabs, or sections to sort your materials. Remove unnecessary items or clutter. Watch what organized people do. Use a graphic organizer to pre-plan your writing.

Time Management: EF Basics Mini-Lesson Series
Supplementary Notes for Lessons

EF and definition	Connection activity ideas	Examples from daily life	Strategy examples
Time Management Estimating how much time you have and how to use it to stay within time limits and deadlines.	*What do you have time for? Mix and match, modify, or simplify. These ideas will get you thinking.* Cover all clocks and remove all watches/ phones. Have everyone stand up and close their eyes. Tell students to sit down quietly and open their eyes after what they believe has been a minute. Everyone will sit down and open their eyes at different times. Ask students to estimate how many times they can do a small, token activity (walk the perimeter of the classroom or playground, write their signature, give handshakes) in one minute. Were estimates way off? Did the group tend to over- or underestimate? Do we have a good sense of time?	*Try to share examples from your own life, but don't feel you have to exaggerate. Be honest and model self-compassion, self-understanding, and self-acceptance.* Knowing you have 45 minutes to complete 10 questions and focusing only on the first question for 20 minutes. Starting a big project on time so you have enough time to finish. Taking too long to get ready to go outside. Having enough time to proofread.	*Keep an open mind and be creative. Students will come up with surprising and unusual strategies that might just work!* Set a timer bell. Ask a group member or teacher for reminders. Work in 5-minute bursts and keep track of what you get done. Wear a watch or sit where you can see a clock. Assign a group time manager.

Goal-Directed Persistence: EF Basics Mini-Lesson Series

Supplementary Notes for Lessons

EF and definition	Connection activity ideas	Examples from daily life	Strategy examples
Goal-Directed Persistence Following through to the completion of your goal without being distracted by competing interests.	*What do you have time for? Mix and match, modify, or simplify. These ideas will get you thinking.* . . . . Give students a yardstick or a ruler and challenge them to learn to balance it on one finger, straight up and down. This will take multiple tries and plenty of persistence. Teach students how to make a "house of cards" by leaning cards against each other to make structures. Invite them to persevere through 10 attempts in a row. Have students write down an individual goal for the day. Before dismissal, circle back and see how many achieved their goals.	*Try to share examples from your own life, but don't feel you have to exaggerate. Be honest and model self-compassion, self-understanding, and self-acceptance.* . . . . Trying to figure out how to use new technology by patiently exploring menus, features, and YouTube videos. Making multiple drafts of an essay. Proofreading or double-checking work. Trying once and then giving up.	*Keep an open mind and be creative. Students will come up with surprising and unusual strategies that might just work!* . . . . Do big assignments in "pomodoros" (or chunks) with short breaks in between. Break your job into steps and check each one as you go along. Work with a partner and encourage each other. Make a goal and see if you can achieve it.

Metacognition: EF Basics Mini-Lesson Series
Supplementary Notes for Lessons

EF and definition	Connection activity ideas	Examples from daily life	Strategy examples
Metacognition Noticing how you're doing. Thinking about how you're thinking.	*What do you have time for? Mix and match, modify, or simplify. These ideas will get you thinking.* Display snapshots of people. These might be shots you already have of your class, or for fun you could use *http://awkwardfamilyphotos.com.* Draw thought bubbles over them and encourage students to complete the thought, "I just realized that I . . ." Give students a cue card and ask them to write advice to next year's students. "If I could do this grade/month/year/class over again, I would . . ."	*Try to share examples from your own life, but don't feel you have to exaggerate. Be honest and model self-compassion, self-understanding, and self-acceptance.* Noticing that you're making the same mistake over and over again. Realizing that you know the answer to a question but just can't remember it right now. Realizing that you've forgotten something important and should find a replacement.	*Keep an open mind and be creative. Students will come up with surprising and unusual strategies that might just work!* Use self-talk: "Okay. What might I be forgetting?" or "How can I improve this?" Think of someone you admire and ask yourself, "How would they have done this differently?"

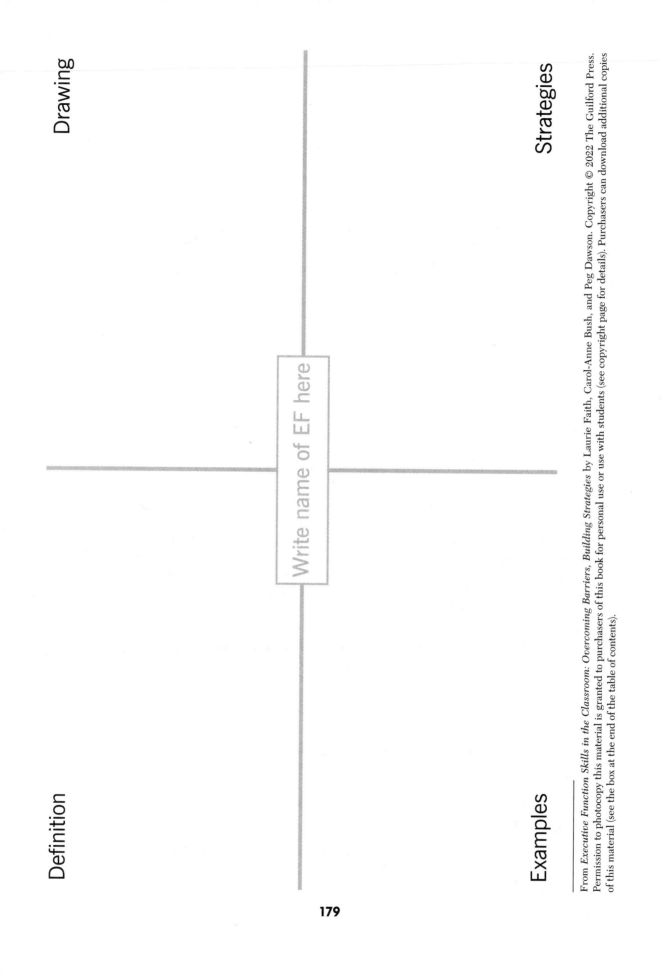

Drawing

Definition

Write name of EF here

Strategies

Examples

APPENDIX C

Mentor Texts for Teaching About Executive Functions

The following is a list of storybooks and novels that relate to EF themes at a range of different grade levels. We hope you will consider incorporating them into your school year somehow. They make great read-alouds to recommend for home reading, to conduct with your class, or to present to your whole school during assembly. We know principals who gather their entire population—students, teachers, parents, and staff—once per month to discuss an EF and read a related story. Using these books, you can create shared experiences with EFs and build rich conceptual understanding. We are grateful to Meg Clements and her colleagues at the Trillium Lakelands District School board, as well as to Amarinder Mehta, a graduate of the University of Toronto Master of Arts in Child Study and Education program, for doing so much of the heavy lifting to create this list.

We know the materials, even as we speak, are continuing to evolve and change in the hands of the many teachers who helped create them and who use them. Now they are yours to expand upon and improve. If you come up with anything interesting, including adaptations or improvements, we'd love for you to share them with our community. Please see the preface for information about where to find us!

MENTOR TEXTS: PREKINDERGARTEN TO GRADE 3

(AR = age range)

Response Inhibition: PreK–3

Cook. J. (2008). *My mouth is a volcano.* Chattanooga, TN: National Center for Youth Issues. AR: 5–8.
Cook, J. (2014). *Decibella.* Boys Town, NE: Boys Town Press. AR: 5–8.
Cook, J. (2016). *That rule doesn't apply to me!* Boys Town, NE: Boys Town Press. AR: 4–6.

Ferrell, S. (2016). *The snurtch.* New York: Atheneum Books for Young Readers. AR: 4–8.

John, J. (2017). *The bad seed.* New York: HarperCollins Children's Books. AR: 4–8.

Jones, C. (2012). *Lacey Walker the non-stop talker.* North Mankato, MN: Picture Window Books. AR: 4–6.

Watt, M. (2009). *Chester.* Toronto, ON: Kids Can Press. AR: 4–8.

Working Memory: PreK–3

Esham, B. (2016). *Last to finish: A story about the smartest boy in math class.* Naperville, IL: Little Pickle Press. AR: 4–10.

Teckentrup, B. (2014). *The memory tree.* London: Orchard Books. AR: 5–8.

Emotional Control: PreK–3

Atwood, M. (2005). *Rude Ramsay and the roaring radishes.* New York: Bloomsbury USA. AR: 4–8.

Baptiste, B. (2004). *My daddy is a pretzel.* Cambridge, MA: Barefoot Books. AR: 4–8.

Bottner, B. (1992). *Bootsie Barker bites.* New York: Scholastic. AR: 4–8.

Cain, J. (2000). *The way I feel.* Seattle, WA: Parenting Press. AR: 2–8.

Cook. J. (2013). *Thanks for the feedback . . . (I think)!* Boys Town, NE: Boys Town Press. AR: 5–8.

Cook, J. (2015). *Lying up a storm.* Chattanooga, TN: National Center for Youth Issues. AR: 5–8.

Cornwall, G. (2017). *Jabari jumps.* Somerville, MA: Candlewick. AR: 4–8.

Desmond, J. (2014). *Eric, the boy who lost his gravity.* Maplewood, NJ: Blue Apple Books. AR: 4–8.

Ferrell, S. (2016). *The snurtch.* New York: Atheneum Books for Young Readers. AR: 4–8.

John, J. (2017). *The bad seed.* New York: HarperCollins Children's Books. AR: 4–8.

Joosse, B. (1991). *Mama, do you love me?* San Francisco, CA: Chronicle Books LLC. AR: 4–8.

Lienas, A. (2015). *The colour monster.* London: Templar Publishing. AR: 3–7.

Manning, J. (2012). *Millie Fierce.* New York: Penguin Group. AR: 3–7.

McCloud, C. (2006). *Have you filled a bucket today?* Brighton, MI: Ferne Press. AR: 4–10.

Parton, D. (2009). *I am a rainbow.* New York: Penguin Young Readers Group. AR: 3–5.

Seuss, Dr. *Many colored days.* New York: Alfred A. Knopf. AR: 3–5.

Tomlinson, J. (1968). *The owl who was afraid of the dark.* Middlesex, UK: Penguin Books. AR: 6–8.

Witek, J. (2014). *In my heart: A book of feelings.* New York: Harry N. Abrams. AR: 3+.

Flexibility: PreK–3

Baptiste, B. (2004). *My daddy is a pretzel.* Cambridge, MA: Barefoot Books. AR: 4–8.

Brown, M. (1947). *Stone soup.* New York: Simon & Schuster. AR: 4–8.

Cook, J. (2011). *I just don't like the sound of no!* Boys Town, NE: Boys Town Press. AR: 5–8.

Cook, J. (2017). *Bubble gum brain: Ready, get mindset . . . grow!* Chattanooga, TN: National Center for Youth Issues. AR: 4–8.

Goodrich, C. (2011). *Say hello to Zorro!* New York: Simon & Schuster Books for Young Readers. AR: 3–8.

John, J. (2017). *The bad seed.* New York: HarperCollins Children's Books. AR: 4–8.

Robinson, M. (2014). *There is a lion in my corn flakes.* London: Bloomsbury Press. AR: 3–7.

Spires, A. (2014). *The most magnificent thing.* Toronto, ON: Kids Can Press. AR: 3–7.

Sustained Attention: PreK–3

Gerstein, M. (2007). *The man who walked between the towers.* New York: Roaring Brook Press. AR: 5–8.

Hohn, N. L. (2018). *Harriet Tubman: freedom fighter.* New York: HarperCollins Publishers. AR: 4–8.

McCully, E. A. (1992). *Mirette on the high wire.* New York: Putnam. AR: 4–8.
Spires, A. (2014). *The most magnificent thing.* Toronto, ON: Kids Can Press. AR: 3–7.
Wild, M. (2017). *The sloth who slowed down.* Sydney, Australia: Allen & Unwin. AR: 4–7.

Task Initiation: PreK–3

Hay, S. (2018). *The star in the jar.* London: Egmont Books. AR: 4–8.
Seuss, Dr. (1954). *Horton hears a who!* New York: Random House Publishing. AR: 5–9.

Planning and Prioritizing: PreK–37

Ferry, B. (2015). *Land shark.* San Francisco, CA: Chronicle Books. AR: 4–8.

Organization: PreK–3

Cook, J. (2015). *I can't find my whatchamacallit!* Chattanooga, TN: National Center for Youth Issues. AR: 4–12.

Time Management: PreK–3

Adler, D. A. (1992). *A picture book of Harriet Tubman.* New York: Holiday House. AR: 6–8.
Paramore, L. (2017). *Anything's possible. Anything goes!* American Fork, UT: Heart Centered Productions. AR: 4–8.

Goal-Directed Persistence: PreK–3

Andreae, G. (2019). *Giraffes can't dance.* New York: Hachette Book Group. AR: 4–8.
Ferry, B. (2015). *Land shark.* San Francisco, CA: Chronicle Books. AR: 4–8.
Gerstein, M. (2007). *The man who walked between the towers.* New York: Roaring Brook Press. AR: 5–8.
Kirk, D. (2007). *Library mouse: A friend's tale.* New York: Abrams Books for Young Readers. AR: 4–8.
McCully, E. A. (1992). *Mirette On the high wire.* New York: Putnam. AR: 4–8.
Piper, W. (2005). *The little engine that could.* New York: Penguin Random House. AR: 3–7.
Santat, D. (2017). *After the fall: How Humpty Dumpty got back up again.* New York: Roaring Books Press. AR: 3–7.
Schoenherr, I. (2006). *Pip and squeak.* New York: HarperCollins. AR: 4–8.
Spires, A. (2014). *The most magnificent thing.* Toronto, ON: Kids Can Press. AR: 3–7.
Sweeney, M. (2016). *How the crayons saved the rainbow.* New York: Simon & Schuster. AR: 3–5.
Vazquez, P. [Blender]. (2016, January 29). *Caminandes 3: Llamigos—Funny 3D animated short* [Video File]. Retrieved from www.youtube.com/watch?v=SkVqJ1SGeL0.
Wilson, K. (2009). *Don't be afraid, little Pip.* New York: Simon & Schuster Children's Publishing. AR: 3–7.
Yahgulanaas, M. (2010). *The little hummingbird.* Vancouver, BC: Greystone Books. AR: 5–6.
Yousafzai, M. (2017). *Malala's magic pencil.* New York: Hachette Book Group. AR: 4–8.

Metacognition: PreK–3

Cook. J. (2013). *Thanks for the feedback (I think)!* Boys Town, NE: Boys Town Press. AR: 5–8.
Fogliano, J. (2013). *If you want to see a whale.* New York: Roaring Brook Press. AR: 4–7.
John, J. (2017). *The bad seed.* New York: HarperCollins Children's Books. AR: 4–8.

John, J. (2019). *The good egg.* New York: HarperCollins Children's Books. AR: 4–8.

Yamada, K. (2014). *What do you do with an idea?* Seattle, WA: Compendium. AR: 5–7.

Yamada, K. (2016). *What do you do with a problem?* Seattle, WA: Compendium. AR: 3–8.

MENTOR TEXTS: GRADES 4 TO 6

(AR = age range)

Response Inhibition: 4–6

Copeland, L. (1998). *Hunter and his amazing remote control.* Chapin, SC: YouthLight. AR: 8–12.

D'Adamo, F. (2005). *Iqbal.* New York: Aladdin. AR: 8–12.

Wishinsky, F. (2004). *What's the matter with Albert?* Toronto, ON: Maple Tree Press. AR: 7–12.

Working Memory: 4–6

Esham, B. (2016). *Last to finish: A story about the smartest boy in math class.* Naperville, IL: Little Pickle Press. AR: 4–10.

Emotional Control: 4–6

Cook, J. (2012). *Wilma Jean the worry machine.* Chattanooga, TN: National Center for Youth Issues. AR: 7–11.

Cook, J. (2014). *The Anti-Test Anxiety Society.* Chattanooga, TN: National Center for Youth Issues. AR: 7–10.

Hunt, L. M. (2017). *Fish in a tree.* London: Puffin Books. AR: 10+.

Pittman, H. C., & Rand, T. (1993). *Once when I was scared.* New York: Penguin Group. AR: 7–10.

Riordan, R. (2010). *Percy Jackson and the Olympians, Book One: The lightning thief.* New York: Hyperion Books for Children. AR: 9+.

Zelinger, L. E., & Zelinger, J. (2011). *Please explain anxiety to me!* Ann Arbor, MI: Loving Healing Press. AR: 6–12.

Flexibility: 4–6

Dahl, R. (2001). *The BFG.* London: Puffin Books. AR: 9–13.

Ellis, D. (2000). *The breadwinner.* Berkeley, CA: Groundwood Books. AR: 9–12.

Mikaelsen, B. (2001). *Touching spirit bear.* New York: HarperCollins Children's Books. AR: 9–12.

Palacio, R. J. (2012). *Wonder.* New York: Alfred A. Knopf. AR: 9–12.

Spinelli, J. (2004). *Stargirl.* New York: Dell Laurel-Leaf. AR: 9–12.

Sustained Attention: 4–6

Baltazar, A. (2017). *Timeless: Diego and the rangers of the Vastlantic.* New York: HarperCollins. AR: 8–12.

Walters, E. (2003). *Run.* Toronto, ON: Penguin Group Canada. AR: 9–12.

Task Initiation: 4–6

Espeland, P. (2008). *See you later, procrastinator.* Minneapolis, MN: Free Spirit Publishing. AR: 8–13.

Planning and Prioritizing: 4–6

Cook, J. (2013). *I just want to do it my way.* Boys Town, NE: Boys Town Press. AR: 8–9.

Cook, J. (2016). *Planning isn't my priority: And making priorities isn't in my plans.* Chattanooga, TN: National Center for Youth Issues. AR: 7–11.

Cook, J. (2016). *Study skilled . . . NOT!* Chattanooga, TN: National Center for Youth Issues. AR: 8–9.

Organization: 4–6

Cook, J. (2015). *I can't find my whatchamacallit!* Chattanooga, TN: National Center for Youth Issues. AR: 4–12.

Fox, J. S. (2017). *Get organized without losing it.* Minneapolis, MN: Free Spirit Publishing. AR: 8–13.

Smith, B. (2018). *It was just right here.* Boys Town, NE: Boys Town Press. AR: 6–12.

Time Management: 4–6

Campbell, N. I. (2005). *Shi-shi-etko.* Toronto, ON: Groundwood Books. AR: 7–9.

Goldish, M. (2009). *Michael Phelps: Anything is possible!* New York: Bearport Publishing. AR: 9–14.

Riordan, R. (2010). *Percy Jackson and the Olympians, Book One: The lightning thief.* New York: Hyperion Books for Children. AR: 9+.

Walters, E. (2003). *Run.* Toronto, ON: Penguin Group Canada. AR: 9–12.

Goal-Directed Persistence: 4–6

Applegate, K. (2012). *The one and only Ivan.* New York: HarperCollins. AR: 8–12.

D'Adamo, F. (2005). *Iqbal.* New York: Aladdin. AR: 8–12.

DiCamillo, K. (2002). *The tale of Despereaux.* Somerville, MA: Candlewick Press. AR: 7–12.

Hiaasen, C. (2002). *Hoot.* New York: Random House Children's Books. AR: 10+.

Jones, J. C. (2017). *Pip and Houdini.* Crows Nest, Australia: A&U Children's. AR: 8–12.

Korman, G. (2009). *Swindle.* Toronto, ON: Scholastic. AR: 9–12.

Poletti, F., & Yee, K. (2017). *The girl who ran: Bobbi Gibb, the first woman to run the Boston Marathon.* Seattle, WA: Compendium. AR: 6–9.

Ridge, Y. (2017). *Inside Hudson Pickle.* Toronto, ON: Kids Can Press. AR: 9–12.

Sachar, L (1998). *Holes.* New York: Random House Children's Books. AR: 10+.

Silverstein, S. (1964). *The giving tree.* New York: HarperCollins. AR: 6–12.

Trottier, M. (2010). *Terry Fox: A story of hope.* Toronto, ON: Scholastic Canada. AR: 9–14.

Weston, C. (2014). *Ava and Pip, volume 1.* Naperville, IL: Sourcebooks Jabberwocky. AR: 9–13.

Wishinsky, F. (2004). *What's the matter with Albert.* Toronto, ON: Maple Tree Press. AR: 7–12.

Metacognition: 4–6

D'Adamo, F. (2005). *Iqbal.* New York: Aladdin. AR: 8–12.

Mikaelsen, B. (2001). *Touching spirit bear.* New York: HarperCollins Children's Books. AR: 9–12.

Silverstein, S. (1964). *The giving tree.* New York: HarperCollins. AR: 4–12.

Zelinger, L. E., & Zelinger, J. (2011). *Please explain anxiety to me!* Ann Arbor, MI: Loving Healing Press. AR: 6–12.

MENTOR TEXTS: GRADES 7 TO 8

(AR = age range)

Response Inhibition: 7–8

George, J. C. (2016). *Julie of the wolves.* New York: HarperCollins. AR: 14+.
O'Dell, S. (2010). *Island of the blue dolphins.* Boston, MA: Houghton Mifflin. AR: 10+.
Paulsen, G. (2000). *Hatchet.* New York: Atheneum Books. AR: 15+.
Pierce, T. (2005). *Alanna (the 1st adventurer).* Toronto, ON: Simon Pulse. AR: 12+.
Thomas, A. (2017). *The hate you give.* New York: HarperCollins. AR: 15+.

Emotional Control: 7–8

George, J. C. (2016). *Julie of the wolves.* New York: HarperCollins. AR: 14+.
Graudin, R. (2015). *Wolf by wolf.* London: Indigo. AR: 15+.
Mathieu, J. (2017). *Moxie.* New York: Roaring Books Press. AR: 14+.
Paulsen, G. (2000). *Hatchet.* New York: Atheneum Books. AR: 15+.
Pierce, T. (2005). *Alanna (the 1st adventurer).* Toronto, ON: Simon Pulse. AR: 12+.

Flexibility: 7–8

O'Dell, S. (2010). *Island of the blue dolphins.* Boston, MA: Houghton Mifflin. AR: 10+.
Pierce, T. (2005). *Alanna (the 1st adventurer).* Toronto, ON: Simon Pulse. AR: 12+.
Thomas, A. (2017). *The hate you give.* New York: HarperCollins. AR: 15+ young adult.

Task Initiation: 7–8

Pierce, T. (2005). *Alanna (the 1st adventurer).* Toronto, ON: Simon Pulse. AR: 12+.

Goal-Directed Persistence: 7–8

Graudin, R. (2015). *Wolf by wolf.* London: Indigo. AR: 15+.
Mathieu, J. (2017). *Moxie.* New York: Roaring Books Press. AR: 14+.
Pierce, T. (2005). *Alanna (the 1st adventurer).* Toronto, ON: Simon Pulse. AR: 12+.
Thomas, A. (2019). *On the come up.* New York: HarperCollins. AR: 15+ young adult.

Metacognition: 7–8

Ciccarelli, K. (2017). *The last Namsara.* New York: Harper Teen. AR: 13+.
Pierce, T. (2005). *Alanna (the 1st adventurer).* Toronto, ON: Simon Pulse. AR: 12+.
Thomas, A. (2019). *On the come up.* New York: HarperCollins. AR: 15+ young adult.

APPENDIX D

Index of EF Barriers and Strategies

Following is a large index of the EF barriers and strategies students may experience across 10 academic skills and nine life (or 21st-century) skills. We include this because no matter how many times we encourage teachers to think of themselves and their students as "strategy experts," we are asked for strategy ideas. We get it. Teachers who are just getting started with EF literacy in the classroom really want to have all the help they can get. We say, "Talk to your students—they will provide you with all of the eccentric and resourceful strategy ideas you could ever want!" and teachers reply, "Great. Oh, and can you please send us a list of strategies?"

So, we have filled many pages with lists of the EF barriers your students may face on a daily basis and a few strategies to overcome each of them. First, you will find a barriers and strategies breakdown for 10 different academic skills. These are organized from the most common, ordinary school skills like reading to more emergent skills like coding. Then you will find barriers and strategies for nine other school skills that relate to 21st-century learning. You will notice that the EF barriers are sometimes clustered together. For example, for mathematical problem solving, we have grouped together barriers related to task initiation and emotional control because they often present themselves together in this context. Only a handful of EF barriers are highlighted for each skill—these are the ones we feel have the greatest impact on the performance of school-aged children. Similarly, only a handful of strategies are provided for each one. These are just a few examples of types of strategies we have learned from children and their teachers over the years. We are grateful to the many educators who shared their insight and experience to help us create this resource. We are especially grateful to Merrick David, a Toronto-based educator, who helped us bring life to this section with additional research, insight, and writing.

Several of the 21st-century skills and one of the academic skills we mention are quite emergent—they are related to new or modern approaches that we are only just beginning to see in schools. In these cases, we were grateful to be able to complement our educational knowledge and experience with the expertise of a few experts. So, the section on *collaborative writing* was written with the input of Jana Sinyor, an Emmy award-winning screenwriter. The section on *designing to specifications* was written with the input of Brian Giesbrecht, a well-established industrial designer. The section on *coding* was written with the input of Arun Ranganathan, who was an engineer at Netscape and has worked in the technology industry at AOL, Mozilla, and Pinterest. Finally, the section on *debate* was written with the input of Jessica Prince, a former Canadian national debate champ and noted Canadian lawyer. Debate isn't really a new skill, but we couldn't resist asking Jessica for a few tricks.

We hope you will enjoy this material. Perhaps you'll sit down and read it from start to finish and make connections to your own school performance, or to the ways EFs continue to affect your life and work. Perhaps you'll navigate to certain pages as you tackle new academic or 21st-century skills. Or maybe you'll share portions of it with your students. Regardless, we hope the practical and tangible examples it provides will breathe even more life into your understanding of an EF-literate classroom. Most of all, we hope you use it primarily as a springboard to launch yourself and your students toward the most valuable strategy of all: the ability to put this book down, roll up your sleeves, and create some weird and wonderful strategies of your own.

INDEX OF ACADEMIC EF BARRIERS AND STRATEGIES

Academic Skill: Listening

	Barriers	Strategies
Response inhibition	Listener is so focused on what he has to say that he is unable to listen to what is being said and blurts out his contribution.	Think of one key "anchor" word that will remind you of the idea for later. Use a small notebook to quickly jot ideas (or just a key anchor word) so you don't lose them. As soon as you realize you have blurted or interrupted say, "I'm so sorry! Please go on."
Working memory	Listener can't hold and contemplate the first, middle, and final ideas simultaneously.	Say, "So what you're saying is . . ." and try to summarize the ideas. Ask, "Can you please repeat that?" Use a notebook to jot small key words or picture cues.
Emotional control	Listener is triggered emotionally, and all relevant EFs are suppressed.	Take deep, slow breaths. Ask to excuse yourself for a moment. Say, "Hang on. I'm interested in what you're saying, but I need a minute to take a breath/calm down."
Flexibility and sustained attention	Listener doesn't shift away from own thoughts in time to catch the beginning of the idea. Listener can't deeply or fully engage with and capture the information.	Say, "I'm sorry, but I missed that. Can you repeat the beginning?" when you realize you're lost. Watch and point to the speaker, and nod and smile as they speak. Actively build connection and engagement while listening by trying to sympathize with, engage in, personally connect to, or share in the perspective presented.
Task initiation	Listener is unable to start the task as she wasn't listening to the instructions. She is unable to gather enough information together to know what to do.	Say, "Can you please repeat that?" Ask if your teacher will always write two to three key "instruction words" on the board.
Metacognition	Listener is partway through a task or response and realizes he must have missed something.	Say, "Hold on a minute. I think I missed something." Find someone who can tell you what you missed.

Academic Skill: Reading—Decoding

	Barriers	Strategies
Emotional control	Reader is discouraged and stops practice. Reader is triggered emotionally, and all relevant EFs are suppressed.	Explore many different combinations of sound. Read in a funny accent. If the emotions are really big, take a 5-minute break to listen to music, go for a walk, or have a snack. Say, "I just need a break and then I'll be okay." Say, "This is hard work. I just need a break, but I know I can do it."
Flexibility	Reader does not quickly access and attempt multiple rules for different phonemes.	Don't be embarrassed to say the word out loud in different ways until it sounds right. Print out a chart reminding you of the different sounds each vowel/vowel team can make.
Response inhibition	Reader is overwhelmed by the other words on the page and can't focus on the one word that is being decoded. Student repeats a simple error, perhaps saying "thick" instead of "think," over and over, seeming to be stuck in a rut.	Block out other words with paper, a ruler, or a hand. When stuck on the same mistake, reset your mouth by making a funny "raspberry" or "lip trill" sound, by saying "blah de blah de blah," or by shaking out your whole body.
Goal-directed persistence	Reader feels hopeless and quits easily when she can't decode a word.	Say, "What strategies have I tried?" Put a list of your favorite strategies on a bookmark, and check it for ideas.
Metacognition	Reader is fatigued and accuracy is affected. Instead of suspecting fatigue, she gets upset, gets frustrated, and says, "I suck at reading!"	Notice when you need a break and take one. Say, "I'm just getting tired. I need a quick break." Hold your place with a finger and refresh your eyes by looking at 10 other things in the room. Move to a different position in the room or change chairs.

Academic Skill: Reading—Comprehension

	Barriers	Strategies
Working memory	Reader can't hold beginning of sentence or paragraph in memory long enough to process it along with the end of the idea. Struggles to make meaning.	Read text aloud and touch each word to boost sensory input. Reduce background noise. Reduce visual clutter by making use of support tools, e.g., highlighting ruler to highlight text or cutting a rectangular shape out of a piece of paper so only the words you want to read are visible. When you make a connection or understand something deeply, write your thoughts on a sticky note and put them right in the book.
Sustained attention	Reader decodes letters mechanically without dedicating full attention to the whole task of reading. Reader is distracted by external/internal stimuli, making it difficult to understand and gain momentum.	Make use of every cue available to you before you even start reading, e.g., book cover, table of contents, or illustrations, or by scanning text, etc. Place index fingers at each end of a line and move eyes across the text, to support tracking and ability to follow punctuation. Make use of support tools, e.g., highlighting ruler to highlight text.
Planning, prioritizing and organization	Reader does not notice or benefit from patterns and structure of sentence, paragraph, section, or whole text.	Figure out what kind of text you're reading before you start—an article, a cartoon, a recipe, a story, a textbook, etc. Scan text before reading to preview patterns and organization.
Goal-directed persistence	Reader struggles with vocabulary and would rather read books that are below his reading grade level and are easy to read than to push on through with a more challenging text.	Skim for unknown words before you start—jot them down or highlight them and then either look them up or ask for clarification. Find a favorite online dictionary, keep it on your desktop, and use it as often as possible. Challenge yourself to look up at least one word every day.
Metacognition	Reader does not notice and correct misunderstandings or build connections.	Pause regularly to check understanding. After each paragraph use self-talk: "Does this make sense?" If not, go back and reread. Find someone to check in with to make sure you're on the right track.

Academic Skill: Reading—Fluency

	Barriers	Strategies
Response inhibition	Reader focuses on going quickly to the exclusion of everything else.	Read as though a little kid is listening or as if you're a YouTube presenter. Read aloud in a fancy accent. Tap twice at periods and once at commas. Listen to a recording of yourself reading too fast, too slow, and just right. Try reading at a turtle's pace.
Working memory and sustained attention and flexibility	Reader cannot manage the quick back and forth between reading and scanning ahead. Reader doesn't recall what was just read.	Read the whole text through once before reading aloud. Slow down the pace and practice prereading each sentence quietly before actually reading it. Try emphasizing several different words in a sentence. Pause to recall personal connections to the text.
Emotional control and task initiation	Reader is anxious and reluctant to read.	Tell your teacher you feel nervous. Ask for a heads up, or time to rehearse before having to read aloud. Breathe and remind yourself that everyone reads differently.
Sustained attention	Reader doesn't focus on punctuation. Reader does not understand the meaning of the text and is not captivated.	Place index fingers at end of each line as you go. Follow the text using an audiobook while reading at the same time. Use a highlighting ruler to spotlight text. Pick up cues from illustrations. Record yourself reading, critique your skills, and pick out one thing to work on the next time.
Goal-directed persistence	Reader knows his reading level is low; he gives up easily or turns to books way below his grade level.	Alternate between harder and more comfortable books, either book by book or day by day. So, if you have 30 minutes to read, you might read a challenging book for 15 and a comfortable book for 15. Keep track of your "pages read."
Metacognition	Reader does not notice making mistakes and plows ahead having said incorrect and confusing words.	Use audiobooks or choral reading to get a feel for how text sounds. Say, "Huh?" if you think you made a mistake. Keep a tally of the number of mistakes you notice. Record yourself and listen to see if you notice anything you could improve upon.

Academic Skill: Writing

	Barriers	Strategies
Response inhibition	Writer is having difficulty starting, and impulsively turns to soothing preoccupations such as snacking, daydreaming, chatting, tidying, or going online.	Use small goals and rewards. Say, "I'm nervous to begin, but I can handle this." It doesn't matter what you write; just get started by putting some words on the page.
Working memory	Writer cannot hold ideas in mind long enough to craft complete and coherent arguments and reasons.	Reread your writing aloud. Use voice-to-text software. Do a "brain dump" without editing or organizing.
Emotional control	Writer is afraid to fail, embarrassed about poor writing skills, or anxious about the time it will take to complete the project. Writer shuts down.	Write after vigorous exercise. Listen to soothing music while writing. Combine writing time with a snack. Write with a partner if that makes it more fun.
Flexibility	Writer does not agree with some or all of the ideas he is responsible for writing about.	Make two or more different outlines. Try writing from different perspectives. Advocate for a topic you care about.
Sustained attention	Writer crafts poorly structured arguments or fails to finish assignment because of loss of attention.	Discuss your connections to the topic. Read your work to a partner. List the work in chunks and check them off.
Task initiation	Writer doesn't shift into starting but rather remains preoccupied with the project guidelines, finding materials, class discussions, or other distractions.	Say, "It is hard to start, but once I get going I'll be fine." Ask a friend or teacher to give you a random first line. Make a start-up checklist: writing materials, comfy seating, etc.
Prioritizing and organization	Writer cannot visualize or understand the sequence of ideas and the flow of arguments.	Plan with a mind map or a flowchart. Take a break and reset; then plan your next break and return to work.
Goal-directed persistence	Writer is overwhelmed and exhausted by the mental effort and stops work without restarting.	Use snack or activity breaks. Make a very small goal. Say, "I needed a break, but now I can get back to work."
Metacognition	Writer is unaware that her writing lacks continuity and is difficult to read.	Find a partner to read your work and ask for three pieces of feedback. Plan to make three small changes and two big changes. Keep track of how much time it takes you to make your first draft, and try to match the time for your edits.

Academic Skill: Mathematical Calculation

	Barriers	Strategies
Response inhibition and attention	Mathematician rushes through work, making a lot of mistakes.	Get in the habit of doing calculations twice, coding the double-checked work with a "DC." Think aloud to self, "Where are my mistakes?" When work is complete, make 10 improvements before handing it in.
Working memory	Mathematician cannot hold a number in memory while preforming an operation, causing multiple errors, confusion, and exhaustion.	Work with a partner. Speak the problem aloud while preforming it to involve auditory memory. Use larger paper and write larger numbers. Use larger paper to allow for more shorthand and jotting down of midways steps such as "carries." Make a sketch or use objects to represent the problem.
Emotional control	Mathematician worries about mastery of multiplication facts, algorithms, or the speed of calculation.	Advocate for, locate, or retrieve number facts charts and lists of steps quickly. Work with a partner. Start short, daily math facts practice, making small goals. Make an achievable goal for the day's work and enjoy a feeling of success. Make a list of all the fact types you already know, e.g., doubles or doubles +1.
Flexibility	Mathematician sticks to favorite approaches, rules, or ideas and avoids trying new ones.	Take a walk around the room to see different ways other students solve problems. Ask yourself, "What is the fastest way to do this? What is the slowest?" Challenge yourself to try one new approach per assignment—mark it with a star.
Planning, prioritizing and organization	Mathematician has difficulty writing numbers and equations clearly enough to work with.	Use larger or graph paper and write larger numbers. Keep a number chart nearby for easy reference. Organize the pace of writing by using a metronome to set a steady speed—try to write only one number per metronome tick.
Metacognition	Mathematician is preoccupied by the mechanics of the arithmetic and forgets the meaning of the numbers. She doesn't notice obvious errors.	Visualize: Get in the habit of imagining silly scenarios for what the numbers and arithmetic symbols mean: 105×3 is the day your baby sister dumped three boxes of crackers on the floor. She did it three times! (She didn't do it once and then add three more single crackers.) Also, make a checklist of common errors and double-check for them.

Academic Skill: Mathematical Problem Solving

	Barriers	Strategies
Response inhibition	Mathematician asks for too much help, rushes, or copies. Mathematician makes conclusions about the answer too soon.	Say, "Let's try a little more before we check the answer." Develop two separate solutions using two different approaches. Set a metronome to tick out a calm pace.
Working memory	Mathematician can't hold all parts of the problem in memory long enough to see patterns and interrelationships.	Highlight important information. Discuss with a partner. Say, "What do we already know? What are we trying to find out?" Make a sketch or use objects to represent the problem.
Flexibility	Mathematician is stuck on one type of solution, which may not work.	Make several different attempts at the solution. Look for three things to improve in the solution.
Sustained attention	Mathematician cannot stay focused long enough to do thoughtful, complete, and accurate work.	Number the different parts of the problem. Work with a partner you enjoy. Make a goal and race to meet it. Exercise before or during the process.
Task initiation and emotional control	Mathematician fears failure or waits for a "perfect start" and delays starting work.	Draw a picture to show what you're thinking about the problem. Get started in the first minute. Say, "This is not a perfect start, but it is good enough." Run up and down the stairs.
Planning, prioritizing and organization	Mathematician can't appreciate the order or sequence of the information given or can't construct an appropriate plan for response.	Review the information in the problem, or your solution idea, across your fingers, saying, "First . . . second . . . third . . ." Make a written "to do" list for the problem.
Goal-directed persistence	Mathematician stalls during longer solutions.	Work in 5-minute bursts. Change seating or position for each new question. Work with an elbow partner.
Metacognition	Mathematician does not double-check thinking or respond to evidence that thinking is flawed.	Find one mistake in each of your solutions. Get in the habit of doing calculations twice, coding the double-checked work with a "DC." Double-check against your elbow partner.

Academic Skill: Long-Term Projects

	Barriers	Strategies
Working memory	Producer feels overwhelmed and confused by the project.	Keep your plan posted, and look at it often. Don't be embarrassed to clarify; say, "Hang on, I'm confused" and get the information you need.
Emotional control	Producer feels stressed about how things are going and feels stuck.	Listen to your gut. Write down your feelings about the way things are going. Prompt yourself by writing, "I am upset. What am I upset about?"
Flexibility	Producer's mind is closed to feedback. He avoids asking for input.	Ask for feedback when you're least stressed, or on a certain day. Force yourself to ask three questions about the feedback.
Sustained attention	Producer loses interest in the work.	Figure out what you like about the project: Talk to a friend; do an online search related to the project to get inspiration and new ideas.
Task initiation	Producer knows what needs to be done but doesn't get started.	Set a 2-minute timer and make a jump start on something small. Start overwhelming tasks with a partner. Make a deadline with a peer. Use stern, commanding, confident self-talk.
Goal-directed persistence	Producer stops when faced with unfamiliar subtasks in the project.	Creative projects are full of unpracticed skills and unfamiliar tasks—get used to it! Say, "I can figure this out. Who can I ask about this? Where can I find this out? What is the first step?" Keep your courage up and your blood pumping.
Metacognition	Producer avoids certain aspects of the project and doesn't realize she's doing it. Producer doesn't act upon feelings of frustration or dissatisfaction.	Keep a journal or have a conversation in which you explore your feelings about the project. Do a daily top-to-bottom assessment of your project plan, noticing your feelings about each part. When you find yourself feeling stressed, depressed, or frustrated, make a list of five possible reasons and circle three that you think are most likely the cause.

Academic Skill: Memorization

	Barriers	Strategies
Task initiation and planning and prioritizing and time management	Despite spending a lot of time worrying about the task of memorization, the time spent on it is minimal and infrequent. All memorization is left to the last minute.	Put ten 5-minute memorization sessions in your calendar, and reward yourself for completion; gradually lengthen the sessions. Bundle your memorizing time with a routine or preferred activity, such as your car/bus ride to school, walking your dog, standing in a lineup, or checking a device. Don't worry about memorizing at other times.
Sustained attention	Memorizer does not attend to the memorization task deeply and strategically enough—material may be read over several times without retention.	For each practice session, test to see what you have not remembered, and target that with extra-intense practice. Try to link new material to information you already know. Use a memorizing technique like using acronyms, mnemonics, or songs. Research memorization techniques to find a good fit.
Goal-directed persistence	Memorizer becomes fatigued and bored while working on memorization.	Work at a standing desk. Make a recording of material to be remembered, and listen to it while walking, running, jumping on a trampoline, or drawing. Work on memorization with a fun partner.
Metacognition	Elements of the information to be memorized are unclear or poorly understood, but the memorizer does not notice or take action to clarify and ends up trying to memorize something that is meaningless.	Do 10 minutes of extra study or Internet searching, or ask a teacher/friend about the material you're meant to memorize. When you have to memorize, get in the habit of asking three clarifying questions before you begin. Say to yourself, "What don't I understand about this information?"

Academic Skill: Computer Coding

	Barriers	Strategies
Response inhibition	Coder is too focused on her desired end result and rushes or fails to code in small, reliable steps.	Before you begin, write down an achievable goal and work toward meeting that goal in the most effective way possible.
Working memory	Coder cannot hold a series of logical steps in mind long enough to understand their relationship and perceive their pattern. Coder does not spend enough time working with code and doesn't achieve fluency with programming languages.	Model the code you have in a flowchart. As you review your lines of code, speak them aloud. Work with a partner. Build fluency and ease with your coding language by practicing regularly on fun and simple projects.
Emotional control	Coder perceives wrong answers or slow progress as failure.	Keep a tally of your successful ideas. Take a break, and do something relaxing, creative, and playful. Tell yourself, "Coding is playful and imaginative work."
Flexibility	Coder gets stuck on one idea and can't let it go in order to explore other options.	Work with a partner and say, "This is fun. Let's try another option." When you run into a problem, put yourself in someone else's shoes and imagine a different solution from their point of view. Ask a partner, "What if we . . . ?"
Sustained attention	Coder attends long enough to discover problems, or detect patterns, but loses attention before applying this learning to a useful conclusion.	Use a big whiteboard to work through problems visually. Work through problems with a partner or talk to yourself. Take frequent, active breaks. Set a timer, and work with maximum effort for a specific, manageable amount of time.
Planning, prioritizing and organization	Coder cannot visualize common or repeating patterns. Coder can't easily visualize the sequence of steps that link faulty outcome to faulty code.	Model the code you have on a large flowchart. Post your flowchart, and talk it through with a partner.
Goal-directed persistence	Coder stops when faced with problems or glitches.	Look for and enjoy each small successful step. Make a tally of each successful step as you make it, and take a short break after every five steps.

21st-Century Skill: Collaboration (in Writing)

	Barriers	Strategies
Working memory	Collaborators struggle to balance the demands of keeping their own train of thought while listening effectively to a partner.	Jot down the basics of good ideas. Before speaking, say, "I have an idea to share with you. Do you need a minute of jot-note time to clear your mind?" and then double-check by asking, "Are you ready?" When your partner is finished sharing an idea, restate it by saying, "So what you're saying is . . ."
Emotional control & flexibility	Collaborators hold back ideas or questions, or have difficulty changing their mind or accepting the ideas of others.	Use cues, such as "Let me critique that . . ." or "Here's an unfinished idea . . ." Say, "This is messy, but it will lead us somewhere interesting." Share at least five critiques and five risky ideas. Ask, "Are we working well? How can we do better?" Build understanding by asking, "Will you tell me more about that?"
Sustained attention	Collaborators cannot focus on the work intently enough to be productive and effective.	Exercise and eat well prior to and during work. Change volume, proximity, furniture, clothing, technology, etc. Speak in an accent. Point to your collaborator while he or she is speaking. Restate your collaborator's ideas.
Planning, prioritizing and organizing	The project is disorganized, incomplete, and overwhelming.	Outline the project on oversized paper. Summarize the idea for the project in three points, then five, and then 10. Make a 10-point checklist.
Time management	Collaborators lose track of time or dwell on one thing.	Make a plan for each session of work and follow it. Finish each session of work by asking, "How did we do? Did we meet our objectives?"
Goal-directed persistence	Collaborators give up when faced with challenges.	Admit "This is frustrating, and I want to give up. Should we take a break and then try again?" Work on a different part of the project for a while. Ask someone else for a fresh perspective.
Metacognition	Collaborators have different inspiration, knowledge, or plans and don't realize it.	Before starting the project, and frequently during the process, ask your partner, "What do you know about this topic? What are we trying to do here? Where are we going with this? What is our intention?"

21st-Century Skill: Presenting

	Barriers	Strategies
Response inhibition	Presenter overresponds to questions or comments and gets off track.	Plan several ways to redirect interrupting questions or comments. For example, the presenter might say, "The short answer is no because x, y, and z, but will you please write down your question, so we can address it more fully at the end of the presentation?"
Working memory and emotional control	Presenter feels overwhelmed, confused, and disorganized.	Do extra practice to make the presentation more automatic. Test all technology well before presentation starts. Meditate or exercise before the presentation. Stop the presentation occasionally to ask for feedback. For example, say, "Show me with thumbs up or down if you understand." Ask an enthusiastic and positive participant for positive feedback during and after the presentation.
Sustained attention	Presenter cannot stay focused for the length of the presentation.	Presenter should vary the pace of the presentation, including regular participant "breakouts" or "turn and talks" to allow for a recharge.
Task initiation, planning, prioritizing and organizing	Presentation was not prepared early enough to allow time for practice and refinement.	Using a detailed calendar, presenter should work backward from the date of the presentation and schedule ample time to do writing, practice, and revision. The presenter must make sure to honor the date planned for the first work session, even if the start is small.
Time management	Presenter loses track of time, and the presentation or certain sections of the presentation are too long or too short.	While planning and practicing the presentation, record and perfect the timing of each section. Put the time allowed for each "slide" or portion of the presentation right on the materials as a reminder. Get a friend to give you timing reminders.
Metacognition	Presentation is so stressful that presenter doesn't want to think about feedback, so doesn't improve.	Gather simple "Best part of presentation/ Next time, try . . ." written feedback at the end of your presentation. Ask a trusted friend to sit down for a casual feedback conversation. Try to plan five ways to improve your presentation skills.

21st-Century Skill: Designing to Specifications

	Barriers	Strategies
Response inhibition and flexibility	Designer starts before understanding the intended use of the finished product.	Ask 10 questions about the project. Make a quick prototype so you can find the weaknesses early in the process. Research designs similar to yours. Use self-talk such as "I am overconfident; there must be aspects of this project I don't understand yet" or "I need to keep an open mind."
Emotional control	Designer is afraid to seem incapable, gets frustrated with partners, or feels rushed and shuts down.	Schedule time to ask questions or collaborate. Say, "Collaboration is hard but necessary for success." Notice your signs of frustration and take action to relax. If you don't have the time or materials you need, advocate for them.
Sustained attention	Designer does not pay close-enough attention to measurements, materials, or careful readjustments.	Find a detail-oriented partner. Take regular breaks for exercise, food, and water. Alternate back and forth between the design task and other, different kinds of tasks, such as planning and tidying. Work on design in novel surroundings, such as outside or at different desks or offices. Speak your thought process aloud.
Task initiation	Designer doesn't start work soon enough to have time to test and repair problems.	Right away, make a 10-point plan for how to complete the project. Include approximate task completion dates. Work with a partner on "start day" to make it more fun and unavoidable. Combine your first day's work with a reward.

21st-Century Skill: Debate

	Barriers	Strategies
Response inhibition	Debater responds too early, with ill-formed ideas or ideas that address only the first opposing point given.	Build responses to three parts before delivering—a beginning, a middle, and an end. Practice saying, "You said . . . ," "but . . . ," "so. . . ." Ask, "Are you finished?" before making a response.
Working memory	Debater cannot hold each part of the argument in memory long enough to express them clearly.	Plan small cue words to prompt argument from beginning to end. Have a list of key ways to juxtapose ideas, such as "only if," "but," "although," or "therefore."
Emotional control and metacognition	Debater takes arguments personally, feels overwhelmed, and shows unhelpful emotion with voice, body language, and facial expression. Debater doesn't notice when a line of thinking is not impressing a judge.	Take deep breaths while hearing the opposing arguments. Do not look at your opponent; look at the judge. Make a list of your biases or emotional "triggers" related to the topic before you debate. Watch the judge's face to get clues about which arguments are most effective and which should be dropped.
Flexibility	Debater focuses on own ideas without fully considering opposing ideas. Debater holds on to one idea, or one aspect of an idea, and is not open to being creative about other possibilities.	Divide a jot pad into two sections: one to jot down the ideas of your opponent and the other to jot your own ideas and responses down. Restate the speaker's point: "So what you're saying is . . ." Practice "flip-flopping" your position by exploring different sides and positions. Concede small points when you can.
Sustained attention	Debater's attention dwindles as opponent is speaking, so he or she misses conclusions or final points. Debater struggles to make connections and to be creative as the arguments accumulate.	Restate the speaker's point. Make jot notes or cue words to capture the beginning, middle, and end of opposing arguments. Keep track of main ideas across your fingers, and practice restating a cue word as you touch each finger. Watch, lean toward, point to, and nod at the speaker while they are speaking.
Planning, prioritizing and organizing	Debater cannot sequence ideas logically, so cannot express a coherent argument.	Practice telling the argument across your fingers, with guiding transition words such as "first," "second," "third," and "finally." Make a numbered list of cue words.

21st-Century Skill: Using Social Media

	Barriers	Strategies
Response inhibition	Individual sends undesirable responses without much thought or proofreading. Individual turns too often to social media for distraction or validation.	Do three offline "soothing" activities before turning to social media, such as spending time with pets, going for a walk, or talking to a friend. Before posting something questionable, 10 ten minutes, take 10 deep breaths, or repeat a personal mantra or set of goals, such as "I am kind, compassionate, and careful" or "I am a leader and my words matter."
Emotional control and flexibility	Individual has difficulty understanding other people's viewpoints and often responds unproductively or with a tone that creates conflict.	When you feel frustrated, upset, or confused by a comment, ask for clarification before replying or reply offline. Try simply to restate the point made by saying, "So what you mean is . . ." Look for one thing you agree with. Be twice as polite online as you are offline. Write and post knowing your grandmother or employer will eventually see it.
Sustained attention	Individual is used to the quick satisfaction of social media and cannot sustain attention on other tasks.	Practice meditation to help strengthen and focus your mind. Reduce the time spent on social media. Plan and schedule time for hobbies that require more sustained attention, such as sports, art, or reading.
Planning, prioritizing and organizing	Productive daily activities are not planned or scheduled, and social media is overused because it fills all the "free" time.	Designate certain times of the day to engage with social media or link social media use to the completion of a daily chore. For example, social media can be accessed at a regular time of day as a reward after finishing homework or tidying up. Or experiment with social media "blackout" times, perhaps going without for 1 or 2 hours.
Time management	Individual lingers on social media for long periods of time, avoiding other important tasks.	Set a timer to limit your use of social media. Start social media 1 hour before a regular activity, so you cannot extend your time frame.
Metacognition	Individual neglects other hobbies, relationships, and work, and does not recognize it.	Make a list of the number of online and offline hobbies and friends you have. Go a week without any online activity to see how life changes. Go offline for a week with a friend and discuss how it felt.
Planning, prioritizing and organizing	Designer dwells on one aspect of the design and doesn't understand others.	Make simple drawings or clay models to understand the whole project. Team up with partners who can help render and build prototypes for your idea. Create a series of sketches of the idea, making three improvements on each sketch.
Goal-directed persistence	Designer stops imagining and creating after first good idea.	Review and modify the plan regularly. Say, "How could we make this even better?" or "What is missing?" Ask a partner for a creative walk 'n chat.
Metacognition	Teacher gives vague instructions, and designers don't know exactly what is expected.	Support the client's (teachers') organization and metacognition. Ask for clarification in the form of specific information, timelines, or examples.

21st-Century Skill: Building Close Relationships

	Barriers	Strategies
Response inhibition	Individual blurts out or acts out in a way that is not productive.	Fully explain what you meant when you blurted out, even if you're not quite ready. Say, "I'm sorry. That doesn't make sense. Let me clarify."
Working memory	Individual is embarrassed or discouraged by conversation because they get confused.	Say, "I'm so interested, but I missed the first part. Can you repeat that?" Restate your friend's main points, saying, "So, let me see if I understand this . . ." Boost engagement by leaning in, making eye contact, etc.
Emotional control	Individual is prone to jealousy, possessiveness, or feeling hurt by passing comments.	Have several close friends. Explore your feelings with a counselor. Get more exercise, sleep, and nutrition. Take a 15-minute walk when you feel upset. Don't be afraid to say sorry. Check in with your friend right away if you suspect a problem. Be a helpful, involved, considerate friend.
Flexibility	Individual cannot see a situation from another's point of view. Individual doesn't match friend's moods.	Watch your friends' faces carefully to understand their moods. Have a code with your friends; for example, level 1 means *let's have fun*, level 2 means *I need to have a calm talk*, level 3 means *I need a very serious talk*, level 4 means *I need sympathy*, and level 5 means *I'm in trouble. I need your support.*
Sustained attention	Individual looks distant, bored, or uncaring during long conversations or activities that are less preferred.	Think about how friend's experiences relate to your own. Ask your friend questions about their feelings. Boost your physical engagement by leaning in, making eye contact, etc. Speak to your friend in a quiet location. Meet with your close friends after a vigorous workout so your energy is high.
Planning and prioritizing	Individual doesn't plan ahead to see close friends, so ends up losing touch or discouraging the friendship. Individual misses meetings, birthdays, or other important commitments.	Make the first of every month a "scheduling" day during which you make 10 social arrangements. Refer to your calendar of dates each morning over breakfast, or during any other regularly scheduled activity.

21st-Century Skill: Communication—Courageous or Difficult Conversations

	Barriers	Strategies
Response inhibition	Individual addresses interpersonal problems by blurting out complaints or criticisms at inopportune times.	Wait 3 slow seconds before responding. Take a long slow breath and make a thoughtful gesture (tapping finger to your chin, scratching your head, or clasping your hands) before responding.
Working memory	Individual feels confused and is not able to gather and express their thoughts clearly, made even worse by the emotional intensity of the conversation.	Make notes to follow during the conversation. Tell the person you're speaking to, "I'm a little nervous and I feel scattered. Please bear with me . . ."
Emotional control	Individual feels overwhelmingly mad, sad, or scared by the problem and avoids dealing with it.	Exercise or meditate, get proper sleep and nutrition, indulge in an upbeat movie or music, and practice with a friend. Say, "I am strong and kind enough to handle this conversation" or "This conversation is important to me."
Flexibility	Individual has difficulty understanding another person's point of view and may feel the problem arose because of ill will.	On your own or with a friend, list the reasons the issue may have arisen. Journal how the issue makes you and the other person feel. Say, "Will you tell me about how you are feeling?"
Planning and prioritizing	Individual cannot sequence the issue clearly enough to understand what has happened.	Practice telling the issue across your fingers, sequencing your ideas in order. Make jot notes to follow during the conversation.
Goal-directed persistence	Individual perceives a problem to be addressed with a courageous conversation but never gets around to planning a meeting.	Plan to have one serious or "courageous" conversation every week or month. Schedule it by writing it down in your calendar. If you don't have a problem to address, use the time to express gratitude.
Metacognition	Individual doesn't connect bad feelings to the problems or people they result from. Or individual doesn't realize they can address their problems with specific action.	Keep a journal in which you explore your feelings. When you find yourself feeling stressed, depressed, or frustrated, have a conversation with someone in which you explore the possible reasons. When you find yourself feeling stressed, depressed, or frustrated, make a list of five possible reasons and circle three that you think are most likely the cause.

21st-Century Skill: Putting Your Best Foot Forward—Grooming, Exercise, and other Self-Care

	Barriers	Strategies
Response inhibition and task initiation	Even if there is enough time for self-care, other, more satisfying, relaxing, or pleasurable activities are done during this time. Individual can't get out of bed.	Write morning routine on a list, post it, and try to follow it in order every day for 9 days straight. Plan a reward for completing self-care jobs. Start with a small, manageable routine. Think of nothing but putting your feet on the floor; don't agonize about getting up.
Emotional control and flexibility	Individual does not feel good about the way he looks and feels discouraged.	Smile at yourself in the mirror. Combine self-care activities related to grooming with meditation and deep breathing. Play encouraging music during morning routine. Find a part of your personal appearance that you like and focus on that. Write an affirmation on the mirror with whiteboard markers. Don't do grooming in front of a mirror.
Task initiation	Individual has time, but the task feels tiring or boring or discouraging so she doesn't get started.	Set a small alarm to mark the start of the morning routine. Start with the smallest, easiest, or most enjoyable part of the routine. Combine a favorite morning treat with the beginning of the routine, such as a delicious drink, a favorite vitamin, or a great song.
Planning and prioritizing	Individual doesn't have the tools or articles needed to properly groom, dress, and prepare for the day.	Plan a fun outing with a friend to get the things you need. You don't have to spend a lot of money—if you are resourceful you can equip yourself quite cheaply using secondhand, thrift, and drugstore finds.
Organizing and time management	Not enough time has been allowed in the morning routine for self-care. There are a vast number of small tasks, and doing them is confusing and overwhelming.	Add 30 minutes to the morning routine with an earlier alarm. Write your morning routine on a list, and post it so it is less confusing to accomplish.
Goal-directed persistence	Individual starts on a new self-care routine or activity but loses interest and gives up.	Don't think of new self-care routines as lifelong commitments. Instead make a 1-month plan, expect to be a little bored with it when the month is over, and look forward to making a new plan at that time.

21st-Century Skill: Sleep

	Barriers	Strategies
Response inhibition	The sleeper has great difficulty stopping her reading or activities on a device.	Make a firm cutoff time for use of devices, and get in the habit of honoring this cutoff time. Don't charge your phone or device in your bedroom. Put your bedside light on a timer.
Emotional control	Sleeper is anxious about the day to come and stays awake to stall its arrival.	Talk over your worries by listening to a bedtime story (online works!), counting sheep, or listening to music. Read. Write down three worries and then forget them. Write down three things you are grateful for. Look at happy images of yourself or others.
Task initiation	Sleeper delays starting on bedtime routine.	Make a firm cutoff time for use of devices, and get in the habit of honoring this cutoff time. Put your bedside light on a timer.
Planning, prioritizing and organizing and time management	Sleeper doesn't know how many hours of sleep he needs. Bedtime is erratically scheduled. Plan for when to go to sleep does not include "wind down" time.	Research sleep requirements for your age and calculate the optimal bed time and wake time. Write down everything you need to do before you go to sleep and allot time realistically and generously. Keep a constant wake-up time using an alarm clock or a light on a timer. In the winter months, consider using a "light therapy box" to reinforce and energize your wake-up schedule.
Goal-directed persistence	Sleeper has a good plan but doesn't execute on the plan regularly.	Cancel activities planned for the evening times, if you are overscheduled. Keep a tally of the number of days you succeed at your sleep plan. Write up a specific sleep plan with a specific and achievable goal—perhaps you will aim to maintain your sleep plan from Monday to Wednesday each week, to start. Discuss your sleep plan with someone and make a goal together.
Metacognition	Sleeper does not make the connection between moody, foggy, exhausted feelings during the day and poor sleep habits.	Make the connection! Ask friends about how sleep affects their mood and productivity. Do some reading about the importance of sleep. Keep a journal in which you score the productivity of your days from 1 to 10 and the quality of your sleep.

References

Aitken, M., Martinussen, R., Childs, R., & Tannock, R. (2017). Profiles of co-occurring difficulties identified through school-based screening. *Journal of Attention Disorders, 24*(9), 1355–1365.

Ajzen, I. (1985). From intentions to actions: A theory of planned behavior. In J. Kuhl & J. Beckmann (Eds.), *Action control.* Berlin: Springer.

Ajzen, I. (1991). The theory of planned behavior. *Organizational Behavior and Human Decision Processes, 50,* 179–211.

Ajzen, I., & Fishbein, M. (2000). Attitudes and the attitude-behavior relation: Reasoned and automatic processes. *European Review of Social Psychology, 11,* 1–33.

Andrews, G. R., & Debus, R. L. (1978). Persistence and the causal perception of failure: Modifying cognitive attributions. *Journal of Educational Psychology, 70,* 154–166.

Arunkumar, R., Midgley, C., & Urdan, T. (1999). Perceiving high or low home-school dissonance: Longitudinal effects on adolescent emotional and academic well-being. *Journal of Research on Adolescence, 9,* 441–466.

Baadte, C., & Kurenbach, F. (2017). The effects of expectancy-incongruent feedback and self-affirmation on task performance of secondary school students. *European Journal of Psychology of Education, 32,* 113–131.

Baartman, L. K. J., Bastiaens, T. J., Kirschner, P. A., & Van der Vleuten, C. P. M. (2006). The wheel of competency assessment: Presenting quality criteria for competency assessment programs. *Studies in Educational Evaluation, 32,* 153–170.

Bakker, A. B., Demerouti, E., & Euwema, M. C. (2005). Job resources buffer the impact of job demands on burnout. *Journal of Occupational Health Psychology, 10,* 170–180.

Bandura, A. (1997). *Self-efficacy: The exercise of control.* New York: Freeman.

Bandura, A., & Locke, E. A. (2003). Negative self-efficacy and goal effects revisited. *Journal of Applied Psychology, 88*(1), 87–99.

Barkley, R. A. (2012). *Executive functions: What they are, how they work, and why they evolved.* New York: Guilford Press.

Barthes, R., & Duisit, L. (1975). An introduction to the structural analysis of narrative author(s). *New Literary History, 6*(2), 237–272.

Bekle, B. (2004). Knowledge and attitudes about attention-deficit hyperactivity disorder (ADHD): A comparison between practicing teachers and undergraduate education students. *Journal of Attention Disorders, 7*(3), 151–161.

Bennett, N., & Kell, J. (1989). *A good start? Four year olds in infant schools.* Oxford, UK: Blackwell.

Berland, L. K., Schwarz, C. V., Krist, C., Kenyon, L., Lo, A. S., & Reiser, B. J. (2016). Epistemologies in practice: Making scientific practices meaningful for students. *Journal of Research in Science Teaching, 57*(3), 1082–1112.

Bermejo-Toro, L., Prieto-Ursúa, M., & Hernández, V. (2016). Towards a model of teacher well-being: Personal and job resources involved in teacher burnout and engagement. *Educational Psychology, 36*(3), 481–501.

Bethell, C., Newacheck, P., Hawes, E., & Halfon, N. (2014). Adverse childhood experiences: Assessing the impact on health and school engagement and the mitigating role of resilience. *Health Affairs, 33*(12), 2016–2115.

Bialik, M., & Fadel, C. (2015). *Skills for the 21st century: What should students learn?* Boston, MA: Centre for Curriculum Redesign.

Bianchi, R., Schonfeld, I. S., & Laurent, E. (2015). Is it time to consider the "Burnout Syndrome" a distinct illness? *Frontiers in Public Health, 3,* 158.

Blair, C., & Razza, R. P. (2007). Relating effortful control, executive function, and false belief understanding to emerging math and literacy ability in kindergarten. *Child Development, 78*(2), 647–663.

Brandstatter, V., Lengfelder, A., & Gollwitzer, P. (2001). Implementation intentions and efficient action initiation. *Journal of Personality and Social Psychology, 81,* 946–960.

Brownlie, F., & King, J. (2011). *The importance of "belonging" in a classroom: Learning in safe schools* (2nd ed.). Markham, Ontario: Pembroke Publishers.

Bussing, R., Gary, F., Leon, C., Garvan, C., & Reid, R. (2002). General classroom teachers' information and perceptions of attention deficit hyperactivity disorder. *Behavioral Disorders, 27*(4), 327–339.

Butler, D. L., Schnellert, L., & Perry, N. E. (2016). *Developing self-regulated learners.* Toronto, Ontario, Canada: Pearson.

Carr, M. (2001). *Assessment in early childhood settings.* London: Sage.

Cerasoli, C. P., Nicklin, J. M., & Ford, M. T. (2014). Intrinsic motivation and extrinsic incentives jointly predict performance: A 40-year meta-analysis. *Psychological Bulletin, 140*(4), 980–1008.

Chang, M. L. (2013). Toward a theoretical model to understand teacher emotions and teacher burnout in the context of student misbehavior: Appraisal, regulation and coping. *Motivation and Emotion, 37,* 799–817.

Chapin, M., & Dyck, D. (1976). Persistence in children's reading behavior as a function of N length and attributional retraining. *Journal of Abnormal Psychology, 85,* 511–515.

Chen, S. S., & Chin, J. (2006). Development of collective efficacy scale for middle school students. *Journal of School Health, 10,* 861–862.

Chmielewski, A. K. (2019). The global increase in the socioeconomic achievement gap, 1964 to 2015. *American Sociological Review, 84*(3), 517–544.

Corbin, C. M., Alamos, P., Lowenstein, A. E., Downer, J. T., & Brown, J. L. (2019). The role of teacher–student relationships in predicting teachers' personal accomplishment and emotional exhaustion. *Journal of School Psychology, 77,* 1–12.

Corno, L. (1993). The best-laid plans: Modern conceptions of volition and educational research. *Educational Research, 22,* 14–22.

Davis, B., & Sumara, D. (2006). *Complexity and education: Inquiries into learning, teaching, and research.* Mahwah, NJ: Lawrence Erlbaum Associates.

Dawson, P., & Guare, R. (2018). *Executive skills in children and adolescents: A practical guide to assessment and intervention* (3rd ed.). New York: Guilford Press.

Deci, E., & Ryan, R. (2000). The "what" and "why" of goal pursuits: Human needs and self-determination of behavior. *Psychological Inquiry, 11*(4), 227–268.

DeLong, M., & Winter, D. (2002). Strategies for motivating students. In *Learning to teach and teaching to learn mathematics: Resources for professional development*. Washington, DC: Mathematical Association of America.

Demerouti, E., Bakker, A. B., Nachreiner, F., & Schaufeli, W. B. (2001). The job demands–resources model of burnout. *Journal of Applied Psychology, 86*, 499–512.

Diamond, A. (2013). Executive functions. *Annual Review of Psychology, 64*, 135–168.

Diamond, A. (2014). Want to optimize executive functions and academic outcomes? Simple, just nourish the human spirit. *Minnesota Symposia on Child Psychology, 37*, 205–232.

Diamond, A., & Ling, D. S. (2020). Review of the evidence on, and fundamental questions about, efforts to improve executive functions, including working memory. In K. Novick, M. F. Bunting, M. R. Dougherty, & R. W. Engle (Eds.), *Cognitive and working memory training: Perspectives from psychology, neuroscience, and human development*. New York: Oxford University Press.

Dignath-van Ewijk, C., Dickhäuser, O., & Büttner, G. (2013). Assessing how teachers enhance self-regulated learning: A multiperspective approach. *Journal of Cognitive Education and Psychology, 12*, 338–358.

Dronek, P. J., & Blessing, S. B. (2006). *The effect of Einstellung on compositional processes*. Paper presented at the 28th annual conference of the Cognitive Science Society, Vancouver, British Columbia, Canada.

Duckworth, A. L., & Seligman, M. E. P. (2005). Self-discipline outdoes IQ in predicting academic performance of adolescents. *Psychological Science, 16*(2), 939–944.

Dweck, C. (2006). *Mindset: The new psychology of success.* New York, NY: Random House.

Dweck, C. (2016). Growth mindset doesn't promise students the world. *The Times Educational Supplement, 5158*.

Dweck, C. S. (1975). The role of expectations and attributions in the alleviation of learned helplessness. *Journal of Personality and Social Psychology, 31*, 674–685.

Elik, N., Wiener, J., & Corkum, P. (2010). Preservice teachers' open-minded thinking dispositions, readiness to learn, and attitudes towards learning and behavioral difficulties in students. *European Journal of Teacher Education, 33*(2), 127–146.

Elliott, E. S., & Dweck, C. S. (1988). Goals: An approach to motivation and achievement. *Journal of Personality and Social Psychology, 54*, 5–12.

Elliott, R. (2003). Executive functions and their disorders: Imaging in clinical neuroscience. *British Medical Bulletin, 65*(1), 49–59.

Espy, K. A., McDiarmid, M. M., Cwik, M. F., Stalets, M. M., Hamby, A., & Senn, T. E. (2004). The contribution of executive functions to emergent mathematic skills in preschool children. *Developmental Neuropsychology, 26*(1), 465–486.

Fadel, C., Bialik, M., & Trilling, B. (2015). *Four-dimensional education: The competencies learners need to succeed.* Boston, MA: The Centre for Curriculum Redesign.

Faith, L. (2018). EFs 2 the Rescue Pedagogy. In P. Dawson & D. Guare (Eds.), *Executive skills in children and adolescents: A practical guide to assessment and intervention* (3rd ed.). New York: Guilford Press.

Farrington, C., Roderick, M., Allensworth, E., Nagaoka, J., Keyes, T., Johnson, D., & Beechum, N. (2012). *Teaching adolescents to become learners: The role of noncognitive factors in shaping school performance; A critical literature review*. Retrieved from Chicago: *https://consortium.uchicago.edu/publications/teaching-adolescents-become-learners-role-noncognitive-factors-shaping-school.*.

Fitzgerald, M., Danaia, L., & McKinnon, D. H. (2019). Barriers inhibiting inquiry-based science teaching and potential solutions: Perceptions of positively inclined early adopters. *Research in Science Education, 49*(2), 543–566.

Fletcher, J. M., & Grigorenko, E. L. (2017). Neuropsychology of learning disabilities: The past and the future. *Journal of the International Neuropsychological Society, 9–10*, 930–940.

Flint, A., Zisook, T., & Fisher, T. E. (2011). Not a one-shot deal: Generative professional development among experienced teachers. *Teaching and Teacher Education, 27*(8), 1163–1169.

Forster, M., & Masters, G. (1996). *Performances: Assessment resource kit.* Camberwell, Australia: Australian Council for Educational Research.

Framework for 21st Century Learning. (2016). *Partnership for 21st century learning.* Retrieved from *www. p21.org/our-work/p21-framework*.

Friedman-Krauss, A., Raver, C. C., Neuspiel, J., & Kinsel, J. (2014). Child behavior problems, teacher executive functions, and teacher stress in head start classrooms. *Early Education Development, 25*(5), 681–702.

Fryer, S. L., Tapert, S. F., Mattson, S. N., Paulus, M. P., Spadoni, A. D., & Riley, E. P. (2007). Prenatal alcohol exposure affects frontal-striatal response during inhibitory control. *Alcoholism, Clinical and Experimental Research, 3*(18), 1415–1424.

Gaier, S. (2015). Understanding why students do what they do: Using attribution theory to help students succeed academically. *Research and Teaching in Developmental Education, 31*(2), 6–19.

García-Madruga, J. A., Elosúa, M. R., Gil, L., Gómez-Veiga, I., Vila, J. Ó., Orjales, I., . . . Duque, G. (2013). Reading comprehension and working memory's executive processes: An intervention study in primary school students. *Reading Research Quarterly, 48*(2), 155–174.

Garet, M. S., Porter, A. C., Desimone, L., Birman, B. F., & Yoon, K. S. (2001). What makes professional development effective? Results from a national sample of teachers. *American Educational Research Journal, 38*(4), 915–945.

Gay, G. (2000). *Culturally responsive teaching: Theory, research, and practice.* New York: Teachers College Press.

Gilmore, C., & Cragg, L. (2014). Teachers' understanding of the role of executive functions in mathematics learning. *Mind, Brain, and Education, 8*(3), 132–136.

Gioia, G. A., & Isquith, P. K. (2004). Ecological assessment of executive function in traumatic brain injury. *Developmental Neuropsychology, 25*, 135–158.

Gollwitzer, P., & Brandstatter, V. (1997). Implementations and effective goal striving. *Journal of Personality and Social Psychology, 73*, 186–199.

Goodwin, C. (1994). Professional vision. *American Anthropologist, 96*, 606–633.

Greene, R. W. (2008). *Lost at school: Why our kids with behavioral challenges are falling through the cracks and how we can help them.* New York: Scribner.

Guskey, T. R. (2002). Professional development and teacher change. *Teachers and Teaching: Theory and Practice, 8*(3/4), 381–391.

Haddad, F. A., Evie Garcia, Y., Naglieri, J. A., Grimditch, M., McAndrews, A., & Eubanks, J. (2003). Planning facilitation and reading comprehension: Instructional relevance of the pass theory. *Journal of Psychoeducational Assessment, 21*(3), 282–289.

Hadfield, C. (2013). *An astronaut's guide to life on Earth: What going to space taught me about ingenuity, determination, and being prepared.* Toronto: Random House Canada.

Hall, G., & Hord, S. (2001). *Implementing change: Patterns, principles, and potholes.* Needham Heights, MA: Allyn and Bacon.

Hall, N. C., Hladkyj, S., Perry, R. P., & Ruthig, J. C. (2004). The role of attributional retraining and elaborative learning in college students' academic development. *Journal of Social Psychology, 144*, 591–612.

Hall, N. C., Perry, R. P., Goetz, T., Ruthig, J. C., Stupnisky, R. H., & Newall, N. E. (2007). Attributional retraining and elaborative learning: Improving academic development through writing-based interventions. *Learning and Individual Differences, 17*, 280–290.

Hammond, Z. (2015). *Culturally responsive teaching and the brain.* Thousand Oaks, CA: Corwin.

Hannesdottir, D. K., Ingvarsdottir, E., & Bjornsson, A. (2017). The OutSMARTers program for children with

ADHD: A pilot study on the effects of social skills, self-regulation, and executive function training. *Journal of Attention Disorders, 21*(4), 353–364.

Hattie, J., & Timperley, H. (2007). The power of feedback. *Review of Educational Research, 77*(1), 81–112.

Haynes, T. L., Ruthig, J. C., Perry, R. P., Stupnisky, R. H., & Hall, N. C. (2006). Reducing the academic risks of over-optimism: The longitudinal effects of attributional retraining on cognition and achievement. *Research in Higher Education, 47,* 755–779.

Heifetz, R. A., & Linsky, M. (2002). *Leadership on the line: Staying alive through the dangers of leading.* Boston, MA: Harvard Business School Press.

Hummer, V. L., Dollard, N., Robst, J., & Armstrong, M. I. (2010). Innovations in implementation of trauma-informed care practices in youth residential treatment: A curriculum for organizational change. *Child Welfare, 89*(2), 79–95.

Ingvarson, L., Meiers, M., & Beavis, A. (2005). Factors affecting the impact of professional development programs on teachers' knowledge, practice, student outcomes and efficacy. *Educational Policy Analysis Archives, 13*(10), 1–28.

Iseman, J. S., & Naglieri, J. A. (2011). A cognitive strategy instruction to improve math calculation for children with ADHD and LD: A randomized controlled study. *Journal of Learning Disabilities, 44*(2), 184–195.

Jones, H., & Chronis-Tuscano, A. (2008). Efficacy of teacher in-service training for attention-deficit/hyperactivity disorder. *Psychology in the Schools, 45*(10), 918–929.

Jones, M. H., Alexander, J. M., & Estell, D. B. (2010). Homophily among peer members' perceived self-regulated learning. *The Journal of Experimental Education, 78*(3), 378–394.

Katz, S., & Dack, L. (2013). *Intentional Interruption: Breaking Down Learning Barriers to Transform Professional Practice.* Thousand Oaks, CA: Corwin Press.

Kazdin, A. (1980). Acceptability of alternative treatments for deviant child behavior. *Journal of Applied Behavior Analysis, 13,* 259–273.

Kenworthy, L., Anthony, L. G., Naiman, D. Q., Cannon, L., Wills, M. C., Luong-Tran, C., . . . Wallace, G. L. (2014). Randomized controlled effectiveness trial of executive function intervention for children on the autism spectrum. *Journal of Child Psychology and Psychiatry, 55*(4), 374–383.

Kersting, N. B., Givvin, K. B., Sotelo, F. L., & Stigler, J. W. (2010). Teachers' analyses of classroom video predict student learning of mathematics: Further explorations of a novel measure of teacher knowledge. *Journal of Teacher Education, 61*(1–2), 172–181.

Kistner, S., Rakoczy, K., Otto, B., Dignath-van Ewijk, C., Büttner, G., & Klieme, E. (2010). Promotion of self-regulated learning in classrooms: Investigating frequency, quality, and consequences for student performance. *Metacognition and Learning, 5*(2), 157–171.

Klusmann, U., Kunter, M., Trautwein, U., Ludtke, O., & Baumert, J. (2008). Teachers' occupational well-being and quality of instruction: The important role of self regulatory patterns *Journal of Educational Psychology, 100*(3), 702–715.

Kramarski, B., & Michalsky, T. (2009). Investigating preservice teachers' professional growth in self-regulated learning environments. *Journal of Educational Psychology, 101*(1), 161–175.

Kusché, C. A., & Greenberg, M. T. (1994). *The PATHS curriculum: Promoting alternative thinking strategies.* Seattle: Developmental Research and Programs.

Lakin, J., & Shannon, D. (2015). The role of treatment acceptability, effectiveness, and understanding in treatment fidelity: Predicting implementation variation in a middle school science program. *Studies in Educational Evaluation, 47,* 28–37.

Lanham, H. J., Leykum, L. K., Taylor, B. S., McCannon, C. J., Lindberg, C., & Lester, R. T. (2013). How complexity science can inform scale-up and spread in health care: Understanding the role of self-organization in variation across local contexts. *Social Science & Medicine, 93,* 194–202.

Le Fevre, D. (2014). Barriers to implementing pedagogical change: The role of teachers' perceptions of risk. *Teaching and Teacher Education, 38,* 56–64.

Liljestrand, J., & Hammarberg, A. (2017). The social construction of the competent, self-governed child in documentation: Panels in the Swedish preschool. *Contemporary Issues in Early Childhood, 18*(1), 39–54.

Linde, C. (1993). *Life Stories: The Creation of Coherence.* New York: Oxford University Press.

Linville, P. W. (1985). Self-complexity and affective extremity: Don't put all of your eggs in one cognitive basket. *Social Cognition: Special Issue on Depression, 3,* 94–120.

Martel, M. M. (2013). Individual differences in attention deficit hyperactivity disorder symptoms and associated executive dysfunction and traits: Sex, ethnicity, and family income. *American Journal of Orthopsychiatry, 83*(2–3), 165–175.

Martinussen, R., Tannock, R., & Chaban, P. (2011). Teachers' reported use of instructional and behavior management practices for students with behavior problems: Relationship to role and level of training in ADHD. *Child & Youth Care Forum, 40*(3), 193–210.

Marzano, R., Pickering, D., & Pollock, J. (2001). *Classroom instruction that works: Research-based strategies for increasing student achievement.* Alexandria, VA: Association for Supervision and Curriculum Development.

Maslach, C., & Jackson, S. E. (1981). The measurement of experienced burnout. *Journal of Occupational Behavior, 2*(2), 99–113.

Maslach, C., Schaufeli, W. B., & Leiter, M. P. (2001). Job burnout. *Annual Review of Psychology, 52,* 397–422.

McCloskey, G., & Perkins, L. (2013). *Essentials of executive functions assessment.* Hoboken, NJ: Wiley & Sons, Inc.

Meltzer, L., Dunstan-Brewer, J., & Krishnan, K. (2018). Learning differences and executive function: Understandings and misunderstandings. In L. Meltzer (Ed.), *Executive function in education: From theory to practice* (2nd ed., pp. 109–141). New York: Guilford Press.

Meltzer, L., Basho, S., Reddy, R., & Kurkul, K. (2015). The role of mentoring in fostering executive function, effort, and academic self-concept. *International Journal for Research in Learning Disabilities, 2*(2), 91–123.

Menec, V. H., Perry, R. P., Struthers, C. W., Schönwetter, D. J., Hechter, F. J., & Eichholz, B. L. (1994). Assisting at-risk college students with attributional retraining and effective teaching. *Journal of Applied Social Psychology, 24,* 675–701.

Michalsky, T., & Schechter, C. (2013). Preservice teachers' capacity to teach self-regulated learning: Integrating learning from problems and learning from successes. *Teaching and Teacher Education, 30,* 60–73.

Moffitt, T., Arseneault, L., Belsky, D., Dickson, N., Hancox, R., Harrington, H., . . . Caspi, A. (2011). A gradient of childhood self-control predicts health, wealth, and public safety. *Proceedings of the National Academy of Sciences, 108*(7), 2693–2698.

Muller, S., Gorrow, T., & Fiala, K. (2011). Considering protective factors as a tool for teacher resiliency. *Education, 131*(3), 545–555.

Mullis, I. V. S., Martin, M. O., Foy, P., & Hooper, M. (2016). *TIMSS 2015 international results in mathematics.* Boston, MA: TIMSS & PIRLS International Study Center, Boston College.

NASEM. (2018). *How people learn II: Learners, contexts, and cultures.* Washington, DC: National Academies Press.

Nash, K., Stevens, S., Greenbaum, R., Weiner, J., Koren, G., & Rovet, J. (2015). Improving executive functioning in children with fetal alcohol spectrum disorders. *Child Neuropsychology, 21*(2), 191–209.

National Scientific Council on the Developing Child. (2004). *Children's emotional development is built into the architecture of their brains: Working paper No. 2.* Retrieved from *www.developingchild.net.*

Naumann, E. (2004). *Love at first sight: The stories and science behind instant attraction.* Chicago: Sourcebooks Casablanca.

Nizielski, S., Hallum, S., Schütz, A., & Lopes, P. N. (2013). A note on emotion appraisal and burnout: The mediating role of antecedent-focused coping strategies. *Journal of Occupational Health Psychology, 18*(3), 363–369.

OECD. (2009). *Chapter 4: Teaching practices, teachers' beliefs and attitudes.* Paris: TALIS Database, OECD Publishing.

OECD. (2017). *PISA 2015 results: Student's well being (Volume III).* Paris: OECD Publishing.

Oettingen, G., & Gollwitzer, P. M. (2010). Strategies of setting and implementing goals: Mental contrasting and implementation intentions. In J. E. Maddux & J. P. Tangney (Eds.), *Social psychological foundations of clinical psychology.* New York: Guilford Press.

Ozonoff, S., & Jensen, J. (1999). Brief report: Specific executive function profiles in three neurodevelopmental disorders. *Autism and Developmental Disorders, 29,* 171–177.

Panadero, E., & Jarvela, S. (2015). Socially shared regulation of learning: A review. *European Psychologist, 20*(3), 190–203.

Patall, E. A. (2013). Constructing motivation through choice, interest, and interestingness. *Journal of Educational Psychology, 105*(2), 522–534.

Penuel, W. R., Sun, M. I. N., Frank, K. A., & Gallagher, H. A. (2012). Using social network analysis to study how collegial interactions can augment teacher learning from external professional development. *American Journal of Education, 119*(1), 103–136.

Perry, N. E., Hutchinson, L., & Thauberger, C. (2008). Talking about teaching self-regulated learning: Scaffolding student teachers' development and use of practices that promote self-regulated learning. *International Journal of Educational Research, 47*(2), 97–108.

Perry, N. E., Phillips, L., & Hutchinson, L. (2006). Mentoring student teachers to support self-regulated learning. *The Elementary School Journal, 106*(3), 237–254.

Perry, N. E., Yee, N., Mazabel, S., Lisaingo, S., & Maatta, E. (2017). Using self-regulated learning as a framework for creating inclusive classrooms for ethnically and linguistically diverse learners in Canada. In N. J. Cabrera & B. Leyendecker (Eds.), *Handbook on positive development of minority children and youth.* (pp. 361–377). New York: Springer.

Perry, R. P., Stupnisky, R. H., Hall, N. C., Chipperfield, J. G., & Weiner, B. (2010). Bad starts and better finishes: Attributional retraining and initial performance in competitive achievement settings. *Journal of Social and Clinical Psychology, 29*(6), 668–700.

Piaget, J. (1952). *The origins of intelligence in children.* New York: International Universities Press.

Pintrich, P. R., & Garcia, T. (1991). Student goal orientation and self-regulated learning in the college classroom. In M. L. Maehr & P. R. Pintrich (Eds.), *Advances in motivation and achievement: Goals and self-regulatory processes* (Vol. 7, pp. 371–402). Greenwich, CT: JAI Press.

Polletta, F., Chen, P. C. B., & Gardner, B. G. (2011). The sociology of storytelling. *Annual Review of Sociology, 37,* 109–130.

Project Zero & Reggio Children. (2011). *Making learning visible.* Reggio Emilia, Italy: Reggio Children.

Quan-McGimpsey, S., Kuczynski, L., & Brophy, K. (2013). Tensions between the personal and the professional in close teacher-child relationships. *Journal of Research in Childhood Education, 27,* 111–126.

Raines, M. L. (2000). Ethical decision making in nurses: Relationships among moral reasoning, coping style, and ethics stress. *JONA's Healthcare Law, Ethics and Regulation, 2*(1), 29–41. Retrieved from *https://journals.lww.com/jonalaw/Fulltext/2000/02010/Ethical_Decision_Making_in_Nurses__Relationships.6.aspx.*

Rees, P. H., Wohland, P., Norman, P., & Lomax, N. (2017). Population projections by ethnicity: Challenges and solutions for the United Kingdom. In D. A. Swanson (Ed.), *The frontiers of applied demography.* Cham, Switzerland: Springer International Publishing.

Reimers, T. M., Wacker, D. P., & Koeppl, G. (1987). Acceptability of behavioral treatments: A review of the literature. *School Psychology Review, 16,* 212–227.

Rimm-Kaufman, S., & Sandilos, L. (2015). Improving students' relationships with teachers to provide essential supports for learning. *American Psychological Association.* Retrieved from *www.apa.org/education/k12/relationships.aspx.*

Rimm-Kaufman, S. E., Fan, X., Chiu, Y. J., & You, W. (2007). The contribution of the responsive classroom approach on children's academic achievement: Results from a three year longitudinal study. *Journal of School Psychology, 45*(4), 401–421.

Robinson, V., Hohepa, M., & Lloyd, C. (2009). *School leadership and student outcomes: Identifying what works and why.* Wellington, New Zealand: Ministry of Education.

Rodríguez-Mantilla, J. M., & Fernández-Díaz, M. J. (2017). The effect of interpersonal relationships on burnout syndrome in Secondary Education teachers. *Psichotema, 29*(3), 370–377.

Rosenberg, M., & McCullough, B. C. (1981). Mattering: Inferred significance and mental health among adolescents. *Research in Community and Mental Health, 2,* 163–182.

Ryan, R. M., & Deci, E. L. (2002). An overview of self-determination theory: An organismic-dialectical perspective. In E. L. Deci & R. M. Ryan (Eds.), *Handbook of self-determination research.* Rochester: The University of Rochester Press.

Schildkamp, K., Lai, M. K., & Earl, L. (2013). *Data-based decision making in education.* Dordrecht, The Netherlands: Springer.

Schulz, M. (2013). Frühpädagogische konstituierung von kindlichen bildungs-und lernprozessen. *Zeitschrift für Soziologie der Erziehung und Sozialisation, 33*(1), 26–41.

Shivers, J., Levenson, C., & Tan, M. (2017). Visual literacy, creativity, and the teaching of argument. *Learning Disabilities: A Contemporary Journal, 15*(1), 67–84.

Skaalvik, E. M., & Skaalvik, S. (2011). Teacher job satisfaction and motivation to leave the teaching profession: Relations with school context, feeling of belonging, and emotional exhaustion. *Teaching and Teacher Education, 27,* 1029–1038.

Southern Education Foundation. (2015). A new majority: Low income students now a majority in the nation's public schools. Retrieved from *www.southerneducation.org/wp-content/uploads/2019/02/New-Majority-Update-Bulletin.pdf.*

Spruce, R., & Bol, L. (2015). Teacher beliefs, knowledge, and practice of self-regulated learning. *Metacognition and Learning, 10*(2), 245–277.

Statistics Canada. (2017). *Immigration and diversity: Population projections for Canada and its regions, 2011 to 2036.* Retrieved from www150.statcan.gc.ca/n1/en/pub/91-551-x/91-551-x2017001-eng.pdf?st=LOHXEDBV.

Stein, J. A., & Krishnan, K. (2018). Nonverbal learning disabilities and executive function: The challenges of effective assessment and teaching. In L. Meltzer (Ed.), *Executive function in education: From theory to practice* (2nd ed.). New York: Guilford Press.

Stigler, J. W., & Hiebert, J. (1999). *The teaching gap.* New York: Free Press.

Swanson, H. L. (1990). Influence of metacognitive knowledge and aptitude on problem solving. *Journal of Educational Psychology* (82), 306–314.

Swing, E. L., Gentile, D. A., Anderson, C. A., & Walsh, D. A. (2010). Television and video game exposure and the development of attention problems. *Pediatrics, 126*(2), 214–221.

Taylor, M. (2014, April 1). Jane Goodall blames "chaotic note taking" for plagiarism controversy. *The Guardian.*

Tomlinson, C. A. (2001). *How to differentiate instruction in mixed-ability classrooms* (2nd ed.). Alexandria, VA: ASCD.

Torgesen, J. K. (1977). Memorization processes in reading-disabled children. *Journal of Educational Psychology, 69*(5), 571–578.

Tough, P. (2016). *Helping children succeed: What works and why.* New York: Houghton Mifflin.

Tunstall, P., & Gipps, C. (1996). Teacher feedback to young children in formative assessment: A typology. *British Educational Research Journal, 22*(4), 389–404.

Tyler, K. M., Uqdah, A. L., Dillihunt, M. L., Beatty-Hazelbaker, R., Conner, T., Gadson, N., . . . Stevens, R. (2008). Cultural discontinuity: Toward a quantitative investigation of a major hypothesis in education. *Educational Researcher, 37*(5), 280–297.

U.S. Census Bureau. (2015). *New census bureau report analyzes U.S. population projections.* Retrieved from *www.prnewswire.com/news-releases/new-census-bureau-report-analyzes-us-population-projections-300044527.html.*

Usher, E. L., Caihong, R. L., Butz, A. R., & Rojas, J. P. (2018). Perseverant grit and self-efficacy: Are both essential for children's academic success? *Journal of Educational Psychology, 111*(1), 877–902.

Van Overwalle, F., & de Metsenaere, M. (1990). The effects of attribution-based intervention and study strategy training on academic achievement in college freshmen. *British Journal of Educational Psychology, 60,* 299–311.

Vansteenkiste, M., Lens, W., & Deci, E. L. (2006). Intrinsic versus extrinsic goal contents in self-determination theory: Another look at the quality of academic motivation. *Educational Psychologist, 41*(1), 19–31.

Veenman, M. V. J., Van Hout-Wolters, B. H. A. M., & Afflerbach, P. (2006). Metacognition and learning: Conceptual and methodological considerations. *Metacognition and Learning, 1,* 3–14.

Vescio, V., Ross, D., & Adams, A. (2008). A review of research on the impact of professional learning communities on teaching practice and student learning. *Teaching and Teacher Education, 24*(1), 80–91.

Visu-Petra, L., Cheie, L., Benga, O., & Miclea, M. (2011). Cognitive control goes to school: The impact of executive functions on academic performance. *Procedia: Social and Behavioral Sciences, 11,* 240–244.

Vygotsky, L. S. (1978). *Mind in society: The development of higher psychological processes.* Cambridge, MA: Harvard University Press.

Watts, T. W., Gandhi, J., Ibrahim, D. A., Masucci, M. D., & Raver, C. C. (2018). The Chicago School Readiness Project: Examining the long-term impacts of an early childhood intervention. *PloS One, 13*(7).

Weiner, B. (1985). An attributional theory of achievement motivation and emotion. *Psychological Review, 92,* 548–573.

Weiner, B. (1995). *Judgments of responsibility: A foundation for a theory of social conduct.* New York: Guilford Press.

Weiner, B. (2006). *Social motivation, justice, and the moral emotions: An attributional approach.* Mahwah, NJ: Lawrence Erlbaum Associates.

White, R. A., Kross, E., & Duckworth, A. L. (2015). Spontaneous self-distancing and adaptive self-reflection across adolescence. *Child Development, 86*(4), 1272–1281.

Wilson, T. D., & Linville, P. W. (1985). Improving the performance of college freshmen with attributional techniques. *Journal of Personality and Social Psychology, 49,* 287–293.

Wimmer, L., Bellingrath, S., & von Stockhausen, L. (2016). Cognitive effects of mindfulness training: Results of a pilot study based on a theory driven approach. *Frontiers in Psychology, 7*(1037). Retrieved from *www.frontiersin.org/articles/10.3389/fpsyg.2016.01037/full.*

Winne, P. H. (1995). Inherent details in self-regulated learning. *Educational Psychologist, 30,* 173–187.

Winne, P. H. (1996). A metacognitive view of individual differences in self-regulated learning. *Learning and Individual Differences, 8,* 327–353.

Winne, P. H. (1997). Experimenting to bootstrap self-regulated learning. *Journal of Educational Psychology, 89,* 397–410.

Winne, P. H. (2010). Bootstrapping learner's self-regulated learning. *Psychological Test and Assessment Modelling, 52*(4), 472–490.

Winne, P. H. (2017). The trajectory of scholarship about self-regulated learning. *Teachers College Record, 119*(13), 1–16.

Winne, P. H., & Perry, N. E. (2010). Measuring self-regulated learning. In M. Boekaerts, P. Pintrich, & M. Zeidner (Eds.), *Handbook of self-regulation* (pp. 532–568). Orlando, FL: Academic Press.

Wolff, C. E., Jarodzka, H., van den Bogert, N., & Boshuizen, H. P. A. (2016). Teacher vision: Expert and novice teachers' perception of problematic classroom management scenes. *Instructional Science, 44,* 243–265.

Wong, B. Y., Butler, D. L., Ficzere, S. A., & Kuperis, S. (1996). Teaching low achievers and students with learning disabilities to plan, write, and revise opinion essays. *Journal of Learning Disabilities, 29*(2), 197–212.

Yenawine, P. (2013). *Visual thinking strategies: Using art to deepen learning across school disciplines.* Cambridge, MA: Harvard.

Yong, Z., & Yue, Y. (2007). Causes for burnout among secondary and elementary school teachers and preventive strategies. *Chinese Education and Society, 40*(5), 78–85.

Zimmerman, B. J. (2002). Becoming a self-regulated learner: An overview. *Theory Into Practice, 41*(2), 64–70.

Index